JET LIBRARY
01270 612538

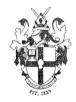

This book is to be returned on or before the
last date stamped below. Overdue charges
will be incurred by the late return of books.

UNIVERSITY COLLEGE
CHESTER

Se Ay 06		
2 7 MAR 2015		

Ocular Tumours

To Frankanne, Erika and Stephen

Ocular Tumours:
Diagnosis and Treatment

Bertil Damato PhD FRCS FRCOphth

Consultant Ophthalmologist and Director of Ocular Oncology Service,
Royal Liverpool University Hospital, Liverpool, UK

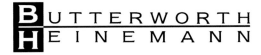

OXFORD AUCKLAND BOSTON JOHANNESBURG MELBOURNE NEW DELHI

Butterworth-Heinemann
Linacre House, Jordan Hill, Oxford OX2 8DP
225 Wildwood Avenue, Woburn, MA 01801-2041
A division of Reed Educational and Professional Publishing Ltd

ℛ A member of the Reed Elsevier plc group

First published 2000

British Library Cataloguing in Publication Data
Damato, Bertil
  Ocular tumours
   1. Eye – tumours
   I. Title
   616.9′92′84

Library of Congress Cataloguing in Publication Data
Damato, Bertil
  Ocular tumours/Bertil Damato.
  p.cm
  Includes bibliographical references and index.
  ISBN 0 7506 2220 2
  1. Eye – tumours.   2. Ophthalmologists.   I. Title.
  [DNLM: 1. Eye Neoplasms.   WW 149 D155o 2000]
  RC280.E9 D36
  616.99′284–dc21
                                    00–020613

ISBN 0 7506 2220 2

Designed and typeset by Keyword Typesetting Services Ltd, Wallington, Surrey
Printed and bound in Spain

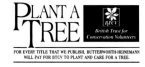

FOR EVERY TITLE THAT WE PUBLISH, BUTTERWORTH-HEINEMANN
WILL PAY FOR BTCV TO PLANT AND CARE FOR A TREE.

Contents

Preface

This book is aimed primarily at general ophthalmologists, optometrists and other specialists who might occasionally need to contribute to the management of patients with ocular tumours. It will also be helpful to trainees in ophthalmology or ocular oncology.

Although there is a growing tendency for patients to be treated by an ocular oncologist, general ophthalmologists continue to play a vital role in diagnosis and follow-up. In this textbook, most emphasis is therefore placed on the diagnosis and differential diagnosis of primary and recurrent disease, with treatment being described in less detail. The reader is referred to published articles for more detailed information on therapeutic outcomes.

As much information as possible is provided in list form, for the sake of brevity and also to facilitate self-assessment. Wherever possible, the layout is designed so that if the reader first covers the page with a sheet of paper then slides the sheet down the page, the topic of the sentence should first appear, providing an opportunity to recall all relevant information before the remaining text is uncovered. Facts are generally listed in order of importance, allowing the reader to ignore relatively minor details. This strategy is preferable to omitting seemingly unimportant information from the text, as this would be detrimental to patients with unusual clinical features. References are cited to encourage further reading and not necessarily to acknowledge original work. When several references are available, the most recent is therefore cited as this should review previous publications.

I would like to acknowledge Wallace S. Foulds, CBE, and William R. Lee, CBE, who were my mentors and teachers at the Tennent Institute of Ophthalmology in Glasgow, where I first trained in ocular oncology. I am indebted to Jack Kanski, for encouraging me to write this book and for providing so much help with its preparation. I am grateful to Anne Currie, Ronnie Jackson and colleagues for the photography, to Keyword Typesetting Services for the artwork and to Mair Pierce Moulton and staff of the library of the Liverpool Medical Institution for retrieval of references. I would like to thank Jane Campbell, Chris Jarvis and their colleagues from Butterworth-Heinemann for producing the book and for being so patient with my numerous revisions. I am also grateful to William R. Lee, Tero Kivelä, Paul Hiscott, Ed Herbert and Jonathan Kim for checking the manuscript and to all those friends and colleagues who have so kindly contributed illustrations from around the world. Such international collaboration has been greatly enhanced by the Ophthalmic Oncology Group (OOG) of the European Organization for Research and Treatment of Cancer (EORTC) and other organizations. Finally, I wish to acknowledge all the referring ophthalmologists, whose collaboration has made this book possible.

INTRODUCTION

Chapter 1

Examination techniques

The assessment of a patient with an ocular tumour follows the same basic principles that apply to general ophthalmology and requires a full history, examination of both eyes and appropriate systemic assessment. A working knowledge of the differential diagnosis is essential (Table 1.1).

SLITLAMP EXAMINATION

In the presence of a conjunctival tumour, it is necessary to inspect the entire bulbar and palpebral conjunctiva. The superior fornix should be examined with gentle double eversion of the upper eyelid using a Desmarres retractor. If this is too painful, the superior fornix can be inspected with the indirect ophthalmoscope, using the condensing lens as a magnifying glass and hooking the upper lid away from the eye with the thumb.

The findings are documented in an annotated drawing, depicting the eye and conjunctiva as a series of concentric rings representing the outer lid margin, inner lid margin, fornix, limbus and pupil respectively (Figure 1.1).

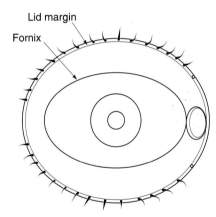

Figure 1.1 Chart for documenting conjunctival lesions

If there is any possibility of regional metastasis, palpate the pre-auricular and submandibular glands, standing behind the patient.

BINOCULAR INDIRECT OPHTHALMOSCOPY

When assessing an intraocular tumour, the following features are noted (see p.5):

Table 1.1 Differential diagnosis of ocular tumours*

	Conjunctiva	Uvea	Retina
Congenital/developmental			
Hereditary	Hereditary intra-epithelial dyskeratosis	Lisch nodules	Multiple CHRPE
			Astrocytic hamartoma
			Haemangioblastoma
			Cavernous angioma
			Dominant exudative vitreoretinopathy
			Norrie's disease
			Incontinentia pigmenti
Non-hereditary	Dermoid	Stromal iris cyst	Solitary CHRPE
	Dermolipoma	Lacrimal gland choristoma	Grouped pigmentation
	Simple choristoma		Racemose angioma
	Complex choristoma		PHPV (vitreous)
			Glioneuroma
Inflammatory			
Infectious	Granuloma (e.g. syphilis)	Granuloma (e.g. TB)	Granuloma (e.g. Toxocara)
Non-infectious	Granuloma (e.g. Sarcoid)	Uveal effusion	
		Posterior scleritis	
Neoplastic			
Benign	Naevus	Naevus/melanocytoma	Retinocytoma
	Papilloma	Haemangioma	Adenoma
	Oncocytoma	Osteoma	Fuchs' adenoma
	PAM without atypia	BDUMP	Benign medulloepithelioma
	Reactive lymphoid hyperplasia	Neurilemmoma	
		Neurofibroma	
		Leiomyoma	
		Mesectodermal leiomyoma	
		Reactive lymphoid hyperplasia	
Pre-malignant	PAM with atypia		
	Actinic keratosis		
	CCIN		
Malignant	Melanoma	Melanoma	Retinoblastoma
Primary	Squamous cell carcinoma		Adenocarcinoma
	Sebaceous carcinoma		Malignant medulloepithelioma
	Kaposi sarcoma		
	Lymphoma		
Secondary	Extraocular tumour spread	Intraocular tumour spread from conjunctiva	Lymphoma
	Leukaemia	Lyphoma	Leukaemia
		Leukaemia	
Metastatic	Metastatic carcinoma/sarcoma	Metastatic carcinoma/sarcoma	Metastatic carcinoma/sarcoma
Traumatic	Implantation cyst	Choroidal haemorrhage	Retinopathy of prematurity
	Foreign body granuloma	Implantation cyst	Retinal detachment
	Pyogenic granuloma	Miotic cyst	Massive reactive gliosis
Degenerative	Retention lacrimal cyst	Disciform lesion	Vasoproliferative tumour
		Sclerochoroidal calcification	
Idiopathic	Lymphangiectatic cyst	Juvenile xanthogranuloma	Coats' disease
			Combined hamartoma
			Iris cysts
			Ciliary epithelial cysts

*Very rare conditions have been omitted

a. Primary tissue involved (i.e., choroid, retinal pigment epithelium, sensory retina).
b. Whether a uveal tumour is directly visible or covered by pigment epithelium.
c. Colour and vascularity of the tumour tissue.
d. Tumour spread (e.g. into subretinal space, retina, vitreous).
e. Changes in RPE overlying or adjacent to a uveal tumour (i.e., drusen, orange pigment, disciform lesion).
f. Retinal changes, such as hard exudates, haemorrhages, detachment.
g. Vitreous deposits (i.e., pigment, melanotic cells, leukocytes, blood, asteroid hyalosis).
h. Distances between tumour margins and optic disc, fovea and limbus.
i. Basal tumour dimensions.

It is essential to examine the entire fundus, with indentation if necessary, to identify any other pathology and to exclude any other tumours, particularly in patients with retinoblastoma.

A retinal chart can be used, preferably one designed to enable estimation of distances from normal landmarks (Figure 1.2).

FUNDUS DRAWING (FIGURE 1.3)

The patient is asked to lie supine on a couch.

1. Place the retinal chart on a tray next to the patient's head or ask the patient to hold the tray below the chin.
2. Hold the indirect lens in your non-dominant hand and a pencil in your dominant hand.
3. Draw symbols for the optic disc and fovea, then look at the fundus and rotate the drawing pad so that the disc and fovea are aligned in the same way as the fundus image.
4. Identify the meridians, in clock hours, of the two lateral margins of the tumour, in relation to disc or fovea, and draw these lines on the chart.

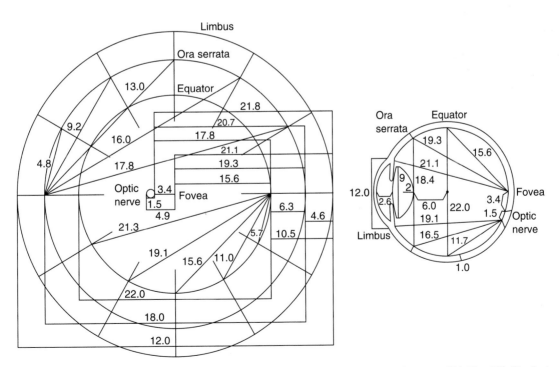

Figure 1.2 Retinal chart for estimating chord lengths in millimetres in an emmetropic eye. (Courtesy of T.A. Rice, MD, Stanford, USA)

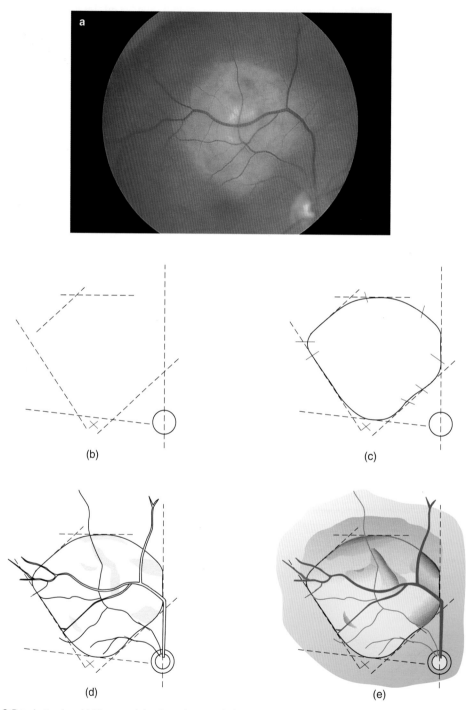

Figure 1.3 Drawing a choroidal tumour: (**a**) colour photograph, inverted to simulate view with binocular indirect ophthalmoscope; (**b**) locating tumour margins with respect to normal landmarks; (**c**) drawing margins; (**d**) adding details and (**e**) adding colour

5. Estimate the distance between posterior tumour margin and disc or fovea and mark that point on the chart.
6. Estimate the location of the anterior tumour margin in relation to equator or ora serrata and mark that point on the chart.
7. Draw the profile of the tumour, using the marks already on the chart as guides.
8. Starting at the tumour and working backwards towards the optic disc, draw the major retinal vessels, placing conspicuous bifurcations and crossings in their correct positions in relation to tumour margins.
9. Fill in details, such as texture, tumour vessels, RPE changes, haemorrhages, exudates and retinal detachment.
10. Ensure that the patient's name and hospital number, the date of the examination and your signature have all been documented.

THREE-MIRROR EXAMINATION

The indications for three-mirror examination are as follows:

a. To identify the cause of raised intraocular pressure.
b. To determine whether a lesion behind the iris is solid or cystic.
c. To find small retinal haemangioblastomas.
d. To note the location of the anterior margin of a pre-equatorial tumour.
e. To measure the circumferential extent of ciliary body or angle involvement by a tumour, aligning the lateral tumour margin with the centre of a mirror and describing the meridian in clock hours or degrees.

TRANSILLUMINATION

Transillumination (also known as 'diaphanoscopy') is ideally performed with a purpose-built transilluminator. There are three methods (Figure 1.4):

1. **Transpupillary transillumination**, which is the most convenient method (Figure 1.4**a**).
2. **Transocular transillumination**. This defines the tumour margins more precisely than transpupillary transillumination, but often requires placement of the probe in the equatorial region of the eye, so that this method can only be used intraoperatively (Figure 1.4**b**).
3. **Trans-scleral transillumination**, placing the light source under the tumour (Figure 1.4**c**) This serves only to determine whether or not the tumour transmits light.

Sources of error in localizing tumour margins include:

a. Overestimation of tumour extent because of subretinal haematoma, normal ciliary body or the penumbra of a thick tumour (Figure 1.4**a**).
b. Underestimation of tumour extent if the tumour is amelanotic or if the uvea is deeply pigmented.

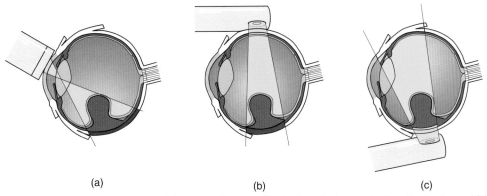

(a)   (b)   (c)

Figure 1.4 Tumour extension, assessed by (**a**) transpupillary transillumination, (**b**) transocular transillumination and (**c**) trans-scleral transillumination

Transillumination has the following limitations:

a. Pigmented tumours, such as melanoma, can transilluminate if cystic.
b. Amelanotic melanoma and other solid tumours can transilluminate brightly.
c. Opaque tumours may be lesions other than melanoma.

FLUORESCEIN ANGIOGRAPHY

The fluorescence of a tumour is related to:

1. **The fluorescein concentration** in the tumour tissue, which depends on the amount leaking from blood vessels in proportion to the amount diffusing into surrounding fluids. A tumour gives brighter fluorescence if there is an overlying serous retinal detachment, in which fluorescein can collect, than if the retina has been perforated by the tumour, in which case the fluorescein diffuses quickly away.
2. **Hyperfluorescent RPE abnormalities**, such as drusen, RPE detachments, serous retinal detachment and choroidal new vessels (Figure 1.5).
3. **Intervening pigments** such as melanin and haemoglobin, which mask underlying fluorescence. Surprisingly little pigment is needed to block fluorescence, because it is not only the incident light that is absorbed but also the fluorescent light. For this reason, a tumour with large blood vessels and extensive intercellular spaces will fluoresce brightly only if it is amelanotic.
4. **Reflections from white tissue** (e.g. retinoblastoma, amelanotic melanoma, exposed sclera), which increase the amount of fluorescent light.
5. **Autofluorescence**, which occurs with drusen of the optic disc.

These principles have certain implications:

a. It is essential to correlate angiographic findings with tumour pigmentation and changes in the overlying RPE.
b. Hypofluorescence of a pigmented tumour does not necessarily indicate that it is benign.
c. Benign choroidal tumours can be hyperfluorescent if they induce secondary degenerative changes in overlying RPE.
d. Hypofluorescence after photocoagulation or radiotherapy may merely be the result of destruction of RPE lesions and choriocapillaris so that the tumour may still be viable (Figure 1.6).

INDOCYANINE GREEN (ICG) ANGIOGRAPHY

The basic principles of fluorescein angiography also apply to indocyanine green angiography, except that the infra-red light is not absorbed by melanin and haemoglobin so that changes in RPE and retina are less conspicuous (Sallet *et al.*, 1995; Shields *et al.*, 1995) (Figure 1.7).

ULTRASONOGRAPHY

Ultrasonography (also known as echography) is invaluable in the management of ocular tumours (Green and Frazier Byrne, 1994).

INDICATIONS

a. To detect an intraocular tumour if the media are opaque, for example, in the presence of a cataract or vitreous haemorrhage.
b. To detect extraocular tumour extension.
c. To define the shape of the tumour. A collarstud configuration is almost pathognomonic of choroidal melanoma.
d. To measure tumour dimensions and distances to the optic disc and lens, thereby aiding treatment selection and planning.
e. To measure tumour change over time, to show whether a tumour is growing or regressing.
f. To demonstrate the internal acoustic reflectivity, which may suggest a particular diagnosis.

BASIC TYPES

1. **A-scan ultrasonography**, performed with a stationary transducer, produces a one-dimensional and parallel beam (Figure 1.8).

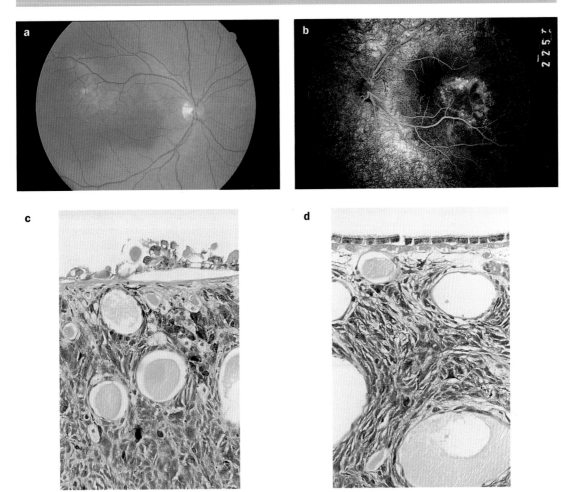

Figure 1.5 Choroidal melanoma in the right eye: (**a**) colour photograph; (**b**) fluorescein angiogram showing central hyperfluorescence and peripheral hypofluorescence relative to the surrounding choroid; (**c**) light micrograph showing drusen in the hyperfluorescent part of the tumour and (**d**) normal pigment epithelium in the hypofluorescent part of the tumour. (From: Damato, B.E. (1992) Tumour fluorescence and tumour-associated fluorescence in choroidal melanomas. *Eye*, **6**, 687–93)

Standardized ultrasonography is performed with an 8 MHz probe, which has been calibrated using a model eye.

2. **B-scan ultrasonography**, performed with an oscillating transducer, produces a two-dimensional beam focused near the retina.

3. **High-frequency ultrasonography**, for examining structures anterior to the ora serrata (Figure 1.9), performed with a water-bath.

4. **Doppler ultrasonography**, which demonstrates blood flow. It is useful in assessing tumour response to radiotherapy (Wolff Kormann *et al.*, 1992).

5. **Three-dimensional imaging** (Shammas *et al.*, 1998) may improve tumour volume measurement (Cusumano *et al.*, 1998) and enhance plaque localization over a tumour (Finger *et al.*, 1998).

Before scanning, find out as much as possible about the patient. Read the case notes and perform detailed examination. Sentinel vessels or localized lens opacities might alert you to the presence of a ciliary body tumour.

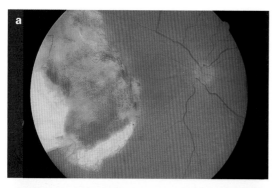

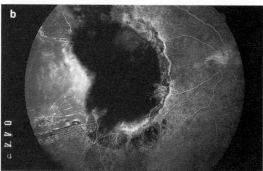

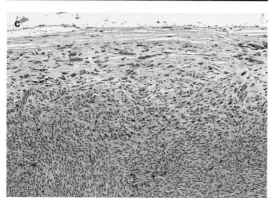

Figure 1.6 Recurrent choroidal melanoma after local resection, treated with photocoagulation: (**a**) colour photograph; (**b**) fluorescein angiogram showing hypofluorescence and (**c**) light micrograph showing viable tumour beneath atrophic RPE and retina. (From Damato, B.E. (1991) Why do choroidal melanomas fluoresce on angiography? In: N. Bornfeld *et al.* (eds), *Tumors of the Eye*, pp. 223–30)

TECHNIQUE

1. Ask the patient to lie supine on a couch.
2. Give the patient a paper tissue for wiping away any gel that might run down the cheek.

3. Sit behind the patient's head with the probe in your dominant hand and the ultrasound machine within reach of your non-dominant hand.
4. Dim the room lighting just enough to view the image clearly.
5. Anaesthetize the eye with drops and warn the patient to be careful when wiping away the gel.
6. Place a drop of methylcellulose or gel onto the tip of the probe.
7. Asking the patient to keep both eyes open, hold the probe against the anaesthetized eyeball, or if this is not possible, against the lower eyelid. Alternatively, place the probe against the closed upper lid with the fellow eye open. Steady the probe by resting your outstretched finger on the patient's cheek.
8. Once the examination is complete, irrigate the eye with sterile saline to prevent discomfort caused by the gel.
9. Sterilize the probe in the same way as a tonometer head (Smith and Pepose, 1999), rinsing in water afterwards and gently drying the probe with tissue paper. Some probes have a delicate tip, which should be rinsed and dried gently.

SCAN POSITIONS

a. **Longitudinal scanning** is performed with the marker pointing towards the limbus, to scan the eye anteroposteriorly (i.e., radially) (Figure 1.10**a**).
b. **Transverse scanning** is performed with the marker rotated 90° from the limbus, to scan the eye circumferentially (Figure 1.10**b**) .
c. **Axial scanning** is performed vertically, horizontally or obliquely, with the eye in the primary position of gaze (Figure 1.10**c** and **d**).

With vertical scans, the marker on the probe is conventionally placed superiorly, so that the superior part of the globe is located right-way-up in the upper part of the image. With horizontal scans, some examiners work with the marker always pointing towards the nose, so that the optic disc is superior to the macula in the image. Others prefer to have the marker positioned so that

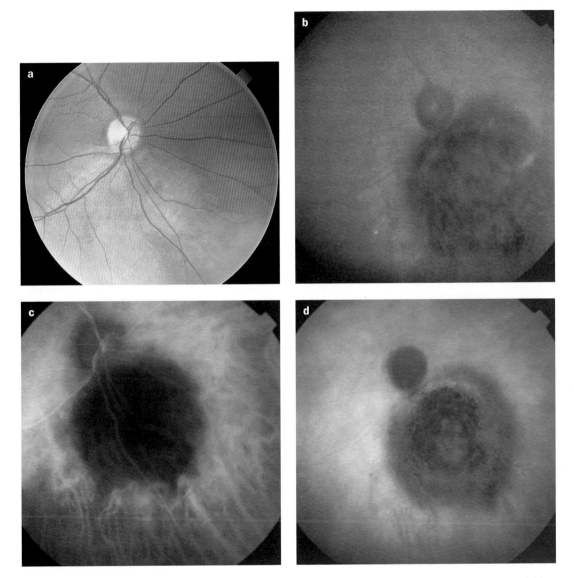

Figure 1.7 ICG of a pigmented choroidal melanoma: (**a**) colour photograph; (**b**) autofluorescence; (**c**) early phase and (**d**) late phase. (Courtesy of B.A. Lafaut, Ghent, Belgium)

the globe is always viewed from below, as with other types of scan.

Probe movements:

- Tilting in one direction.
- 'Flapping' by tilting backwards and forwards.
- Sliding the tip along the surface of the eye.
- Twisting around its axis.

To search for a nasal tumour, ask the patient to look nasally with that eye. Perform a transverse scan of the macular region with the probe placed at the temporal limbus, then slide the tip of the probe backwards to the equator, simultaneously tilting the probe anteriorly until the ciliary body is seen (Figure 1.11). If screening the whole eye, perform the same procedure for each of the eight

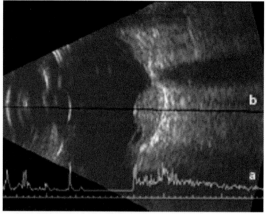 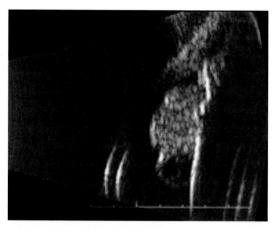

Figure 1.8 Choroidal haemangioma, assessed by (**a**) A-scan ultrasonography and (**b**) B-scan ultrasonography

Figure 1.9 High-frequency ultrasonography demonstrating an iris melanoma with an adjacent cyst

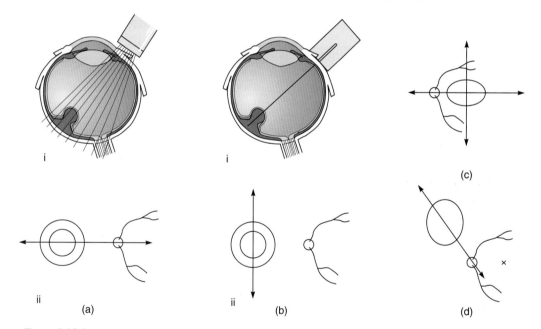

Figure 1.10 B-scan ultrasonography, performed with (**a**) longitudinal, (**b**) transverse, (**c**) axial and (**d**) oblique scans

principal directions of gaze, and then repeat the entire process, performing longitudinal scans.

Distortion of the beam by the lens can give a false impression of thickening in the peripheral fundus (i.e., Baum's bumps).

To measure tumour thickness:

a. Make sure that the scan is taken through the thickest part of the tumour (Figure 1.12**A**).

b. Ensure that the probe is at right-angles to the tumour surface by asking the patient to look in the direction of the tumour (e.g. up and to the left for a supero-temporal tumour in the left eye). An oblique cut may exaggerate tumour thickness (Figure 1.12B).

c. Take account of any overlying retinal detachment, which should not be included in the

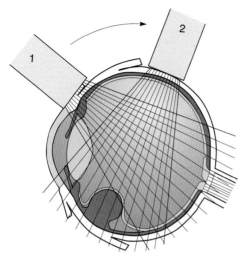

Figure 1.11 Screening for an intraocular tumour by sliding the tip of the probe posteriorly while tilting the probe anteriorly from position 1 to position 2

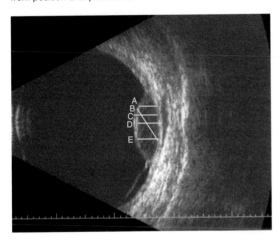

Figure 1.12 Errors in estimating tumour thickness include (A) missing thickest part of tumour, (B) oblique cut, (C) measuring retinal detachment and (D) measuring sclera; (E) correct scan

measurement (Figure 1.12C). Reduce the gain to enhance resolution.

d. Try to identify the inner scleral surface, which is where the basal caliper should be placed (Figure 1.12D). Increase the contrast and ensure that the probe is at right-angles to the scleral surface. If you still cannot recognize the inner scleral surface, place the caliper on the outer surface and record this fact so that sequential measurements can be performed consistently.

To measure the largest basal tumour diameter:

a. Start by looking at the fundus or a photograph, to identify the orientation of the tumour.
b. Flap the probe backwards and forwards, simultaneously twisting it until the greatest width is found.
c. Remember that the basal tumour diameter might be underestimated if the tumour margins are tapering or overestimated if there is overlying retinal detachment.
d. Beware that some ultrasound machines may give spurious longitudinal readings with more anterior tumours. This is recognized by comparing measurements with the eye in the primary position with those obtained with the eye turned towards the tumour.

To measure distance between tumour and disc:

a. First look at the fundus or a photograph to get an idea of the relationship between tumour and disc.
b. Twist the probe until the marker is in approximately the same meridian as an imaginary line drawn between tumour and disc.
c. Flap the probe backwards and forwards. The tumour and optic nerve should appear and disappear at the same time; if not, twist the probe until this happens.

To assess inward spread:

a. Assess tumour surface and retina by reducing the gain to improve resolution.
b. Next, examine the vitreous for opacities by increasing the gain to enhance sensitivity.

To assess extraocular spread:

a. Reduce the gain to differentiate tumour from fat.
b. Scan transversely and longitudinally to differentiate a tumour nodule from extraocular muscle (Figure 1.13).

To assess internal acoustic reflectivity:

a. Ensure that the probe is at right-angles to the surface of the tumour.
b. Reduce the gain to improve resolution.
c. Alter contrast as appropriate.
d. Note whether the sound attenuation is marked or gradual.

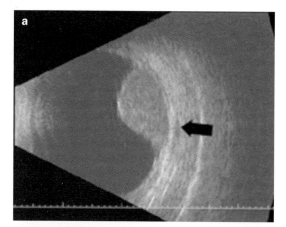

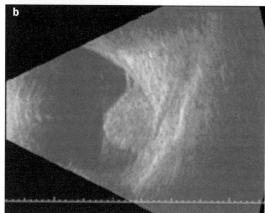

Figure 1.13 Extraocular muscle simulating extraocular tumour extension on transverse scan (**a**) but not on longitudinal scan (**b**)

e. Note whether the reflectivity is homogenous or irregular.

f. Look for spontaneous movement, for example, shimmering or vibrating echoes due to blood flow.

g. Look for echo mobility by asking patient to move the eye to the side and back again.

When performing sequential measurements of tumour thickness, false impressions can occur for the following reasons:

a. Inconsistent placement of calipers at apex or base of tumour.

b. Failure to measure thickest part of tumour at each examination.

c. Oblique scans.

d. Increase or decrease of retinal detachment.

e. A change of machine.

COMPUTERIZED TOMOGRAPHY

As with any radiograph, computerized tomography (CT) measures differential radiational absorption, which is greatest with bone and calcium (Figure 1.14). CT is not useful for tissue diagnosis (Zimmerman, 1980), but is helpful in demonstrating calcification in retinoblastoma (Weber and Mafee, 1992). Although CT also demonstrates bone in a choroidal osteoma, similar information can be obtained less expensively with ultrasonography.

Helical CT provides overlapping axial scans, which can then be reconstructed in any desired plane. Compared to conventional CT, helical CT is quicker, requires less radiation exposure and produces better images (Lakits *et al.*, 1998).

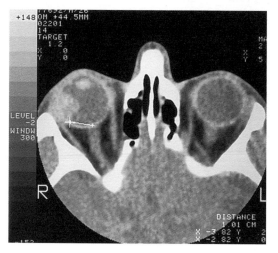

Figure 1.14 Computerized tomography showing a temporal choroidal melanoma in the right eye

MAGNETIC RESONANCE IMAGING

Magnetic resonance imaging (MRI) of ocular tumours is useful in selected cases (De Potter *et al.*, 1995). T1 weighted images demonstrate the behaviour of hydrogen atoms after termination of a pulse of radiofrequency energy and T2 weighted images demonstrate hydrogen atoms during a sustained pulse of this energy (Figure 1.15).

The T1 and T2 signals are described as being hyper-intense, iso-intense or hypo-intense with respect to vitreous. Table 1.2 demonstrates some of the more important signal intensities.

T1 weighted images have a high resolution and extraocular structures are well silhouetted against bright fat. T2 weighted images have a poorer resolution, but intraocular structures are better shown up against the bright vitreous.

Interference by the brightness of fat is diminished by fat suppression, which is performed using a variety of techniques.

Gadolinium contrast agent shortens the relaxation times of adjacent hydrogen atoms, increasing signal intensity in T1 weighted images. This enhancement demonstrates vascularity and breakdown of blood barriers.

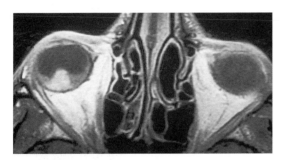

Figure 1.15 T1 weighted MRI scan of a choroidal melanoma with secondary retinal detachment. (Courtesy of P. De Potter, Brussels, Belgium)

Table 1.2 MRI signal intensities

	T1	T2
Fat	+++++	++++
Melanin	+++ (++)	+ (+++)
Haemorrhage	++++	+
Nerve	+++	+++
Muscle	+++	+++
Vitreous	++	+++++
Cortical bone	+	+
Calcification	+	+
Air	—	—

CONJUNCTIVAL IMPRINT CYTOLOGY

Imprint cytology avoids conjunctival scarring and potential seeding of tumour cells into subconjunctival tissues; however, it is more difficult for the pathologist or cytologist to interpret (Paridaens *et al.*, 1992). Furthermore, it only provides information on the most superficial layers of the conjunctival epithelium.

To obtain a sample, a 3 mm disc of cellulose acetate filter paper (Millipore) is placed on the conjunctiva for about 10 seconds, then peeled off gently and immersed in formalin.

CONJUNCTIVAL EXFOLIATIVE CYTOLOGY

The conjunctiva is scraped with a glass rod or the blunt edge of a scalpel. The sample is smeared onto a glass slide, which is fixed with spray and stained with Giemsa or other stains.

CONJUNCTIVAL INCISIONAL BIOPSY

Multiple conjunctival incisional biopsies are useful in the following circumstances:

a. To determine the degree of atypia in primary acquired melanosis (PAM).
b. To establish the diagnosis of conjunctival and corneal intra-epithelial neoplasms.
c. To define the approximate extent of a tumour, by taking multiple specimens.
d. To detect tumour recurrence after treatment.

The conjunctiva is grasped with fine-toothed forceps and an ellipse of tissue is excised with spring scissors (e.g. Vannas scissors). The excision should be no more than 5 mm long to avoid the need for suturing. The specimen is gently placed on a piece of paper, which after a short pause is immersed in formalin fixative.

Care should be taken not to cause crush artefact. Hold the tissue at one point only and do not spread the specimen forcibly on the tissue paper.

Each biopsy is placed in a separate container. The precise location of each biopsy should be identified on the container, on the pathology request form and in the case records.

The risk of transferring malignant cells from one site to another is minimized by taking samples from apparently normal areas after the tumour is removed, either on the same occasion using a different set of instruments or, preferably, on another occasion once the eye has healed.

Scarring with symblepharon or pseudopterygium formation can follow extensive conjunctival excision.

FINE NEEDLE ASPIRATION BIOPSY (FNAB)

FNAB (Augsburger and Shields, 1984; Midena *et al.*, 1985; Shields *et al.*, 1993) has the following indications:

a. Uncertain diagnosis despite full clinical assessment.
b. Patient request for tissue diagnosis before treatment is started.
c. Collection of tumour tissue for prognostication, for example, possibly detecting monosomy 3 in a uveal melanoma.

> FNAB is contraindicated for retinoblastoma, with a few rare exceptions, such as orbital extension.

The procedure is performed with the following:

a. A 25-gauge needle (as a larger needle increases the risk of tumour seeding).
b. A 10 syringe for suction, although some authors stress that suction is not necessary as the cutting action of the needle is sufficient.
c. Flexible tubing between the needle and syringe to improve control of the needle, if suction is applied.
d. A skilled cytopathologist to examine the specimen, preferably at the operating theatre, thereby ensuring that an adequate sample has been obtained. Immunohistochemistry and flow cytometry can be performed where appropriate.

The approach depends on the location of the tumour (Figure 1.16):

a. A choroidal tumour is reached through the opposite pars plana, or, intraoperatively, through the adjacent sclera if immediate plaque radiotherapy is to be given.

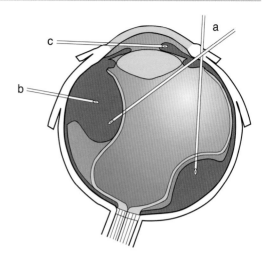

Figure 1.16 Fine needle aspiration biopsy approaches, which are (**a**) transvitreal for a choroidal or ciliary body tumour, (**b**) trans-scleral for a choroidal or ciliary body tumour and (**c**) translimbal for an anterior chamber tumour or a ciliary body tumour in an aphakic eye

b. An iris lesion is approached through the limbus, keeping the needle over the iris to avoid lens.
c. A ciliary body tumour in an aphakic eye is reached through the opposite limbus.

COMPLICATIONS

a. Non-diagnosis, which can be due to a poor yield of cells (e.g. because of cohesive cells in a naevus or melanoma), sampling of necrotic tissue, lysis of tumour cells (e.g. lymphoma) and uncertain cytopathology (e.g. metastasis).
b. Misdiagnosis, if cytopathology is not skilfully performed.
c. Incorrect prognostication, because a non-representative part of tumour is sampled (Folberg *et al.*, 1985).
d. Retinal detachment, which is rare despite retinal perforation.
e. Vitreous haemorrhage, which may complicate placement of a plaque if localization has not already been performed.
f. Seeding of cells to the entry site or episclera (Karcioglu *et al.*, 1985), which is the reason for not performing FNAB if retinoblastoma is

suspected. Although recurrence of melanoma is generally considered unlikely, prophylactic cryotherapy to the scleral puncture site has been advocated.

UVEAL INCISIONAL BIOPSY

In some centres, incisional biopsy is preferred to FNAB, either because the pathologist is not confident with needle biopsy specimens or because the surgeon is concerned about potential ocular complications (see above) (Foulds, 1992).

The surgical techniques are similar to those described for local resection (Chapter 24).

COMPLICATIONS

a. Misdiagnosis, which is less likely to occur if properly fixed tissue is examined instead of frozen sections, and if immunohistochemistry is used.
b. Tumour seeding into the orbit, which may occur with poor technique or uncontrolled haemorrhage.
c. Tumour growth through the scleral defect. If the proposed treatment is by proton beam radiotherapy or enucleation, the wound should be sutured tightly and sealed with tissue glue, and treatment should be completed as soon as possible. If plaque radiotherapy is the treatment of choice then this is started immediately even though there is a possibility of administering unnecessary radiation to a benign lesion.
d. Dehiscence of the scleral wound if radiotherapy delays healing. This is avoided by using non-absorbable sutures.

UVEAL EXCISIONAL BIOPSY

In effect, excisional biopsy is appropriate when there is diagnostic uncertainty and when local resection is the treatment of choice (in any case). Ciliary body tumours are more likely than choroidal tumours to be lesions other than melanoma, so that it is prudent to warn patients of this possibility prior to surgery.

REFERENCES

Augsburger, J.J. and Shields, J.A. (1984) Fine needle aspiration biopsy of solid intraocular tumors: indications, instrumentation and techniques. *Ophthalmic Surg.*, **15**, 34–40.

Cusumano, A., Coleman, D.J., Silverman, R.H., Reinstein, D.Z., Rondeau, M.J., Ursea, R., Daly, S.M. and Lloyd, H.O. (1998) Three-dimensional ultrasound imaging. Clinical applications. *Ophthalmology*, **105**, 300–6.

Damato, B.E. (1992) Tumour fluorescence and tumour-associated fluorescence of choroidal melanomas. *Eye*, **6**, 587–93.

De Potter, P., Shields, J. A. and Shields, C.L. (1995) *MRI of the Eye and Orbit.* Philadelphia: J.B. Lippincott Co.

Finger, P.T., Romero, J.M., Rosen, R.B., Iezzi, R., Emery, R. and Berson, A. (1998) Three-dimensional ultrasonography of choroidal melanoma: localization of radioactive eye plaques. *Arch. Ophthalmol.*, **116**, 305–12.

Folberg, R., Augsburger, J.J., Gamel, J.W., Shields, J.A. and Lang, W.R. (1985) Fine-needle aspirates of uveal melanomas and prognosis. *Am. J. Ophthalmol.*, **100**, 654–7.

Foulds, W.S. (1992) The uses and limitations of intraocular biopsy. *Eye*, **6**, 11–27.

Green, R.L. and Frazier Byrne, S. (1994) Diagnostic ophthalmic ultrasound. In: S.J. Ryan (ed.), *Retina.* St Louis: Mosby, Vol. 1, Ch. 17, pp. 217–309.

Karcioglu, Z.A., Gordon, R.A. and Karcioglu, G.L. (1985) Tumor seeding in ocular fine needle aspiration biopsy. *Ophthalmology*, **92**, 1763–7.

Lakits, A., Prokesch, R., Scholda, C., Bankier, A., Weninger, F. and Imhof, H. (1998) Multiplanar imaging in the preoperative assessment of metallic intraocular foreign bodies. Helical computed tomography versus conventional computed tomography. *Ophthalmology*, **105**, 1679–85.

Midena, E., Segato, T., Piermarocchi, S. and Boccato, P. (1985) Fine needle aspiration biopsy in ophthalmology. *Surv. Ophthalmol.*, **29**, 410–22.

Paridaens, A.D.A., McCartney, A.C.E., Curling, O.M., Lyons, C.J. and Hungerford, J.L. (1992) Impression cytology of conjunctival melanosis and melanoma. *Br. J. Ophthalmol.*, **76**, 198–201.

Sallet, G., Amoaku, W.M., Lafaut, B.A., Brabant, P. and De Laey, J.J. (1995) Indocyanine green angiography of choroidal tumors. *Graefes. Arch. Clin. Exp. Ophthalmol.*, **233**, 677–89.

Shammas, H.J., Dunne, S. and Fisher, Y.L. (1998) *Three-dimensional Ultrasound Tomography of the Eye.* NovaCoast, Ontario.

Shields, C.L., Shields, J.A. and De Potter, P. (1995) Patterns of indocyanine green videoangiography of choroidal tumours. *Br. J. Ophthalmol.*, **79**, 237–45.

Shields, J.A., Shields, C.L., Ehya, H., Eagle, R.C. Jr. and De Potter, P. (1993) Fine-needle aspiration biopsy of suspected intraocular tumors. The 1992 Urwick Lecture. *Ophthalmology*, **100**, 1677–84.

Smith, C.A. and Pepose, J.S. (1999) Disinfection of tonometers and contact lenses in the office setting: are current techniques adequate? *Am. J. Ophthalmol.*, **127**, 77–84.

Weber, A.L. and Mafee, M.F. (1992) Evaluation of the globe using computed tomography and magnetic resonance imaging. *Isr. J. Med. Sci.*, **28**, 145–52.

Wolff-Kormann, P.G., Kormann, B.A., Riedel, K.G., Hasenfratz, G.C., Stefani, F.H., Spengel, F.A. and Lund, O.E. (1992) Quantitative color Doppler imaging in untreated and irradiated choroidal melanoma. *Invest. Ophthalmol. Vis. Sci.*, **33**, 1928–33.

Zimmerman, L.E. (1980) Pathology and computed tomography. *Ophthalmology*, **87**, 602–5.

CONJUNCTIVAL TUMOURS

Chapter 2

Melanotic conjunctival lesions

Melanotic conjunctival lesions include naevus, melanosis, melanocytosis and melanoma. Melanosis generally refers to increased melanin pigmentation, which can be due to increased melanin production or an abnormal melanocytic proliferation. Melanocytosis indicates a congenital over-population of melanocytes. Melanosis can be congenital or acquired, epithelial or sub-epithelial, primary or secondary, unilateral or bilateral, and benign or malignant.

Naevus

Conjunctival naevi are uncommon, and usually small and inconspicuous. They tend to become apparent in the first two decades of life.

PATHOLOGY

Naevi tend to evolve through three stages (Folberg *et al.*, 1989):

a. Intra-epithelial naevus, consisting of a nest of round melanocytes near the junction between epithelium and stroma.
b. Compound naevus, with some melanocytes infiltrating the stroma.

c. Mature sub-epithelial naevus, with no abnormal cells in the conjunctival epithelium, all the cells having migrated to the stroma (Figure 2.1).

SIGNS

*   Location usually in the bulbar conjunctiva (Figure 2.2**a**), caruncle (Figure 2.2**b**), plica semilunaris (Figure 2.2**c**) or lid margin (Figure 2.2**d**),

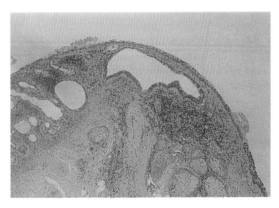

Figure 2.1 Light micrograph of a conjunctival naevus showing cysts

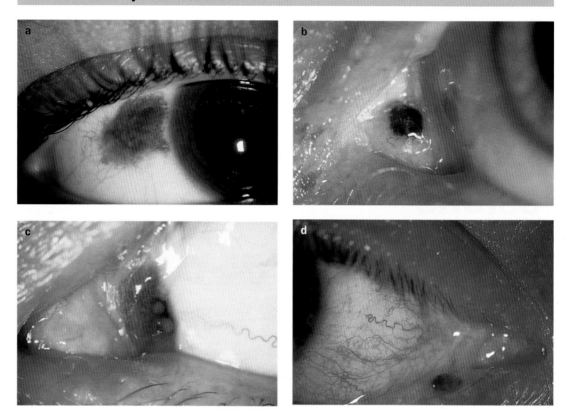

Figure 2.2 Conjunctival naevi affecting (**a**) the bulbar conjunctiva, (**b**) caruncle, (**c**) plica semilunaris and (**d**) lower eyelid. Note the cyst formation

and only rarely in palpebral conjunctiva, fornix or cornea (Gerner *et al.*, 1996).

- Relatively distinct margins.
- Mobility over the scleral surface.
- Grey, brown or black pigmentation in the majority of cases, although a few are non-pigmented (Figure 2.3).
- Cystic spaces, consisting of epithelial inclusions. These are typical and may enlarge, giving the impression of growth at the time of puberty.
- Lack of dilated feeder vessels, except in children (Figure 2.3).

DIFFERENTIAL DIAGNOSIS

1. **Conjunctival melanoma** if small can be very similar to naevus. Any recurrence of a pigmented lesion after excision may indicate malignancy.

2. **Extraocular extension of uveal melanoma**, which is subconjunctival and fixed to the globe (Figure 2.4).

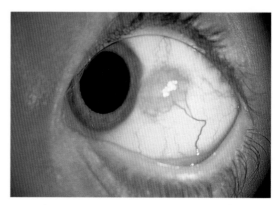

Figure 2.3 Amelanotic conjunctival naevus in a child. Note the dilated feeder vessels

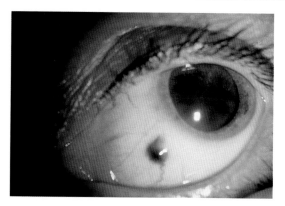

Figure 2.4 Extraocular extension of a ciliary body melanoma (which was not visible ophthalmoscopically)

3. **Axenfeld's nerve loop** occurs 4 mm from the limbus and is fixed to the globe.
4. **Subconjunctival foreign body** may be present without the patient remembering the causative injury (Figure 2.5).

MANAGEMENT

Some ophthalmologists excise all naevi, (i) to obtain histological proof of the benign diagnosis, (ii) to minimize the risk of malignant transformation and (iii) to remove the cosmetic blemish. Others prefer to keep their patients under observation.

Congenital epithelial melanosis

Congenital epithelial melanosis is due to an increased melanin production by a normal population of melanocytes. It occurs as a discrete lesion (i.e., freckle) or, in dark skinned individuals, as 'racial melanosis', which tends to involve exposed, bulbar conjunctiva, usually bilaterally and asymmetrically (Figure 2.6).

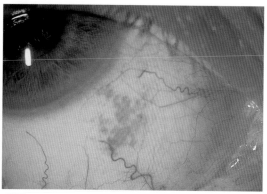

Figure 2.6 Racial melanosis

Congenital sub-epithelial melanocytosis

Congenital sub-epithelial melanocytosis consists of an increased population of melanocytes in the uvea, sclera and episclera (Figure 2.7), sometimes

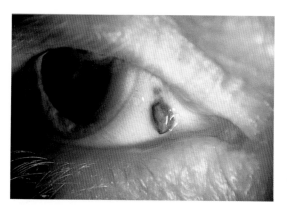

Figure 2.5 Subconjunctival slate fragment mimicking a conjunctival tumour

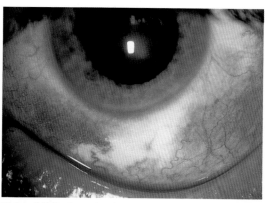

Figure 2.7 Ocular melanocytosis. The pigmentation is deep to normal conjunctiva

with cutaneous involvement (i.e., 'oculodermal melanosis' or 'naevus of Ota') (Figure 2.8). Ocular melanocytosis can be bilateral and asymmetrical. Ocular melanocytosis is associated with an increased incidence of uveal but not conjunctival melanoma.

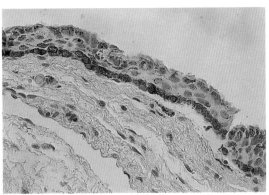

Figure 2.9 Light micrograph of primary acquired melanosis without atypia

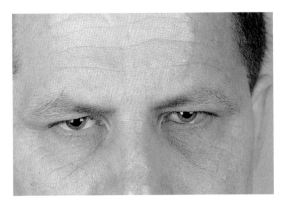

Figure 2.8 Naevus of Ota. Note the subtle pigmentation in the skin around the left eye, together with the episcleral pigmentation and the iris heterochromia. The patient presented with a choroidal melanoma (Figure 7.1)

Primary acquired melanosis (PAM)

PATHOLOGY

Primary acquired melanosis without atypia is a benign, neoplastic proliferation of melanocytes characterized by:

  a. Normal cytology, having long, dendritic processes supplying pigment to adjacent cells.
  b. Normal location of melanocytes in the basal layer of the epithelium (Figure 2.9) (Folberg and McLean, 1986).

PAM with atypia is a pre-invasive, malignant, neoplastic condition characterized by:

  a. Atypical, sometimes epithelioid, melanocytes without dendritic processes.
  b. Abnormal melanocyte distribution usually within all layers of the epithelium (Figure 2.10) and in severe cases with complete replacement of normal epithelial cells by

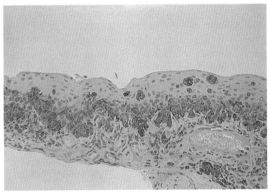

Figure 2.10 Light micrograph of primary acquired melanosis with atypia. The malignant cells are identified by immunohistochemistry using S-100. (Courtesy of P. Hiscott, Liverpool, UK)

melanoma cells. Some prefer the term 'melanoma *in situ*' (Ackerman *et al.*, 1991).

'PAM *sine pigmento*' is a rare variant, in which most of the malignant melanocytes are non-pigmented and therefore clinically invisible. This gives rise to particularly aggressive melanoma, with a poor prognosis, partly because of late diagnosis and late or inadequate treatment (Paridaens *et al.*, 1992b; Jay and Font, 1998).

HISTOPATHOLOGICAL INVESTIGATION

Since PAM without atypia cannot clinically be distinguished from PAM with atypia, multiple incisional micro-biopsies must be taken from representative parts of the conjunctiva. The recognition of melanocytes can be enhanced by immunohistochemistry, in which melanocytes are stained with an antibody such as S-100. Melanocytic proliferation can be assessed by staining proliferating cell nuclear antigen (PCNA) with PC-10 antibody, and Ki-67 antigen with MIB-1 antibody (Seregard, 1993; Chowers *et al.*, 1998). Immunohistochemistry with HMB-45 does not reliably distinguish between benign and malignant conjunctival melanocytes.

PRESENTATION

PAM without atypia can present at any age in adulthood but PAM with atypia is usually seen after the age of 45 years.

SIGNS

The clinical features of PAM with or without atypia are identical (Figure 2.11):

- Unilateral location in almost all cases.
- Irregular, flat, brown pigmentation, often with a granular appearance.
- Skip lesions, in many cases.
- Possible spread to cornea, fornices, palpebral conjunctiva and skin.
- 'Waxing and waning' of the pigmentation.

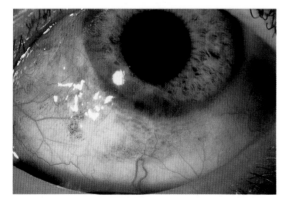

Figure 2.11 Primary acquired melanosis

MANAGEMENT

1. PAM without atypia does not progress to melanoma and therefore does not require treatment.
2. PAM with atypia has a high risk of malignant transformation (i.e. almost 50%, usually within five years (Folberg *et al.*, 1985b). Complete eradication of the transformed melanocytes is therefore desirable, although this can be difficult to achieve. A small area of melanosis can be treated by local excision with adjunctive cryotherapy (Jakobiec *et al.*, 1988) or radiotherapy. If the disease is too extensive for local excision, then the patient can be treated with cryotherapy alone or with mitomycin C drops (Frucht-Pery and Pe'er, 1996).

Secondary acquired melanosis

Bilateral secondary acquired epithelial melanosis can be caused by Addison's disease, or neurofibromatosis. Unilateral lesions may develop in dark skinned individuals in association with epithelial tumours such as cysts, scars, papillary tumours, actinic keratosis and carcinoma.

Melanoma

Conjunctival melanomas are rare (Seregard, 1998). They can arise from primary acquired melanosis with atypia, conjunctival naevi or *de novo*.

HISTOPATHOLOGY

a. Atypical melanocytes, which can be large-epithelioid, small polyhedral, or spindle-shaped (Jakobiec *et al.*, 1989).
b. Invasion of the stroma (Figure 2.12), possibly along nerves and into orbit.
c. Pagetoid spread (i.e., within epithelium) and seeding to other parts of the conjunctiva, occasionally also to nasolacrimal duct and nose (Paridaens *et al.*, 1992c).

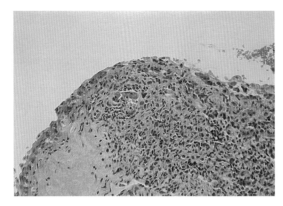

Figure 2.12 Light micrograph of invasive conjunctival melanoma. (Courtesy of P. Hiscott, Liverpool, UK)

Conjunctival melanoma can be associated with the dysplastic naevus syndrome (McCarthy *et al.*, 1993). This is characterized by:

a. Autosomal dominant inheritance.
b. Dysplastic naevi (i.e. irregular, brown and >5 mm wide).
c. Multiple cutaneous melanomas, which develop at a younger age than usual.

SIGNS

- Grey (Figure 2.13**a**) or black colour (Figure 2.13**b**), with some being amelanotic and pink.
- Nodular (Figure 2.13**c**) or diffuse growth (Figure 2.13**d**).
- Location in bulbar or palpebral conjunctiva.
- Fixation of bulbar tumours to episclera.
- Dilated feeder vessels (Figure 2.13**a** and 2.13**c**).

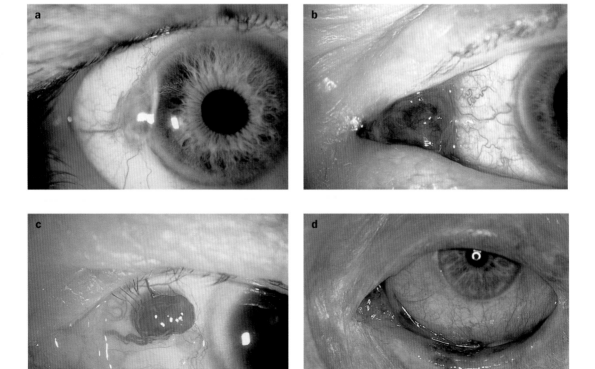

Figure 2.13 Conjunctival melanoma: (**a**) lightly pigmented tumour on the bulbar conjunctiva, (**b**) deeply pigmented tumour arising in caruncle, (**c**) pedunculated bulbar melanoma, (**d**) diffuse melanoma extending all around fornices

DIFFERENTIAL DIAGNOSIS

1. **Naevus** can appear to grow after puberty and mimic a melanoma. Unlike melanoma, limbal naevus does not involve the cornea.
2. **Blue naevus** is rare (Blicker *et al.*, 1992). It is located in the stroma not epithelium and can therefore be blue, brown or black in colour. It is mobile over the eye and not associated with cysts. It may be unrecognized if associated with an overlying epithelial naevus (Crawford *et al.*, 1999).
3. **Carcinoma** can be pigmented in dark skinned individuals (Salisbury *et al.*, 1983).
4. **Pyogenic granuloma** is a rapidly growing, pink–red mass consisting of dilated capillaries and inflammatory cells (i.e., inflamed granulation tissue). It is nearly always associated with previous trauma, such as surgery (e.g., incision and curettage of a chalazion) (Figure 2.14), and can resemble recurrence after excision of a conjunctival melanoma (Figure 2.15). Treatment is by excision of the lesion with cautery to the base.

MANAGEMENT

Circumscribed conjunctival melanoma is excised with wide clearance margins and adjunctive cryotherapy or radiotherapy to prevent local recurrence (Lommatzsch *et al.,* 1990; Shields *et al.,* 1997) (Chapter 24).

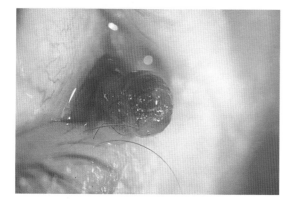

Figure 2.14 Pyogenic granuloma

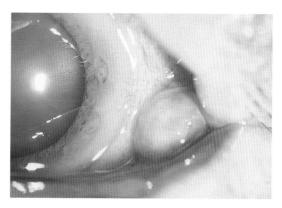

Figure 2.15 Pyogenic granuloma mimicking recurrent conjunctival melanoma after treatment

If radiotherapy is administered, the usual dose is about 100 Gy. There are various possible modes of delivery.

a. The strontium applicator is convenient for epibulbar tumours.
b. An unshielded iodine plaque or a cobalt plaque emits radiation from both surfaces and may be suitable for tumours in the fornix.
c. Proton beam radiotherapy can reach less accessible sites, such as the caruncle (Zografos *et al.,* 1994).
d. External beam radiotherapy is suitable for the orbital cavity, after exenteration.

Conjunctival melanoma with a diffuse component is treated by surgical excision of nodules followed by cryotherapy or topical mitomycin C (Frucht-Pery and Pe'er, 1996; Finger *et al.,* 1998). Radiotherapy has been advocated as a primary procedure (Lederman *et al.,* 1984). Treatment of extensive disease may result in a painful, blind eye.

Orbital recurrence is treated by local resection, possibly with adjunctive radiotherapy. Exenteration does not improve survival and is therefore performed only if there is extensive and aggressive disease that cannot be controlled by less radical methods (Paridaens *et al.,* 1994a). A lid-splitting technique may be used to reduce morbidity if the eyelids are not involved.

After treatment of melanoma or primary acquired melanosis with atypia, lifelong follow-up is indicated. Recurrent disease can be amelanotic (Figure 2.16) and may be invisible on slitlamp

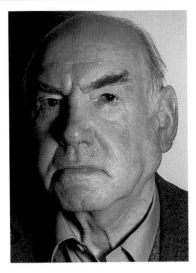

Figure 2.16 Conjunctival melanoma metastasizing to pre-auricular lymph nodes

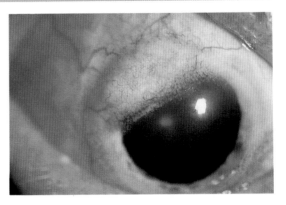

Figure 2.17 Amelanotic recurrence after treatment of conjunctival melanoma

examination so that in high risk cases some workers perform micro-biopsies or impression cytology (Paridaens *et al.*, 1992a). After mitomycin C treatment (Salomao *et al.*, 1999) or cryotherapy, reactive changes may mimic atypia on histology.

METASTATIC DISEASE

The overall rates of metastatic death are approximately 12% at 5 years and 24% at 10 years. Prognostic factors reported to indicate an increased risk of metastatic disease are:

a. Pagetoid spread or multifocal tumours (Paridaens *et al.*, 1994b; Folberg *et al.*, 1985a).
b. Involvement of caruncle, fornix, or palpebral conjunctiva (Jeffrey *et al.*, 1986; Jakobiec *et al.*, 1988; Fuchs *et al.*, 1989; Robertson *et al.*, 1989).
c. Immunoreactivity for proliferating cell nuclear antigen (Seregard, 1993).
d. Tumour thickness greater than 1 mm if location is unfavourable (Paridaens *et al.*, 1994b).
e. Lymphatic invasion (Paridaens *et al.*, 1994b).
f. Local tumour recurrence after treatment (De Potter *et al.*, 1993).
g. Orbital spread.

The main sites of metastasis are regional nodes, lung, brain and liver.

Involvement of regional lymph nodes (Figure 2.17) is managed by surgical excision of enlarged nodes, with adjuvant external beam radiotherapy (Ang *et al.*, 1990).

The systemic treatment and prognosis of metastatic conjunctival melanoma are the same as for cutaneous melanoma (Nathan and Mastrangelo, 1998).

REFERENCES

Ackerman, A.B., Sood, R. and Koenig, M. (1991) Primary acquired melanosis of the conjunctiva is melanoma *in situ. Mod. Pathol.*, **4**, 253–63.

Ang, K.K., Byers, R.M., Peters, L.J., Maor, M.H., Wendt, C.D., Morrison, W.H., Hussey, D.H. and Goepfert, H. (1990) Regional radiotherapy as adjuvant treatment for head and neck malignant melanoma. Preliminary results. *Arch. Otolaryngol. Head Neck Surg.*, **116**, 169–72.

Blicker, J.A., Rootman, J. and White, V.A. (1992) Cellular blue nevus of the conjunctiva. *Ophthalmology*, **99**, 1714–17.

Chowers, I., Livni, N., Solomon, A., Zajicek, G., Frucht-Pery, J., Folberg, R. and Pe'er, J. (1998) MIB-1 and PC-10 immunostaining for the assessment of proliferative activity in primary acquired melanosis without and with atypia. *Br. J. Ophthalmol.*, **82**, 1316–19.

Crawford, J.B., Howes, E.L. Jr. and Char, D.H. (1999) Combined nervi of the conjunctiva. *Arch. Ophthalmol.*, **117**, 1121–7.

De Potter, P., Shields, C.L., Shields, J.A. and Menduke, H. (1993) Clinical predictive factors for development of recurrence and metastasis in conjunctival melanoma: a review of 68 cases. *Br. J. Ophthalmol.*, **77**, 624–30.

Finger, P.T., Czechonska, G. and Liarikos, S. (1998) Topical mitomycin C chemotherapy for conjunctival melanoma and PAM with atypia. *Br. J. Ophthalmol.*, **82**, 476–9.

Folberg, R., Jakobiec, F.A., Bernardino, V.B. and Iwamoto, T. (1989) Benign conjunctival melanocytic lesions. Clinicopathologic features. *Ophthalmology*, **96**, 436–61.

Folberg, R. and McLean, I.W. (1986) Primary acquired melanosis and melanoma of the conjunctiva: terminology, classification and biologic behavior. *Hum. Pathol.*, **17**, 652–4.

Folberg, R., McLean, I.W. and Zimmerman, L.E. (1985a) Malignant melanoma of the conjunctiva. *Hum. Pathol.*, **16**, 136–43.

Folberg, R., McLean, I.W. and Zimmerman, L.E. (1985b) Primary acquired melanosis of the conjunctiva. *Hum. Pathol.*, **16**, 129–35.

Frucht-Pery, J. and Pe'er, J. (1996) Use of Mitomycin C in the treatment of conjunctival primary acquired melanosis with atypia. *Arch. Ophthalmol.*, **114**, 1261–4.

Fuchs, U., Kivelä, T., Liesto, K. and Tarkkanen, A. (1989) Prognosis of conjunctival melanomas in relation to histopathological features. *Br. J. Cancer*, **59**, 261–7.

Gerner, N., Nørregaard, J.C., Jensen, O.A. and Prause, J.U. (1996) Conjunctival naevi in Denmark 1960–1980. A 21-year follow-up study. *Acta Ophthalmol. Scand.*, **74**, 334–7.

Jakobiec, F.A., Folberg, R. and Iwamoto, T. (1989) Clinicopathologic characteristics of premalignant and malignant melanocytic lesions of the conjunctiva. *Ophthalmology*, **96**, 147–66.

Jakobiec, F.A., Rini, F.J., Fraunfelder, F.T. and Brownstein, S. (1988) Cryotherapy for conjunctival primary acquired melanosis and malignant melanoma. Experience with 62 cases. *Ophthalmology*, **95**, 1058–70.

Jay, V. and Font, R.L. (1998) Conjunctival amelanotic malignant melanoma arising in primary acquired melanosis sine pigmento. *Ophthalmology*, **105**, 191–4.

Jeffrey, I.J.M., Lucas, D.R., McEwan, C. and Lee, W.R. (1986) Malignant melanoma of the conjunctiva. *Histopathology*, **10**, 363–78.

Lederman, M., Wybar, K. and Busby, E. (1984) Malignant epibulbar melanoma: natural history and treatment by radiotherapy. *Br. J. Ophthalmol.*, **68**, 605–17.

Lommatzsch, P.K., Lommatzsch, R.E., Kirsch, I. and Fuhrmann, P. (1990) Therapeutic outcome of patients suffering from malignant melanomas of the conjunctiva. *Br. J. Ophthalmol.*, **74**, 615–19.

McCarthy, J.M., Rootman, J., Horsman, D. and White, V.A. (1993) Conjunctival and uveal melanoma in the dysplastic nevus syndrome. *Surv. Ophthalmol.*, **37**, 377–86.

Nathan, F.E. and Mastrangelo, M.J. (1998) Systemic therapy in melanoma. *Semin. Surg. Oncol.*, **14**, 319–27.

Paridaens, A.D.A., McCartney, A.C.E., Curling, O.M., Lyons, C.J. and Hungerford, J.L. (1992a) Impression cytology of conjunctival melanosis and melanoma. *Br. J. Ophthalmol.*, **76**, 198–201.

Paridaens, A.D.A., McCartney, A.C.E. and Hungerford, J.L. (1992b) Multifocal amelanotic conjunctival melanoma and acquired melanosis sine pigmento. *Br. J. Ophthalmol.*, **76**, 163–5.

Paridaens, A.D.A., McCartney, A.C.E., Lavelle, R.J. and Hungerford, J.L. (1992c) Nasal and orbital recurrence of conjunctival melanoma 21 years after exenteration. *Br. J. Ophthalmol.*, **76**, 369–71.

Paridaens, A.D.A., McCartney, A.C.E., Minassian, D.C. and Hungerford, J.L. (1994a) Orbital exenteration in 95 cases of primary conjunctival malignant melanoma. *Br. J. Ophthalmol.*, **78**, 520–8.

Paridaens, A.D.A., Minassian, D.C.E., McCartney, A.C.E., and Hungerford, J.L. (1994b) Prognostic factors in primary malignant melanoma of the conjunctiva: a clinicopathological study of 256 cases. *Br. J. Ophthalmol.*, **78**, 252–9.

Robertson, D.M., Hungerford, J.L. and McCartney, A. (1989) Pigmentation of the eyelid margin accompanying conjunctival melanoma. *Am. J. Ophthalmol.*, **108**, 435–9.

Salomo, D.R., Mathers, W.D., Sutphin, J.E., Cuevas, K. and Folberg, R. (1999) Cytologic changes in the conjunctiva mimicking malignancy after topical mitomycin C chemotherapy. *Ophthalmology*, **106**, 1756–60.

Salisbury, J.A., Szpak, C.A. and Klintworth, G.K. (1983) Pigmented squamous cell carcinoma of the conjunctiva. A clinicopathologic ultrastructural study. *Ophthalmology*, **90**, 1477–81.

Seregard, S. (1993) Cell proliferation as a prognostic indicator in conjunctival malignant melanoma. *Am. J. Ophthalmol.*, **116**, 93–7.

Seregard, S. (1996) Cell growth and p53 expression in primary acquired melanosis and conjunctival melanoma. *J. Clin. Pathol.*, **49**, 338–42.

Seregard, S. (1998) Conjunctival melanoma. *Surv. Ophthalmol.*, **42**, 321–50.

Shields, J.A., Shields, C.L. and De Potter, P. (1997) Surgical management of conjunctival tumors. The 1994 Lynn B. McMahan Lecture. *Arch. Ophthalmol.*, **115**, 808–15.

Zografos, L., Uffer, S., Bercher, L. and Gailloud, C. (1994) Chirugie, cryocoagulation et radiothérapie combinée pour le traitement des mélanomes de la conjunctive. *Klin. Monatsbl. Augenheilkd.*, **204**, 385–90.

Chapter 3

Squamous conjunctival tumours

Squamous conjunctival tumours are rare in temperate climates but relatively common in hot, sunny parts of the world (Lee and Hirst, 1995).

Squamous papilloma

PATHOLOGY

Squamous papillomas are usually filiform (i.e., like cauliflowers) and consist of squamous non-keratinized epithelium over fibrovascular tissue (Figure 3.1), with dysplasia in some cases. Rare varieties of papilloma of the conjunctiva include 'inverted conjunctival papillomas' similar to tumours in the nasal sinuses and lacrimal sac (Streeten *et al.*, 1979), and 'benign inverted mucoepidermoid papillomas' (Jakobiec *et al.*, 1987).

Conjunctival papillomas can be caused by the human papilloma virus (HPV) types 6 and 11, and may develop in infants born to mothers with genital HPV infection (Egbert and Kersten, 1997).

SIGNS

- Irregular surface.
- Pedunculated (Figure 3.2**a**) or sessile (Figure 3.2**b**) configuration.
- Translucent pink colour.
- Red dots, representing stromal blood vessels.
- Location anywhere in the conjunctiva, with pedunculated tumours occurring mostly at the inferior fornix and the sessile tumours usually developing at the limbus.

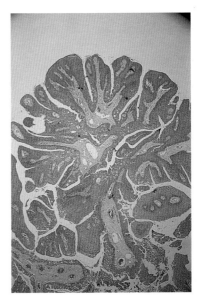

Figure 3.1 Light micrograph of a conjunctival papilloma

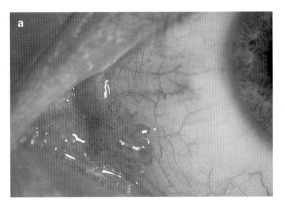
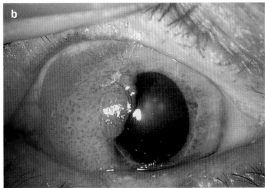

Figure 3.2 Conjunctival papilloma, which can be (**a**) pedunculated or (**b**) sessile

- Variable number, with pedunculated tumours tending to be multiple, affecting one or both eyes. Sessile tumours are usually solitary.

In children, the papillomas tend to be multiple, small and pedunculated, often resolving spontaneously. In adults, papillomas are usually solitary, sessile, juxta-corneal and can become massive if untreated.

MANAGEMENT

The mainstay of treatment has been complete excision with wide clearance margins and adjunctive cryotherapy or photocoagulation to the base (Chapter 24). There is a high recurrence rate. Other therapeutic methods include interferon-alpha (Lass *et al.*, 1987), oral cimetidine (Shields *et al.*, 1999), mitomycin C (Hawkins, *et al.*, 1999) and laser photocoagulation (Jackson *et al.*, 1987).

Actinic keratosis

This lesion consists of conjunctival epithelial acanthosis with cellular atypia, parakeratosis and elastotic degeneration of the underlying stroma. It is caused by prolonged exposure to solar ultraviolet light and occurs as a circumscribed interpalpebral lesion (Mauriello Jr *et al.*, 1995).

Conjunctival and corneal intra-epithelial neoplasia (CCIN)

PATHOLOGY

Neoplastic cells, which may be spindle, epithelioid or both, develop in the basal layers. They later spread superficially, and eventually infiltrate the entire thickness of the epithelium (i.e., carcinoma *in situ*). With increasing de-differentiation the cells lose their polarity in the epithelium and develop larger and more pleomorphic nuclei. By definition, invasion of the stroma is absent.

The development of CCIN (Lee and Hirst, 1995) is associated with the following factors:

a. Ultra-violet radiation.
b. Smoking.
c. HPV types 16 and 18.
d. Immunodeficiency (e.g., HIV infection).

SIGNS

- Gelatinous, 'papilliform' opalescent thickening of the conjunctiva.
- Frosted irregularity of corneal surface if there is extension across the limbus (Figure 3.3).
- Location at nasal limbus in most patients.
- Spontaneous regression, which is very rare (Morsman, 1989).

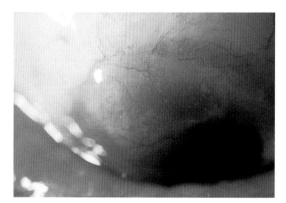

Figure 3.3 Conjunctival and corneal intra-epithelial neoplasia

DIFFERENTIAL DIAGNOSIS

Sebaceous carcinomas, which may develop Pagetoid spread, clinically resemble CCIN (Chapter 4). Histological differentiation between these two conditions is difficult without using lipid stains or immunohistochemistry.

MANAGEMENT

Complete surgical excision is difficult to achieve because of the diffuse nature of CCIN (Erie *et al.*, 1986). Adjunctive cryotherapy using a liquid nitrogen cryoprobe reduces the recurrence rate to about 10% (Fraunfelder and Wingfield, 1983). Treatment with topical mitomycin C at a dose of 0.02–0.04%, four times daily, for two weeks, has been advocated for primary and recurrent lesions (Frucht-Pery *et al.*, 1997).

Encouraging results have also been reported with topical 1% 5-fluorouracil four times daily for two weeks (Yeatts *et al.*, 1995) and topical interferon alpha-2b (Vann and Karp, 1999). Recurrent lesions have also been treated by excision with adjunctive beta irradiation (Jones *et al.*, 1991).

Invasive squamous cell carcinoma

PATHOLOGY

Invasive squamous cell carcinoma has a multifactorial aetiology, which includes exposure to solar ultra-violet radiation, HIV infection and possibly HPV-16 infection (Newton, 1996; Waddell *et al.*, 1996). Histological examination shows atypical epithelial cells with mitotic figures and keratin formation (Figure 3.4). If the tumour arises from actinic keratosis it tends to show leukoplakia and is usually exophytic. If it develops from CCIN it is more likely to invade the eye and orbit. Metastatic disease is rare unless the patient is immunodeficient. Spindle cell carcinoma is a rare variant, which behaves aggressively (Schubert *et al.*, 1995; Seregard and Kock, 1995).

Orbital invasion is a serious complication, which can lead to extension into the cranial cavity and paranasal sinuses as well as metastasis to regional lymph nodes.

Special histological techniques include:

a. Biopsy, for diagnosis and follow-up.
b. Immunohistochemistry using antikeratin antibodies and other epithelial markers, to differentiate spindle cell carcinoma from other spindle cell tumours (e.g., amelanotic melanoma, fibrosarcoma) (Huntington *et al.*, 1990).

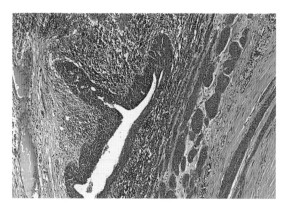

Figure 3.4 Light micrograph of squamous cell carcinoma at the superior fornix, showing scleral invasion

SYMPTOMS

Patients usually present with redness, irritation, or both.

SIGNS

• Location in interpalpebral area, especially if arising from actinic keratosis.

- Multinodular, vascular, gelatinous tumour or superficial diffuse lesion (Figure 3.5).
- Leukoplakia, if arising from actinic keratosis.
- Prominent feeder vessels.
- Intraocular spread, especially if incompletely excised, causing glaucoma and pseudo-uveitis.
- Spread to regional nodes.
- Systemic metastatic disease, rarely.
- Pigmentation in dark skinned individuals (Figure 3.6).
- Massive growth if the tumour is untreated (Figure 3.7).

DIFFERENTIAL DIAGNOSIS

1. **Keratotic plaque** can resemble invasive squamous cell carcinoma with leukoplakia. Histologically, there is hyperkeratosis (i.e.,

leukoplakia) overlying an area of acanthosis (i.e., thickening of the middle epithelial layer). This condition has a variety of causes, such as vitamin A deficiency (i.e., 'Bitôt spot'), and has no malignant potential.

2. **Melanotic tumours** can be mimicked by papillomas and squamous cell carcinoma, which can be pigmented in dark skinned individuals (Kremer *et al.,* 1992) (Figure 3.6).

3. **Granulomata** of the conjunctiva have a wide variety of causes, such as foreign material (e.g. caterpillar hair, golf-ball granuloma), mycobacteria, fungi (*Coccidioides immitis*), parasites, rheumatoid arthritis and sarcoidosis (Figure 3.8).

4. **Reactive epitheliomatous hyperplasia** (pseudoepitheliomatous hyperplasia), which

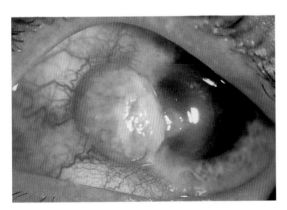

Figure 3.5 Squamous cell carcinoma

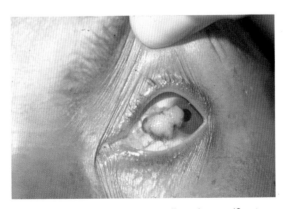

Figure 3.6 Pigmented squamous cell carcinoma. (Courtesy of A. H. Mahomed, Natal, South Africa)

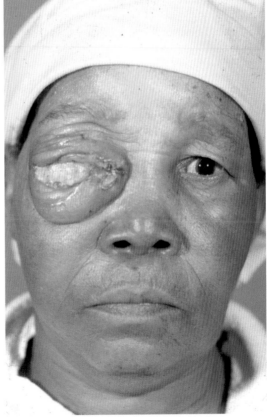

Figure 3.7 Advanced conjunctival carcinoma. (Courtesy of A. H. Mahomed, Natal, South Africa)

presents as a rapidly growing, white, hyper-keratotic mass with indistinct margins. It is usually related to concurrent or previous inflammation.

5. **Mucoepidermoid carcinoma** (Carrau *et al.*, 1994), which is a highly aggressive tumour composed of squamous and mucus-secreting cells. The histological diagnosis is assisted by the use of mucin stains. This tumour tends to recur after local resection and may require enucleation or exenteration to improve survival.

6. **Inverted follicular keratosis**, in which pro-liferating epithelium invaginates connective tissue.

7. **Keratoacanthoma**, which rarely develops in conjunctiva (Coupland *et al.*, 1998).

8. **Hereditary intra-epithelial dyskeratosis**, giving rise to multiple raised plaques near the limbus of both eyes. It is an autosomal dominant disease usually occurring in North America (Dithmar *et al.*, 1998).

9. **Pingueculum and pterygium**, which tend to originate on the bulbar conjunctiva adjacent to the limbus (Figure 3.9).

10. **Conjunctival lymphoid proliferation**, which develops as a smooth, pink tumour (Chapter 20).

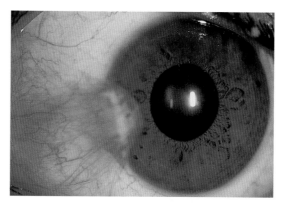

Figure 3.9 Pterygium

MANAGEMENT

Treatment of conjunctival squamous cell carci-noma is by surgical excision with wide margins and careful histological assessment of clearance, ideally examining frozen sections at the time of surgery (Tunc *et al.*, 1999). Bowman's layer should be conserved, if possible, as it is a barrier to intraocular invasion. Adjunctive cryotherapy or radiotherapy (Zehetmayer *et al.*, 1993) is advo-cated. Topical 5-FU may be useful for intra-epithelial disease (Yeatts *et al.*, 1995). Topical chemotherapy is ineffective for invasive disease.

Extensive disease may require autologous scleral, conjunctival or limbal grafts (Copeland and Char, 1990). Localized intraocular invasion may be treatable by local resection but enuclea-tion is required if there is diffuse spread. Orbital invasion is treated by exenteration, with radio-therapy if necessary (Johnson *et al.*, 1997).

Follow-up should be life-long as recurrences are common and can occur after a delay of several years (Tabin *et al.*, 1997).

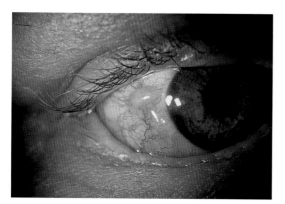

Figure 3.8 Conjunctival sarcoid nodules

REFERENCES

Carrau, R.L., Stillman, E. and Canaan, R.E. (1994) Mucoepidermoid carcinoma of the conjunctiva. *Ophthal. Plast. Reconstr. Surg.*, **10**, 163–8.

Copeland, R.A. Jr. and Char, D.H. (1990) Limbal auto-graft reconstruction after conjunctival squamous cell carcinoma. *Am. J. Ophthalmol.*, **110**, 412–15.

Coupland, S.E., Heimann, H., Kellner, U., Bornfeld, N., Foerster, M.H. and Lee, W.R. (1998) Kerato-acanthoma of the bulbar conjunctiva. *Br J. Ophthalmol.*, **82**, 586.

Dithmar, S., Stulting, R.D. and Grossniklaus, H.E. (1998) Hereditäre benigne intraepitheliale Dyskeratose. *Ophthalmaloge.*, **95**, 684–6.

Egbert, J.E. and Kersten, R.C. (1997) Female genital tract papillomavirus in conjunctival papillomas of infancy. *Am. J. Ophthalmol.*, **123**, 551–2.

Erie, J.C., Campbell, R.J. and Liesegang, T.J. (1986) Conjunctival and corneal intraepithelial and invasive neoplasia. *Ophthalmology*, **93**, 176–83.

Fraunfelder, F.T. and Wingfield, D. (1983) Management of intraepithelial conjunctival tumors and squamous cell carcinomas. *Am. J. Ophthalmol.*, **95**, 359–63.

Frucht-Pery, J., Sugar, J., Baum, J., Sutphin, J.E., Pe'er, J., Savir, H., Holland, E.J., Meisler, D.M., Foster, J.A., Folberg, R. and Rozenman, Y. (1997) Mitomycin C treatment for conjunctival-corneal intraepithelial neoplasia. *Ophthalmology*, **104**, 2085–93.

Hawkins, A.S., Yu, J., Hamming, N.A. and Rubinstein, J.B. (1999) Treatment of recurrent conjunctival papillomatosis with mitomycin C. *Am. J. Ophthalmol.*, **128**, 638–40.

Huntington, A.C., Langloss, J.M. and Hidayat, A.A. (1990) Spindle cell carcinoma of the conjunctiva. An immunohistochemical and ultrastructural study of six cases. *Ophthalmology*, **97**, 711–17.

Jackson, W.B., Beraja, R. and Codère, F. (1987) Laser therapy of conjunctival papillomas. *Can. J. Ophthalmol.*, **22**, 45–7.

Jakobiec, F.A., Harrison, W. and Aronian, D. (1987) Inverted mucoepidermoid papillomas of the epibulbar conjunctiva. *Ophthalmology*, **94**, 283–7.

Johnson, T.E., Tabbara, K.F., Weatherhead, R.G., Kersten, R.C., Rice, C. and Nasr, A.M. (1997) Secondary squamous cell carcinoma of the orbit. *Arch. Ophthalmol.*, **115**, 75–8.

Jones, D.B., Wilhelmus, K.R. and Font, R.L. (1991) Beta radiation of recurrent corneal intraepithelial neoplasia. *Trans. Am. Ophthalmol. Soc.*, **89**, 285–98.

Kremer, I., Sandbank, J., Weinberger, D., Rotem, A. and Shapiro, A. (1992) Pigmented epithelial tumours of the conjunctiva. *Br. J. Ophthalmol.*, **76**, 294–6.

Lass, J.H., Foster, C.S., Grove, A.S., Rubenfeld, M., Lusk, R.P., Jenson, A.B. and Lancaster, W.D. (1987) Interferon-alpha therapy of recurrent conjunctival papillomas. *Am. J. Ophthalmol.*, **103**, 294–301.

Lee, G.A. and Hirst, L.W. (1995) Ocular surface squamous neoplasia. *Surv. Ophthalmol.*, **39**, 429–50.

Mauriello, J.A. Jr, Napolitano, J. and McLean, I. (1995) Actinic keratosis and dysplasia of the conjunctiva: a clinicopathological study of 45 cases. *Can. J. Ophthalmol.*, **30**, 312–16.

Morsman, C.D. (1989) Spontaneous regression of a conjunctival intraepithelial neoplastic tumor. *Arch. Ophthalmol.*, **107**, 1490–1.

Newton, R. (1996) A review of the aetiology of squamous cell carcinoma of the conjunctiva. *Br. J. Cancer*, **74**, 1511–13.

Schubert, H.D., Farris, R.L. and Green, W.R. (1995) Spindle cell carcinoma of the conjunctiva. *Graefes Arch. Clin. Exp. Ophthalmol.*, **233**, 52–5.

Seregard, S. and Kock, E. (1995) Squamous spindle cell carcinoma of the conjunctiva. Fatal outcome of a pterygium-like lesion. *Acta Ophthalmol. Scand.*, **73**, 464–6.

Shields, C.L., Lally, M.R., Singh, A.D., Shields, J.A. and Nowinski, T. (1999) Oral cimetidine (Tagamet) for recalcitrant, diffuse conjunctival papillomatosis. *Am. J. Ophthalmol.*, **128**, 362–4.

Streeten, B.W., Carrillo, R., Jamison, R., Brownstein, S., Font, R.L. and Zimmerman, L.E. (1979) Inverted papilloma of the conjunctiva. *Am. J. Ophthalmol.*, **88**, 1062–6.

Tabin, G., Levin, S., Snibson, G., Loughnan, M. and Taylor, H. (1997) Late recurrences and the necessity for long-term follow-up in corneal and conjunctival intraepithelial neoplasia. *Ophthalmology*, **104**, 485–92.

Tunc, M., Char, D.H., Crawford, B. and Miller, T. (1999) Intraepithelial and invasive squamous cell carcinoma of the conjunctiva: analysis of 60 cases. *Br. J. Ophthalmol.*, **83**, 98–103.

Vann, R.R. and Karp, C.L. (1999) Perilesional and topical interferon alfa-2b for conjunctival and corneal neoplasia. *Ophthalmology*, **106**, 91–7.

Waddell, K.M., Lewallen, S., Lucas, S.B., Atenyi-Agaba, C., Herrington, C.S. and Liomba, G. (1996) Carcinoma of the conjunctiva and HIV infection in Uganda and Malawi. *Br. J. Ophthalmol.*, **80**, 503–8.

Yeatts, R.P., Ford, J.G., Stanton, C.A. and Reed, J.W. (1995) Topical 5-fluorouracil in treating epithelial neoplasia of the conjunctiva and cornea. *Ophthalmology*, **102**, 1338–44.

Zehetmayer, M., Menapace, R. and Kulnig, W. (1993) Combined local excision and brachytherapy with ruthenium-106 in the treatment of epibulbar malignancies. *Ophthalmologica*, **207**, 133–9.

Chapter 4

Miscellaneous conjunctival tumours

Cysts

1. **Simple cysts** are lined by conjunctival epithelium. These are common.
2. **Retention cysts** can occur in the lacrimal gland in the superior fornix (i.e., dacryops).
3. **Implantation cysts** can develop after trauma and surgery. If troublesome, they are treated by complete excision or marsupialization.
4. **Lymphangiectatic cysts** are dilated lymphatics, which arise spontaneously or after inflammation. They can become filled with blood (Scott *et al.,* 1991).

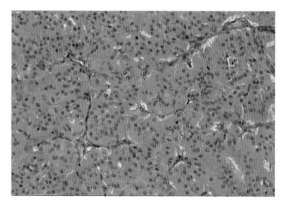

Figure 4.1 Light micrograph of an oncocytoma

Oncocytoma

Oncocytoma, also known as oxyphil cell adenoma, is composed of eosinophilic cells filled with abnormal mitochondria (Orcutt *et al.,* 1992) (Figure 4.1).

This tumour arises from oncocytes present in ductal epithelium. It usually occurs in the caruncle after the age of 50 years (Chang *et al.,* 1995) although it may develop from the principal or accessory lacrimal glands.

Clinically, it presents as a yellow–pink, cystic mass.

Rarely, oncocytoma is malignant, especially if it occurs away from the caruncle.

Treatment is by local excision.

Sebaceous gland carcinoma

Sebaceous gland carcinoma tends to occur in older individuals and is more common in women. In Asia, this tumour accounts for a higher proportion of eyelid and conjunctival tumours (Hayashi *et al.,*

1994). It has been associated with human papilloma virus (HPV) infection (Hayashi *et al.,* 1994).

PATHOLOGY

The tumour is composed of sebaceous cells containing intra-cytoplasmic vacuoles filled with lipid. Histological differentiation from squamous cell carcinoma, basal cell carcinoma and even chalazion can be difficult without lipid stains (e.g. Oil Red O; see Figure 4.2) or immunohistochemistry (Johnson *et al.,* 1999).

When a patient is referred with tumour recurrence, the ocular oncologist may wish to review the histology of the original tumour to ensure that the initial diagnosis was correct.

The tumour usually spreads in a Pagetoid fashion from its origin in a meibomian or Zeiss gland in the eyelid, but it may rarely arise in the conjunctiva *de novo* (Margo and Grossniklaus, 1995).

SIGNS

- Unilateral.
- Diffuse redness and thickening of the conjunctiva (Figure 4. 3).
- Possibly multicentric.

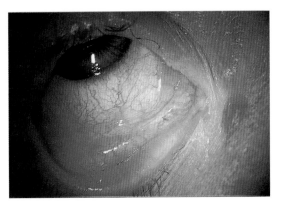

Figure 4.3 Diffuse sebaceous gland carcinoma arising in conjunctiva. (Courtesy of W.S. Foulds, Glasgow, UK)

DIFFERENTIAL DIAGNOSIS

1. **Chalazion**, so that biopsy is mandatory if any presumed chalazion recurs after incision and curettage (Figure 4.4).
2. **Blepharoconjunctivitis**, which is usually bilateral.
3. **Sebaceous adenoma**, which occurs as part of the Muir–Torre syndrome. This is an autosomal dominant disease, which gives rise to visceral malignancy (Jacobiec, 1974; Schwartz and Torre, 1995).

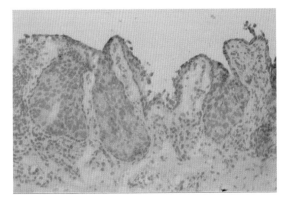

Figure 4.2 Conjunctival sebaceous carcinoma staining positively with Oil Red O stain. (Courtesy of T. Kivelä, Helsinki, Finland)

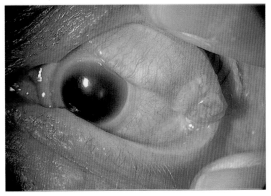

Figure 4.4 Recurrent nodular sebaceous carcinoma after incision and curettage

TREATMENT

Treatment of localized disease is by excision with wide margins and adjunctive cryotherapy. Histological assessment of clearance is useful. Sebaceous carcinoma is not very sensitive to radiotherapy (Nunery *et al.,* 1993). Frequent postoperative examinations are required, because recurrences can grow rapidly.

Exenteration is necessary if the tumour involves most of the conjunctiva or invades the orbit.

Lymph node involvement requires histological confirmation and aggressive treatment.

PROGNOSIS

About 20% of patients develop metastases in the preauricular, cervical, or submandibular nodes. The overall 5-year mortality is approximately 15% (Kass and Hornblass, 1989). Adverse prognostic factors for survival (Rao *et al.,* 1982) include:

- Vascular, lymphatic, lid or orbital invasion.
- Tumour diameter over 10 mm.
- Pagetoid spread.
- De-differentiation.

Kaposi sarcoma

PATHOLOGY

This malignant tumour is caused by human herpesvirus 8 (Li *et al.,* 1998). It tends to occur in immunosuppressed individuals, such as those suffering from the Acquired Immune Deficiency Syndrome (AIDS), in whom it can be the presenting feature.

Histologically, Kaposi sarcoma is composed of dilated vascular channels and pleomorphic spindle cells, which predominate (Figure 4.5).

SIGNS

Conjunctival Kaposi sarcoma has the appearance of a blue–red, nodular or diffuse lesion resembling a subconjunctival haemorrhage, pyogenic granuloma or a foreign body granuloma (Figure 4.6).

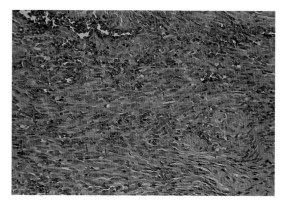

Figure 4.5 Light micrograph of Kaposi sarcoma. (Courtesy of W.H. Spencer, San Francisco, USA)

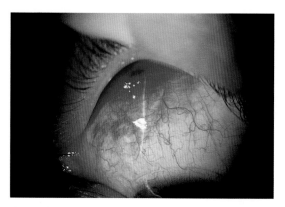

Figure 4.6 Kaposi sarcoma in superior fornix, resembling haemorrhage. (Courtesy of W.H. Spencer, San Francisco, USA)

MANAGEMENT

The tumour is treated if it is progressive and symptomatic. It usually responds to external beam radiotherapy at a dose of 8 Gy in a single fraction (Ghabrial *et al.,* 1992). Other treatments include interferon (Hummer *et al.,* 1993), cryotherapy (Dugel *et al.,* 1992), surgical excision (Dugel *et al.,* 1992) and systemic liposomal daunorubicin (Khan and Dhillon, 1999). If the patient is to receive systemic anti-viral treatment, perhaps for newly diagnosed AIDS, it may be reasonable to withhold local treatment as the tumour may regress.

Choristomas

Choristomas are benign tumours containing tissues not normally present at the site where the tumour is present (Mansour *et al.,* 1989). There are several types, clinically distinguished by their colour, consistency and location.

1. **Dermoids** are composed of fibrous tissue covered by epithelium. They tend to be light brown and located at the infero-temporal limbus or on the cornea (Figure 4.7).
2. **Dermolipomas** (or lipodermoids) are similar to dermoids but contain larger amounts of fat. Clinically, they are more yellow than dermoids and are located supero-temporally (Figure 4.8).

3. **Single tissue choristomas** contain mesoectodermal tissue such as lacrimal gland, nerve, cartilage, or bone (i.e., osseous choristomas). The latter are usually white, hard, and located about 8 mm from the limbus (Figure 4.9).
4. **Complex choristomas** contain structures of different origins, such as lacrimal gland and muscle (Hayasaka *et al.,* 1989).

Choristomas can form part of certain syndromes, such as:

a. Goldenhar's syndrome (oculoauriculovertebral dysplasia);
b. Treacher–Collins syndrome (mandibulofacial dysostosis);
c. Naevus sebaceous syndrome (naevus sebaceous of Jadassohn) (Kruse *et al.,* 1998), which is characterized by naevus sebaceous (linear

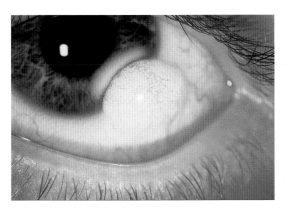

Figure 4.7 Limbal dermoid. (Courtesy of S. Seregard, Stockholm, Sweden)

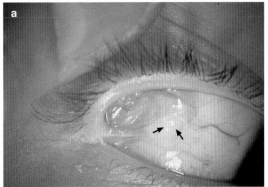

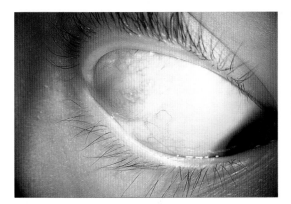

Figure 4.8 Dermolipoma

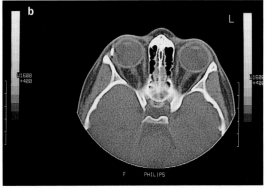

Figure 4.9 Osseous choristoma: (**a**) colour photograph and (**b**) CT scan. (Courtesy of S. Seregard, Stockholm, Sweden)

or otherwise), temporal alopecia, facial melanocytic naevi, seizures, mental retardation and a wide variety of ocular abnormalities (Duncan *et al.,* 1998).

MANAGEMENT

Troublesome limbal choristomas may be excised by lamellar dissection. The surgeon must be prepared to perform corneal or scleral grafting and avoiding damage to adjacent structures. Excision of dermolipoma should be avoided if possible because it may be followed by ptosis, dry eye and limitation of eye movement due to scar tissue. If treatment is necessary, minimal excision should be performed, taking care to identify adjacent structures (Beard, 1990; Fry and Leone Jr, 1994).

Secondary tumours

The conjunctiva may be involved by direct extension of tumours from the following:

a. Inside the eye (i.e., melanoma, retinoblastoma, medulloepithelioma).
b. The eyelids (i.e., basal cell, squamous cell, and sebaceous carcinomas).
c. The orbit (i.e., rhabdomyosarcoma).

Conjunctival metastases are rare (Chapter 19).

REFERENCES

Beard, C. (1990) Dermolipoma surgery, or, 'an ounce of prevention is worth a pound of cure'. *Ophthal. Plast. Reconstr. Surg.,* **6,** 153–7.

Chang, W.J., Nowinski, T.S. and Eagle, R.C. Jr (1995) A large oncocytoma of the caruncle. *Arch. Ophthalmol.,* **113,** 382.

Doxanas, M.T. and Green, W.R. (1984) Sebaceous gland carcinoma. Review of 40 cases. *Arch. Ophthalmol.,* **102,** 245–9.

Dugel, P.U., Gill, P.S., Frangieh, G.T. and Rao, N.A. (1992) Treatment of ocular adnexal Kaposi's sarcoma in acquired immune deficiency syndrome. *Ophthalmology,* **99,** 1127–32.

Duncan, J.L., Golabi, M., Fredrick, D.R., Hoyt, C.S., Hwang, D.G., Kramer, S.G., Howes, E.L. Jr and

Cunningham, E.T. Jr. (1998) Complex limbal choristomas in the linear nevus sebaceous syndrome. *Ophthalmology,* **105,** 1459–65.

Fry, C.L. and Leone, C.R. Jr. (1994) Safe management of dermolipomas. *Arch. Ophthalmol.,* **112,** 1114–16.

Ghabrial, R., Quivey, J.M., Dunn, J.P. Jr and Char, D.H. (1992) Radiation therapy of acquired immunodeficiency syndrome-related Kaposi's sarcoma of the eyelids and conjunctiva. *Arch. Ophthalmol.,* **110,** 1423–6.

Hayasaka, S., Sekimoto, M. and Setogawa, T. (1989) Epibulbar complex choristoma involving the bulbar conjunctiva and cornea. *Pediatr. Ophthalmol. Strabismus.,* **26,** 251–3.

Hayashi, N., Furihata, M., Ohtsuki, Y. and Ueno, H. (1994) Search for accumulation of p53 protein and detection of human papillomavirus genomes in sebaceous gland carcinoma of the eyelid. *Virchows Arch.,* **424,** 503–9.

Hummer, J., Gass, J.D. and Huang, A.J. (1993) Conjunctival Kaposi's sarcoma treated with interferon alpha-2a. *Am. J. Ophthalmol.,* **116,** 502–3.

Jakobiec, F.A. (1974) Sebaceous adenoma of the eyelid and visceral malignancy. *Am. J. Ophthalmol.,* **78,** 952–60.

Johnson, J.S., Lee, J.A., Cotton, D.W.K., Lee, W.R. and Parsons, M.A. (1999) Dimorphic immunohistochemical staining in ocular sebaceous neoplasms: a useful diagnostic aid. *Eye,* **13,** 104–8.

Kass, L.G. and Hornblass, A. (1989) Sebaceous carcinoma of the ocular adnexa. *Surv. Ophthalmol.,* **33,** 477–90.

Khan, M.A. and Dhillon, B. (1999) Epiphora due to Kaposi's sarcoma of the nasolacrimal duct. *Br. J. Ophthalmol.,* **83,** 501–2.

Kruse, F.E., Rohrschneider, K., Burk, R.O. and Völcker, H.E. (1998) Nevus sebaceus of Jadassohn associated with macro optic discs and conjunctival choristoma. *Arch. Ophthalmol.,* **116,** 1379–81.

Li, N., Anderson, W.K. and Bhawan, J. (1998) Further confirmation of the association of human herpesvirus 8 with Kaposi's sarcoma. *J. Cutan. Pathol.,* **25,** 413–19.

Mansour, A.M., Barber, J.C., Reinecke, R.D. and Wang, F.M. (1989) Ocular choristomas. *Surv. Ophthalmol.,* **33,** 339–58.

Margo, C.E. and Grossniklaus, H.E. (1995) Intraepithelial sebaceous neoplasia without underlying invasive carcinoma. *Surv. Ophthalmol.,* **39,** 293–301.

Nunery, W.R., Welsh, M.G. and McCord, C.D. Jr. (1983) Recurrence of sebaceous carcinoma of the eyelid after radiation therapy. *Am. J. Ophthalmol.,* **96,** 10–15.

Orcutt, J.C., Matsko, T.H. and Milam, A.H. (1992) Oncocytoma of the caruncle. *Ophthal. Plast. Reconstr. Surg.,* **8,** 300–2.

Rao, N.A., Hidayat, A.A., McLean, I.W. and

Zimmerman, L.E. (1982) Sebaceous carcinomas of the ocular adnexa: a clinicopathologic study of 104 cases, with five year follow-up data. *Hum. Pathol.*, **13**, 113–22.

Schwartz, R.A. and Torre, D.P. (1995) The Muir–Torre syndrome: a 25-year retrospect. *J. Am. Acad. Dermatol.*, **33**, 90–104.

Scott, K.R., Tse, D.T. and Kronish, J.W. (1991) Hemorrhagic lymphangiectasia of the conjunctiva. *Arch. Ophthalmol.*, **109**, 286–7.

UVEAL TUMOURS

Chapter 5

Naevus

A naevus is a hamartoma consisting of melanocytic cells derived from the neural crest.

Choroidal naevus

Choroidal naevi occur in about 5–10% of Caucasians (Sumich *et al.,* 1998), but many are not detected clinically (Naumann, 1970). They are not seen at birth and rarely present in Africans and Asians.

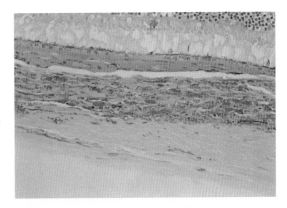

Figure 5.1 Light micrograph of a choroidal naevus

PATHOLOGY

Choroidal naevus cells are of four types:

a. Spindle shaped cells, with variable degrees of pigmentation (Figure 5.1).
b. Deeply pigmented, polyhedral cells with a small nucleus (i.e., 'melanocytoma cells').
c. Dendritic cells, with long branches, large nuclei, prominent nucleoli and variable pigmentation.
d. Large, non-pigmented cells with a foamy cytoplasm (i.e., balloon cells).

Choroidal naevi can cause the following secondary changes in surrounding tissues (Naumann *et al.,* 1971; Damato and Foulds, 1990):

a. Narrowing of the choriocapillaris, without tumour infiltration.
b. RPE degeneration and proliferation, with only small amounts of lipofuscin formation.
c. Serous retinal detachment with photoreceptor damage.
d. Choroidal neovascularization.

SYMPTOMS

Naevi are usually asymptomatic unless the fovea is involved by tumour or subretinal fluid, in which case the patient may complain of metamorphopsia.

SIGNS

TYPICAL NAEVUS

- A grey surface, which is featureless if the RPE is normal (Figure 5.2**a**) but which may contain drusen (Figure 5.2**b**). Rarely, a neovascular membrane can develop on the tumour surface (Mines *et al.*, 1985) (Figure 5.3).
- Ill-defined margins.
- Location anywhere in the choroid, but post-equatorially in about 90% of cases (Naumann, 1970).
- Diameter usually less than 3 mm.
- Thickness usually less than 1 mm.

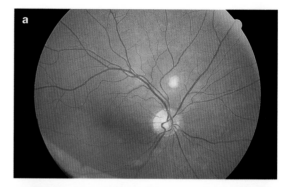

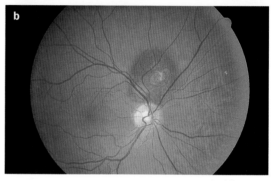

Figure 5.3 Choroidal naevi: (**a**) with active neovascular membrane and (**b**) with regressed neovascular membrane

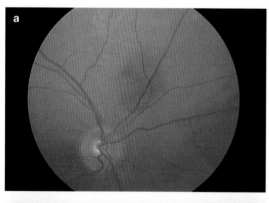

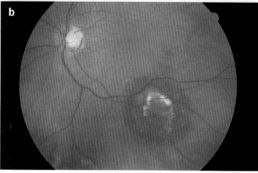

Figure 5.2 Choroidal naevi: (**a**) without surface change, (**b**) with overlying drusen

SUSPICIOUS NAEVUS

Choroidal naevi are regarded as 'suspicious' (i.e. of malignancy) (Shields *et al.*, 1995; The Collaborative Ocular Melanoma Study Group, 1997) if they have any of the following features:

- Thickness greater than 1 mm.
- Diameter greater than 5 mm.
- Flecks of confluent 'orange pigment' at the level of the RPE, consisting of macrophages containing lipofuscin (Figure 5.4).
- Overlying serous retinal detachment.
- Symptoms, such as metamorphopsia or photopsia.
- Absence of drusen on the surface of a thick lesion.
- Absence of an area of RPE change at the tumour margin.
- Margin touching the optic disc.
- Observed growth, as this is rare without histological evidence of malignancy.

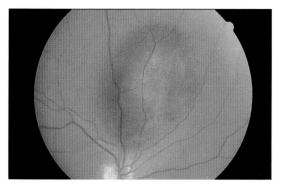

Figure 5.4 Suspicious choroidal naevus in the right eye of a 64-year-old man. The tumour had a thickness of 2.0 mm and orange pigment. No growth has been observed after eight years

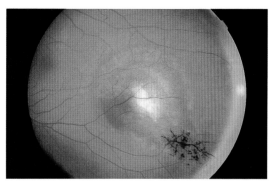

Figure 5.6 Comet's tail

Some naevi (called 'halo naevi') are surrounded by a pale zone, which resembles choroidal atrophy but which histologically consists of balloon-cell degeneration in the tumour cells (Rodriguez and Shields, 1976; Green, 1986) (Figure 5.5). Occasionally, the RPE anterior to the naevus becomes atrophic, with pigment clumping in the retina and a bone spicule appearance, presumably due to ischaemia (Figure 5.6). Retinal pigment epithelial disturbances can also occur below the tumour, as a result of fluid leakage (Haut *et al.*, 1984) (Figure 5.7).

A small minority of choroidal naevi are amelanotic (Brown *et al.*, 1981) (Figure 5.8).

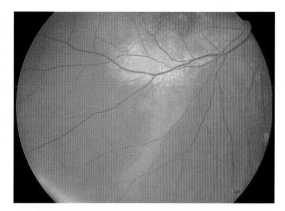

Figure 5.7 Hour-glass tail

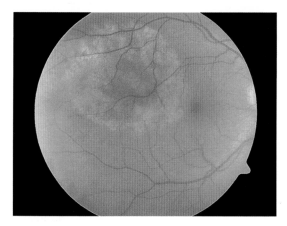

Figure 5.5 Halo naevus

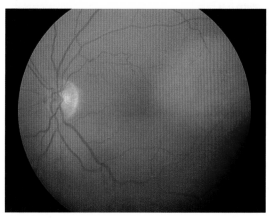

Figure 5.8 Presumed amelanotic naevus

INVESTIGATIONS

VISUAL FIELD EXAMINATION

Choroidal naevi tend to cause relative visual field defects. An absolute scotoma can occur, which does not necessarily indicate malignancy.

FLUORESCEIN ANGIOGRAPHY

Choroidal naevi are mostly hypofluorescent relative to the surrounding choroid (Figure 5.9). Areas of hyperfluorescence may represent drusen, serous retinal detachment and choroidal neovascular membrane formation. Multiple pinpoint areas of hyperfluorescence predict future growth (Butler, 1994).

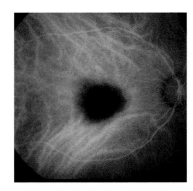

Figure 5.10 ICG angiogram of a choroidal naevus. (Courtesy of B.A. Lafaut, Ghent, Belgium)

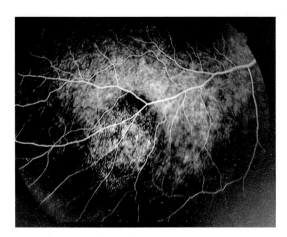

Figure 5.9 Fluorescein angiogram of a choroidal naevus showing masking of choroidal fluorescence and hyperfluorescent drusen

INDOCYANINE GREEN ANGIOGRAPHY

Choroidal naevi are hypofluorescent relative to the surrounding choroid (Figure 5.10).

ULTRASONOGRAPHY

Ultrasonography is useful for documenting the tumour thickness, but measurement of basal dimensions is only approximate because tapering margins are difficult to localize. A low internal acoustic reflectivity suggests malignancy (Butler *et al.,* 1994).

DIFFERENTIAL DIAGNOSIS

1. **Melanoma** (Chapter 7).
2. **Melanocytoma**, which can be clinically indistinguishable (Chapter 6).
3. **Congenital hypertrophy of the RPE** (Chapter 14).
4. **Combined hamartoma of the RPE and retina** (Chapter 15).

MANAGEMENT

Suspicious choroidal naevi should be observed indefinitely, first every 3–6 months and then annually. Slitlamp or ophthalmoscopic appearances should be compared with baseline photographs (Figure 5.11) and sequential ultrasonography performed if increasing thickness is suspected.

It is not unusual for patients to be referred to an ocular oncology centre with an advanced melanoma years after being discharged by their ophthalmologist with an incorrect diagnosis of a naevus, sometimes after a long period of observation.

Monitoring of suspicious naevi should be life-long.

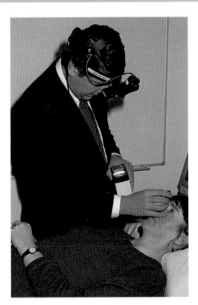

Figure 5.11 Monitoring of a suspicious choroidal naevus by comparing ophthalmoscopic appearances with baseline photographs using a hand-held, illuminated viewer

In patients with symptoms caused by serous retinal detachment, photocoagulation applied to points of leakage has been followed by apparent growth of tumour through defects in Bruch's membrane, suggesting malignancy (Erie *et al.,* 1990). If there is sufficient space between the tumour and the fovea, some authorities prefer to apply a row of burns at the posterior tumour margin, creating a waterproof barrier (Shields, 1994).

Iris naevus

PATHOLOGY

Iris naevi may contain cells that are large and multinucleated.

SYMPTOMS

Most iris naevi are asymptomatic and either present as a cosmetic blemish or are detected on routine examination. Rarely, visual loss occurs because of secondary glaucoma.

SIGNS

Common iris naevi can have any of the following features:

- Diameter of up to 3–4 mm if the tumour is circumscribed (Figure 5.12).
- Thickness of less than 2 mm.
- Yellow, white, grey or brown colour.
- Rough or smooth surface.
- Minimal or no visible vascularity.
- Circumscribed or diffuse configuration.
- Round, irregular or sectorial shape.
- Discrete or indistinct margins.
- Inferior location in most cases.
- Seeding of pigment or growth into the angle.
- Ectropion uveae (Figure 5.13).

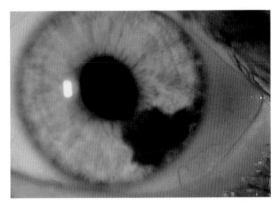

Figure 5.12 Iris naevus

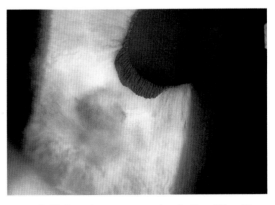

Figure 5.13 Ectropion uveae associated with a diffuse iris naevus

- Rarely, multiple gelatinous nodules giving a 'tapioca' appearance.
- Cyst formation at the pupil margin.

An iris naevus can show apparent growth, especially after puberty, in the teenage years.

A sectorial iris naevus may be associated with a posterior uveal melanoma in the same sector of the eye (Shields and Shields, 1992) (Figure 5.14).

COMPLICATIONS

- Glaucoma, which is rare, occurring either with diffuse iris naevi (Nik *et al.*, 1981) or as a result of pigment scatter.
- Localized lens opacities.

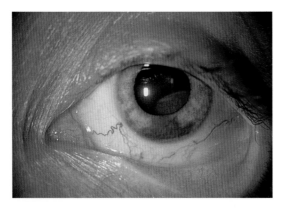

Figure 5.14 Sectorial iris naevus (histologically confirmed) anterior to a choroidal melanoma

INVESTIGATIONS

FLUORESCEIN ANGIOGRAPHY

Fluorescence of iris naevi depends mostly on the degree of pigmentation and is not useful in differentiating a benign tumour from melanoma.

DIFFERENTIAL DIAGNOSIS

1. **Freckles**, which are collections of hypertrophic melanocytes that do not disturb normal architecture (Figure 5.15) .

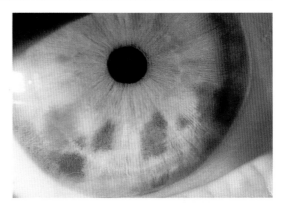

Figure 5.15 Iris freckles

2. **Small melanomas**, which are more likely to show tumour vascularity, localized lens opacities, trans-scleral extension, and growth in adulthood (Territo *et al.*, 1988).
3. **Lisch nodules**, which are multiple, gelatinous, yellow–brown tumours in the iris, up to 2 mm in diameter (Figure 5.16). They occur in over 90% of patients with neurofibromatosis type 1 after the age of six years. Histologically, they are indistinguishable from naevi.
4. **Iris mammillations** (Ragge *et al.*, 1996) (Figure 5.17), also known as 'diffuse iris nodular naevi' (Ticho *et al.*, 1995). These may be (i) unilateral or bilateral; (ii) sporadic or inherited in an autosomal dominant fashion; and (iii) isolated or associated with other

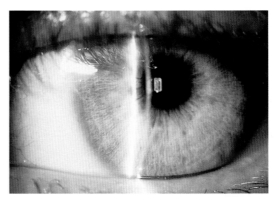

Figure 5.16 Lisch nodules. (Courtesy of J.A. Augsburger, Cincinnati, USA)

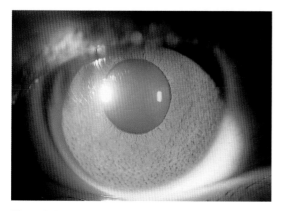

Figure 5.17 Iris mammillations

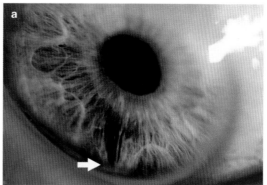

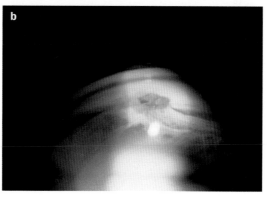

Figure 5.18 Intraocular foreign body: (**a**) slitlamp appearance and (**b**) three-mirror appearance

abnormalities, such as oculodermal melanosis, Axenfeld anomaly and Peters anomaly.

5. **Cogan–Reese syndrome** is caused by downgrowth of an abnormal endothelium across the trabecular meshwork. It causes glaucoma, corneal oedema, ectropion uveae, progressive iris atrophy and nodular or diffuse, pigmented iris lesions (Levy *et al.,* 1995). It forms part of the spectrum of diseases known as the iridocorneal endothelial (ICE) syndrome, which also includes Chandler's syndrome and progressive iris atrophy. Cases have been reported in which an iris naevus has been associated with peripheral anterior synechiae, endothelial downgrowth and glaucoma (Jakobiec *et al.,* 1977).

6. **Intraocular foreign body**, present after a forgotten injury (Figure 5.18).

7. **Iris cysts** may resemble naevus at the pupil margin, in the stroma or in the anterior chamber angle, where they may settle after becoming dislodged (Chapter 16).

MANAGEMENT

As with choroidal naevi, suspicious iris naevi need to be monitored indefinitely, comparing the slit-lamp appearances with baseline photographs.

If biopsy of an iris tumour is indicated, FNAB would be the simplest surgical procedure to perform. If this fails to provide a diagnosis, then incisional or excisional biopsy may be considered.

REFERENCES

Brown, G.C., Shields, J.A. and Augsburger, J.J. (1981) Amelanotic choroidal nevi. *Ophthalmology,* **88**, 1116–21.

Butler, P., Char, D.H., Zarbin, M. and Kroll, S. (1994) Natural history of indeterminate pigmented choroidal tumors. *Ophthalmology,* **101**, 710–16.

Damato, B.E. and Foulds, W.S. (1990) Tumour-associated retinal pigment epitheliopathy. *Eye,* **4**, 382–7.

Erie, J.C., Robertson, D.M. and Mieler, W.F. (1990) Presumed small choroidal melanomas with serous macular detachments with and without surface laser photocoagulation treatment. *Am. J. Ophthalmol.,* **109**, 259–64.

Green, W.R. (1986) Uveal tract. In: W.H. Spencer (ed.), *Ophthalmic Pathology.* Philadelphia: Saunders.

Haut, J., Sobel Martin, A., Dureuil, J., Larricart, P. and Sarnikowski, C. (1984) Atrophies 'like flows' of the retinal pigment epithelium: a neuroepithelium-draining method of the posterior pole. *Ophthalmologica,* **189**, 121–7.

Jakobiec, F.A., Yanoff, M., Motwani, M.V., Mottow, L., Anker, P. and Jones, I.S. (1977) Solitary iris nevus associated with peripheral anterior synechiae and iris endothelialization. *Am. J. Ophthalmol.*, **83**, 884–91.

Levy, S.G., McCartney, A.C.E., Baghai, M.H.B.M.C. and Moss, J. (1995) Pathology of the iridocorneal-endothelial syndrome. *Invest. Ophthalmol. Vis. Sci.*, **36**, 2592–601.

Mines, J.A., Freilich, D.B., Friedman, A.H. and Lazar, M. (1985) Choroidal (subretinal) neovascularization secondary to choroidal nevus and successful treatment with argon laser photocoagulation: case reports and review of literature. *Ophthalmologica*, **190**, 210–18.

Naumann, G. (1970) Pigmentierte Naevi der Aderhaut und des Ciliarkörpers. *Adv. Ophthalmol.*, **23**, 187–272.

Naumann, G.O.H., Hellner, K. and Naumann, L.R. (1971) Pigmented nevi of the choroid. Clinical study of secondary changes in the overlying tissues. *Trans. Am. Acad. Ophthalmol. Otolaryngol.*, **75**, 110–23.

Nik, N.A., Hidayat, A., Zimmerman, L.E. and Fine, B.S. (1981) Diffuse iris nevus manifested by unilateral open angle glaucoma. *Arch. Ophthalmol.*, **99**, 125–7.

Ragge, N.K., Acheson, J. and Murphree, A.L. (1996) Iris mammillations: significance and associations. *Eye*, **10**, 86–91.

Rodriguez, M.M. and Shields, J.A. (1976) Malignant melanoma of the choroid with balloon cells. A clinicopatholoic study of three cases. *Can. J. Ophthalmol.*, **11**, 208–16.

Shields, J.A. (1994) The expanding role of laser photocoagulation for intraocular tumors. The 1993 H. Christian Zweng Memorial Lecture. *Retina*, **14**, 310–22.

Shields, J.A. and Shields, C.L. (1992) *Intraocular Tumors. A Text and Atlas.* Philadelphia: W.B. Saunders, pp. 62–3.

Shields, C.L., Shields, J.A., Kiratli, H., De Potter, P. and Cater, J.R. (1995) Risk factors for growth and metastasis of small choroidal melanocytic lesions. *Ophthalmology*, **102**, 1351–61.

Sumich, P., Mitchell, P. and Wang, J.J. (1998) Choroidal nevi in a white population. The Blue Mountains Study. *Arch. Ophthalmol.*, **116**, 645–50.

Territo, C., Shields, C.L., Shields, J.A., Augsburger, J.J. and Schroeder, R.P. (1988) Natural course of melanocytic tumors of the iris. *Ophthalmology*, **95**, 1251–5.

The Collaborative Ocular Melanoma Study Group (1997) Factors predictive of growth and treatment of small choroidal melanoma. COMS report no. 5. *Arch. Ophthalmol.*, **115**, 1537–44.

Ticho, B.H., Rosner, M., Mets, M.B. and Tso, M.O.M. (1995) Bilateral diffuse iris nodular nevi. Clinical and histopathologic characterization. *Ophthalmology*, **102**, 419–25.

Chapter 6

Melanocytoma

Melanocytoma is a distinctive type of naevus, which merits a separate section. The tumour is rare in Caucasians and relatively common in dark skinned people (Joffe *et al.*, 1979). The incidence is slightly higher in females.

The true incidence of choroidal and ciliary body melanocytomas is probably underestimated, because they may be mistaken for more common naevi and melanomas (Char and Miller, 1995).

PATHOLOGY

Melanocytomas consist of deeply pigmented, large polyhedral cells or small spindle cells with a small nucleus (Zimmerman and Garron, 1962; Juarez and Ts'o, 1980) (Figure 6.1). They are most often clinically diagnosed at the optic nerve head but can occur anywhere in the uveal tract.

Melanocytomas have a tendency to undergo necrosis, inflammation and oedema. At the optic nerve head this can cause nerve fibre compression, vascular obstruction, retinal haemorrhages, macular oedema (Zimmerman, 1965) and neovascular glaucoma (Croxatto *et al.*, 1983). Necrosis can also cause pigment dispersion, which may reach the anterior chamber (Yamaguchi *et al.*, 1987).

Ciliary body melanocytomas can extend into the anterior chamber and extraocularly. Necrosis

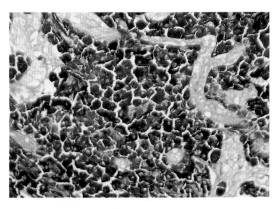

Figure 6.1 Light micrograph of a melanocytoma showing deeply pigmented, plump cells with small nuclei (H&E)

can cause uveitis, pigment dispersion and glaucoma (Fineman *et al.*, 1998).

Malignant transformation can occur, but this is rare (Roth, 1978; Shields *et al.*, 1990) (Figure 6.2).

SYMPTOMS

Most patients are asymptomatic, unless the tumour causes optic nerve damage, uveitis, or glaucoma.

SIGNS

OPTIC DISC

- Black or grey colour (Figure 6.3**a**–**c**).
- Feathery anterior margin within the retinal nerve fibre layer.

- Size varying from a small fraction of the optic disc area to about 2 mm, sometimes completely obscuring the disc.
- Inferior location in most cases (Joffe *et al.*, 1979).
- Slow growth in a small proportion of patients (Mansour *et al.*, 1989).

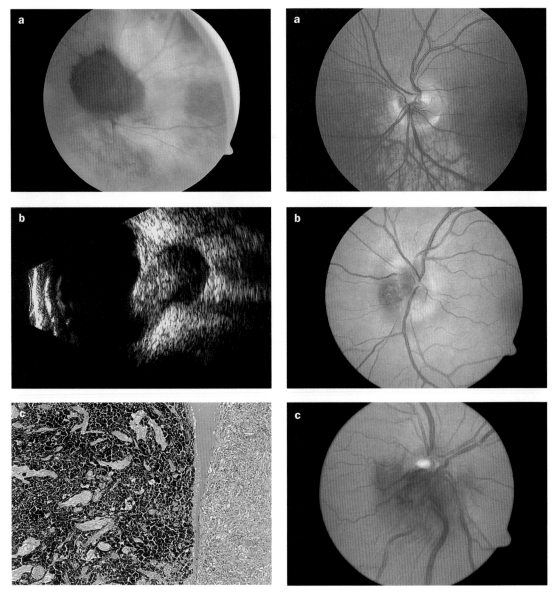

Figure 6.2 Optic disc melanocytoma associated with malignant transformation and massive extraocular extension: (**a**) fundus photograph, (**b**) ultrasonography and (**c**) light micrograph showing melanocytoma to left and melanoma to right (H&E)

Figure 6.3 Melanocytoma of the optic disc: (**a**) confined to disc, (**b**) with flat extension into adjacent choroid and (**c**) with minimal retinal involvement

- An afferent pupillary defect in a minority of patients. This does not indicate malignancy (Osher *et al.*, 1979).
- Swelling of the adjacent optic disc.
- Ocular melanosis and naevi, which are more common in eyes with melanocytoma (Joffe *et al.*, 1979).

CHOROID

Choroidal melanocytomas are clinically indistinguishable from large naevi and small melanomas. A rare, diffuse variety has been described resembling diffuse melanoma (Haas *et al.*, 1986).

CILIARY BODY AND IRIS

Ciliary body melanocytomas can extend into the anterior chamber and extraocularly, to mimic malignant invasion by melanoma (Figure 6.4) (Adenis *et al.*, 1983; Rummelt *et al.*, 1994). As with melanoma, cystoid spaces may be present (Croxatto *et al.*, 1984), which are demonstrable with high-frequency ultrasonography.

INVESTIGATIONS

CLINICAL

Optic nerve head melanocytomas can be diagnosed by ophthalmoscopy. Baseline colour photography enables subtle growth to be detected more reliably.

PATHOLOGICAL

If sufficient material is obtained by fine needle aspiration biopsy, then melanocytoma should be distinguishable from melanoma. Incisional biopsy of a ciliary body or iris tumour would provide a better specimen for microscopy. Excisional biopsy should also prevent the complications of melanocytoma. When performing the histology, bleaching of the melanin with hydrogen peroxide allows cellular detail to be examined.

DIFFERENTIAL DIAGNOSIS

1. **Melanoma**, which is more likely to demonstrate growth, but which may be clinically

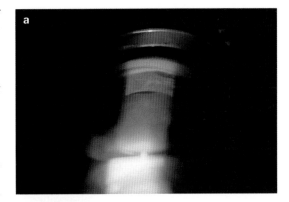

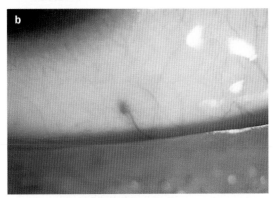

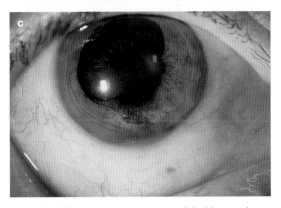

Figure 6.4 Ciliary body melanocytoma: (**a**) with extension to anterior chamber and (**b**) episclera; (**c**) same patient after excision biopsy and plaque radiotherapy, with vision of 6/5 more than one year postoperatively

indistinguishable, even with imaging (see Figure 6.2) (Chapter 7).
2. **Congenital hypertrophy of the RPE**, which does not extend over the disc (Chapter 14).

3. **Combined hamartoma of the retina and RPE**, which causes contracture of the retina similar to an epiretinal membrane (Chapter 15).
4. **RPE adenoma and adenocarcinoma** (Chapter 17).

MANAGEMENT

OPTIC DISC MELANOCYTOMA

As with suspicious naevi, life-long observation is required, aided by colour photography and ultrasonography.

CILIARY BODY MELANOCYTOMA

If a ciliary body melanocytoma can be differentiated from melanoma with certainty, the patient should be kept under observation, although at some risk of uveitis, pigment dispersion, glaucoma and malignant transformation. The author has dealt with this problem by performing iridocyclectomy with adjunctive plaque radiotherapy (Figure 6.4**c**).

PROGNOSIS

The prognosis for survival is excellent unless there is malignant transformation. Visual loss due to optic nerve damage is usually permanent (Wiznia and Price, 1974).

REFERENCES

Adenis, J.P., Loubet, A., Leboutet, M.J., Loubet, R. and Robin, A. (1983) Mélanocytome de l'iris, du corps ciliaire et tumeurs pigmentées multiples. Etude ultrastructurale. *J. Fr. Ophtalmol.*, **6**, 257–65.

Char, D.H. and Miller, T. (1995) Accuracy of presumed uveal melanoma diagnosis before alternative therapy. *Br. J. Ophthalmol.*, **79**, 692–6.

Croxatto, J.O., Ebner, R., Crovetto, L. and Morales, A.G. (1983) Angle closure glaucoma as initial manifestation of melanocytoma of the optic disc. *Ophthalmology*, **90**, 830–4.

Croxatto, J.O., Malbran, E.S. and Lombardi, A.A. (1984) Cavitary melanocytoma of the ciliary body. *Ophthalmologica*, **189**, 130–4.

Fineman, M.S., Eagle, R.C. Jr., Shields, J.A., Shields, C.L. and De Potter, P. (1998) Melanocytomalytic glaucoma in eyes with necrotic iris melanocytoma. *Ophthalmology*, **105**, 492–6.

Haas, B.D., Jakobiec, F.A., Iwamoto, T., Cox, M., Bernacki, E.G. and Pokorny, K.L. (1986) Diffuse choroidal melanocytoma in a child. A lesion extending the spectrum of melanocytic hamartomas. *Ophthalmology*, **93**, 1632–8.

Joffe, L., Shields, J.A., Osher, R.H. and Gass, J.D. (1979) Clinical and follow-up studies of melanocytomas of the optic disc. *Ophthalmology*, **86**, 1067–83.

Juarez, C.P. and Ts'o, M.O.M. (1980) An ultrastructural study of melanocytomas (magnocellular nevi) of the optic disc and uvea. *Am. J. Ophthalmol.*, **90**, 48–62.

Mansour, A.M., Zimmerman, L.E., La Piana, F.G. and Beauchamp, G.R. (1989) Clinico-pathological findings in a growing optic nerve melanocytoma. *Br. J. Ophthalmol.*, **73**, 410–15.

Osher, R.H., Shields, J.A. and Layman, P.R. (1979) Pupillary and visual field evaluation in patients with melanocytoma of the optic disc. *Arch. Ophthalmol.*, **97**, 1096–9.

Roth, A.M. (1978) Malignant change in melanocytomas of the uveal tract. *Surv. Ophthalmol.*, **22**, 404–12.

Rummelt, V., Naumann, G.O., Folberg, R. and Weingeist, T.A. (1994) Surgical management of melanocytoma of the ciliary body with extrascleral extension. *Am. J. Ophthalmol.*, **117**, 169–76.

Shields, J.A., Shields, C.L., Eagle, R.C., Jr, Lieb, W.E. and Stern, S. (1990) Malignant melanoma associated with melanocytoma of the optic disc. *Ophthalmology*, **97**, 225–30.

Wiznia, R.A. and Price, J. (1974) Recovery of vision in association with a melanocytoma of the optic disk. *Am. J. Ophthalmol.*, **78**, 236–8.

Yamaguchi, K., Shiono, T. and Mizuno, K. (1987) Pigment deposition in the anterior segment caused by melanocytoma of the optic disc. *Ophthalmologica*, **194**, 191–3.

Zimmerman, L.E. (1965) Melanocytes, melanocytic nevi and melanocytomas. *Invest. Ophthalmol. Vis. Sci.*, **4**, 11–40.

Zimmerman, L.E. and Garron, L.K. (1962) Melanocytoma of the optic disc. *Int. Ophthalmol. Clin.*, **2**, 431–40.

Chapter 7

Uveal melanoma

Uveal melanoma is by far the commonest primary intraocular malignancy in adults and is therefore discussed more fully than other tumours.

EPIDEMIOLOGY

The overall incidence of uveal melanoma is 6–7 per million per year (Egan *et al.*, 1988; Scotto *et al.*, 1976). It increases with age from about 2.5 per million between the ages of 15 and 44 years to 25 per million after the age of 65 years (Seddon and Egan, 1993). The tumour is extremely rare in children. There is no significant sex difference. Uveal melanoma is much more common in Caucasians than in Africans or Asians (Margo *et al.*, 1998). Familial cases are rare (Singh *et al.*, 1996).

Epidemiological studies suggest that intraocular melanoma is 2–3 times more common in blue/grey than in brown eyes (Egan *et al.*, 1988). The importance of sunlight is uncertain.

ASSOCIATIONS

1. **Ocular melanocytosis**, which consists of an increased population of melanocytes within the uvea and episclera (Singh *et al.*, 1998) (Figure 7.1).

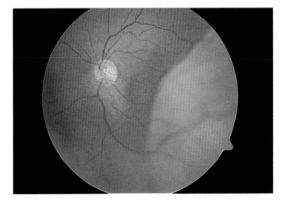

Figure 7.1 Uveal melanoma in an eye with oculodermal melanocytosis. (This is the same patient as shown in Figure 2.8)

2. **Oculodermal melanocytosis** (naevus of Ota), which also involves the periocular skin and meninges. Ocular and oculodermal melanocytosis are associated with a lifetime incidence of uveal melanoma of approximately one in 400 (Singh *et al.*, 1998).

3. **Simple and dysplastic cutaneous naevi and cutaneous melanomas**, which are more common in patients with uveal melanoma (Bataille *et al.*, 1995)

4. **Neurofibromatosis type 1**, which is associated with an increased incidence of uveal naevi (Wiznia *et al.,* 1978) and rarely of uveal melanoma (Friedman and Margo, 1998).

There is no significant increase in the incidence of other cancers (Holly *et al.,* 1991).

PATHOLOGY

Uveal melanomas are different from conjunctival and cutaneous melanomas. They arise in the choroid (80%), ciliary body (12%) and iris (8%).

CELL TYPES

a. Spindle B cells, which are long and fusiform, with an oval nucleus and a prominent nucleolus (Figure 7.2**a**).
b. Epithelioid cells, which are large and round, with abundant eosinophilic cytoplasm and a large nucleus containing a conspicuous nucleolus (Figure 7.2**b**).
c. Intermediate cells, having features of both spindle cells and epithelioid cells.

Spindle A cells are now regarded as being benign.

MODIFIED CALLENDER CLASSIFICATION (McLean *et al.,* 1983)

Uveal melanomas are categorized as:

a. Spindle cell (45%), containing only spindle cells, with a small proportion described as *fascicular* because of the way in which the cells are orientated parallel to each other.
b. Epithelioid (5%), consisting of only epithelioid cells.
c. Mixed (45%), having variable proportions of the two cell types.
d. Necrotic (5%), which are unclassifiable because of extensive necrosis.

NOTABLE HISTOLOGICAL FEATURES

a. Pigmentation, which tends to be greater in dark skinned individuals.
b. Lymphocytic infiltration, which is prominent in about 12% of tumours (de la Cruz Jr. *et al.,* 1990).
c. Mitotic rate, usually about 3 per 40 high power fields.
d. Necrosis, which is present in a small proportion of cases.
e. Vascularity, with both microvascular density and pattern having prognostic significance. Nine microvascular patterns have been described, of which closed vascular loops have the worst prognosis (Rummelt *et al.,* 1994) (Figure 7.3).

SPECIAL TECHNIQUES

a. Masson–Fontana stain, to label melanosomes in amelanotic melanomas.
b. Permanganate or hydrogen peroxide bleach (Kivelä, 1995) to allow cellular detail to be studied in deeply pigmented tumours.

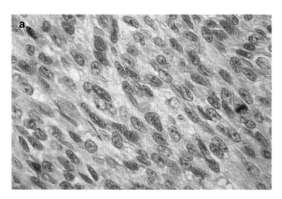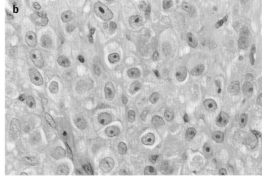

Figure 7.2 Light micrographs of uveal melanoma showing (**a**) spindle B cells and (**b**) epithelioid cells

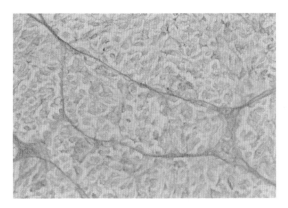

Figure 7.3 Closed vascular loops in a uveal melanoma

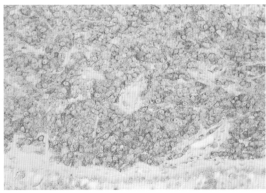

Figure 7.4 Immunohistochemical staining of uveal melanoma with HMB-45, which is often helpful in differentiating amelanotic melanoma from a non-melanomatous metastasis

c. PAS without counterstain, to analyse micro-vascular patterns.

d. Immunohistochemistry, to detect expression of melanoma associated antigens (MAA), such as S100 protein and HMB-45 (Figure 7.4). Proliferation markers such as Ki-67 and PC-10 (Seregard *et al.,* 1996) provide an indication of cell turnover.

e. Chromosome studies on tumour samples, which may show monosomy of chromosome 3 and multiplication of chromosome 8q, especially in ciliary body melanomas (Figure 7.5).

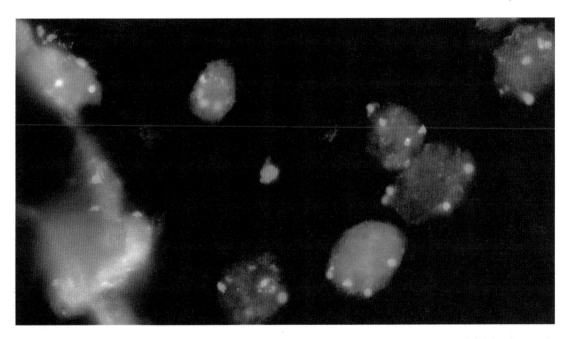

Figure 7.5 Monosomy 3 (green) and trisomy 8 (red) demonstrated with fluorescence in-situ hybridization (FISH) in a fine needle aspirate of a uveal melanoma. (Courtesy of J.E.M.M. de Klein, Rotterdam, The Netherlands)

Choroidal melanoma

PATHOLOGY

SECONDARY CHANGES (Damato and Foulds, 1990) (Figure 7.6)

a. Disruption of the choriocapillaris.
b. Destruction of Bruch's membrane.
c. Proliferation, multilayering and atrophy of the RPE.
d. Pigment epithelial detachments.
e. Accumulation of hard drusen, soft drusen and lipofuscin ('orange pigment').
f. Rarely, choroidal neovascularization.

Amelanotic melanomas may falsely appear pigmented because of RPE proliferation (Figure 7.7).

SECONDARY CHANGES IN SENSORY RETINA

a. Photoreceptor degeneration, causing visual field loss and an afferent pupillary defect.
b. Serous retinal detachment, which eventually becomes extensive and bullous. Separation of the retina from the choriocapillaris causes retinal ischaemia, which contributes to the development of rubeosis and neovascular glaucoma.
c. Cystoid macular oedema, even with peripheral tumours.

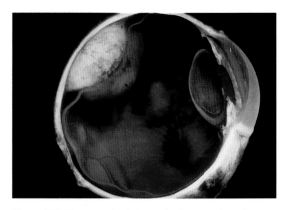

Figure 7.7 Macroscopic photograph of an enucleated eye showing an amelanotic melanoma covered by a proliferated pigment epithelium

PATTERNS OF TUMOUR SPREAD

a. Rupture of Bruch's membrane and RPE, with herniation into the subretinal space, usually with the development of a 'collar-stud' shape (Figure 7.8).
b. Perforation of the retina, with vitreous seeding (Dunn *et al.,* 1988) and haemorrhage.
c. Invasion of vortex veins, causing metastasis.
d. Extension into the orbit, usually via scleral openings for blood vessels and nerves.
e. Invasion of the optic nerve in a small proportion of cases (Shields *et al.,* 1987), usually in blind and glaucomatous eyes (Spencer, 1975).

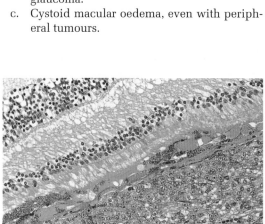

Figure 7.6 Multilayering, atrophy and drusen formation in RPE over a choroidal melanoma demonstrated by light microscopy (H&E)

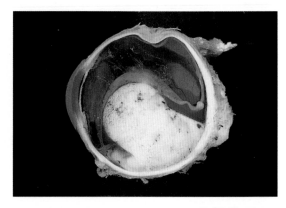

Figure 7.8 Collar-stud melanoma. (Courtesy of W.R. Lee, Glasgow, UK)

f. Spread along retina (Kirelä and Summanen, 1997).

About 5% of all melanomas are diffuse and infiltrate the uvea widely without significant increase in choroidal thickness (Figure 7.9). These tumours are particularly aggressive and often extend extraocularly by the time of diagnosis (Shields *et al.*, 1996).

Tumours that are large or diffuse tend to undergo necrosis, which may cause severe uveitis and episcleritis. Tumour recurrence and metastatic disease can follow spontaneous regression.

SYMPTOMS

a. Blurred vision, caused by retinal detachment, posterior tumour location, or vitreous haemorrhage.
b. Visual field loss, caused usually by the retinal detachment and sometimes by the tumour itself.
c. Floaters, from vitreous haemorrhage.
d. Photopsia, which differ from those of vitreoretinal traction in that they are described as a ball of light moving across the visual field over several seconds, more noticeably in subdued lighting.
e. Pain secondary to neovascular glaucoma or uveitis.

Many patients are asymptomatic and the tumour is detected on routine fundus examination performed for other reasons.

SIGNS

- RPE multilayering over a choroidal melanoma gives the tumour a grey–brown colour. This appearance occurs whether or not the tumour itself is pigmented. The abnormal RPE is recognizable by the presence of drusen, orange pigment, and other secondary changes (Figure 7.10). Where the RPE is absent, the tumour itself is visible as a white, yellow, tan, brown, grey or black mass (Figure 7.11).
- A collar-stud shape, if present, is usually easily recognized, unless the tumour is large and anterior. Large intra-tumoral vessels are nearly always visible if the tumour is amelanotic (Figure 7.12**a**) but not if the tumour is deeply pigmented (Figure 7.12**b**).
- In the early stages, retinal detachment is present only over the tumour surface. Later, the

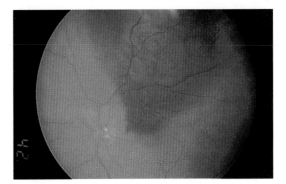

Figure 7.10 Sub-RPE choroidal melanoma, showing confluent orange pigment

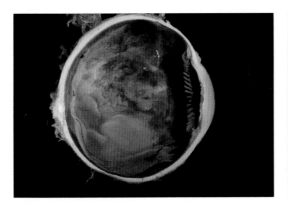

Figure 7.9 Diffuse choroidal melanoma. (Courtesy of W.R. Lee, Glasgow, UK)

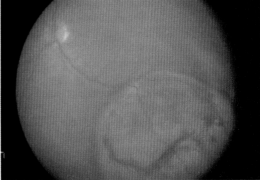

Figure 7.11 Atrophy of the RPE over a choroidal melanoma, showing amelanotic nature of tumour

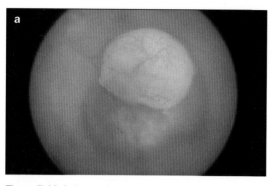
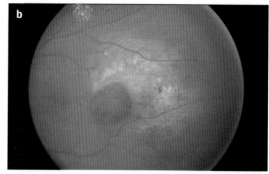

Figure 7.12 Collar-stud melanomas, which can be (**a**) amelanotic and (**b**) melantotic, with tumour vasculature visible only in the amelanotic tumours

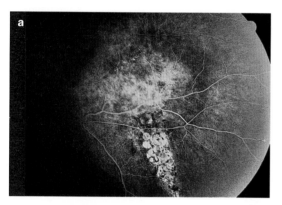
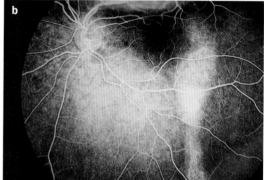

Figure 7.13 (**a**) Comet's tail and (**b**) hour-glass RPE degeneration peripheral to melanoma

subretinal fluid shifts inferiorly, to cause a small bullous detachment, resembling retinoschisis. The exudative detachment gradually becomes more extensive and eventually total. Unlike rhegmatogenous retinal detachment, the subretinal fluid shifts with ocular movement and gravity. Rarely, there is no retinal detachment, particularly if a collar-stud tumour has perforated the retina.

- Melanomas and suspicious naevi can interfere with the choroidal circulation to cause a straight line of cobblestone degeneration pointing outwards from the posterior pole (i.e, 'comet's tail'). This is usually associated with 'bone spicules' (Figure 7.13**a**).
- Leakage of fluid from the tumour to the inferior equatorial region of the globe may cause an 'hour-glass' pattern of RPE stippling (Figure 7.13**b**) (Haut *et al.*, 1984).

- Diffuse melanomas show extensive, flat, grey, irregular discoloration of the fundus and retinal detachment (Figure 7.14). If the optic nerve is invaded, central retinal vein occlusion may

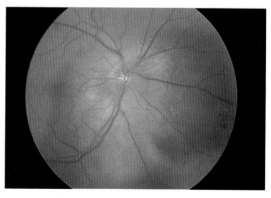

Figure 7.14 Diffuse choroidal melanoma surrounding optic disc

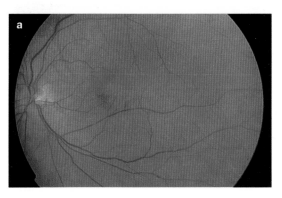
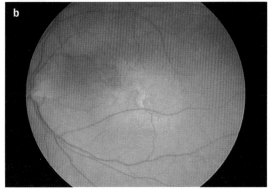

Figure 7.15 Rapid growth of a choroidal melanoma: (**a**) small, pigmented tumour at the left macula and (**b**) 13 months later. (Courtesy of D.J. Mooney, Dublin, Republic of Ireland)

occur. Extraocular extension is relatively common, even with small tumours.

- Most choroidal melanomas grow slowly, over months or years. Rarely, dramatic growth occurs, even if the tumour is small (Figure 7.15).

DIFFERENTIAL DIAGNOSIS

- **Naevus** (Chapter 5).
- **Melanocytoma** (Chapter 6).
- **Metastasis** (Chapter 19).
- **Choroidal haemangioma** (Chapter 8).
- **Choroidal neovascular membranes** with secondary haemorrhage and exudation usually develop at the macula (i.e., 'disciform macular lesion') but they can occur anywhere in the fundus (i.e., 'eccentric disciform lesion'). These lesions are more likely to be associated with hard exudates and subretinal haemorrhage than melanomas of equivalent size (Figure 7.16a). On ultrasonography, they tend to show more irregular reflectivity (Figure 7.16b). They are also more likely to cause vitreous haemorrhage. Unlike melanoma, however, sequential ultrasonography shows contraction instead of growth. The vitreous eventually clears to reveal a typical disciform scar (Figure 7.17).
- **Choroidal osteoma** (Chapter 9).
- **Congenital hypertrophy of the RPE** (Chapter 14).

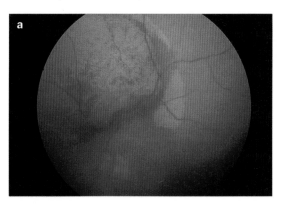
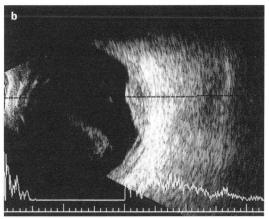

Figure 7.16 Macular subretinal haemorrhage arising from age-related choroidal neovascularization. Note the fresh haemorrhage and exudation, which are unusual with melanoma: (**a**) colour photograph; (**b**) ultrasound scan

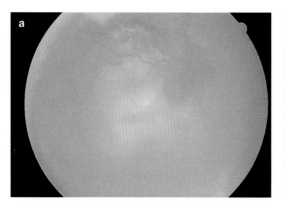
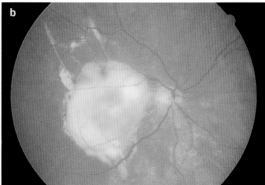

Figure 7.17 Macular neovascular membrane (**a**) obscured by vitreous haemorrhage and (**b**) a few months later, when typical features of a disciform scar are recognizable

- **Combined hamartoma of the retina and RPE** (Chapter 15).
- **Choroidal haemorrhage** tends to be covered by a normal RPE, often with folds radiating to vortex vein insertions in the sclera. This lesion tends to resolve spontaneously (Figure 7.18).
- **Posterior scleritis** (Chapter 8).
- **Choroidal granuloma** (Figure 7.19), due to conditions such as tuberculosis, syphilis and sarcoidosis. The disease may be diagnosed by PCR testing on aqueous humour samples (Sarvananthan *et al.,* 1998).
- **Paraneoplastic melanocytic proliferation** may resemble diffuse melanoma (Chapter 22).
- **Ocular compression** by an extraocular tumour changes position with eye movement and is not discoloured.

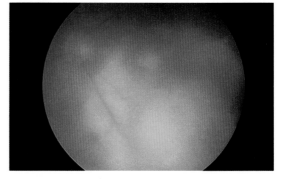

Figure 7.19 Choroidal granuloma, which on biopsy contained numerous eosinophils

Uveal melanoma can regress briefly with steroid therapy, mimicking an inflammatory mass (Simpson, 1999).

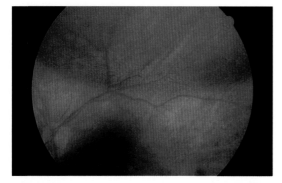

Figure 7.18 Choroidal haematoma after lens extraction. Note the smooth RPE with a fold radiating from the vortex vein insertion

Ciliary body melanoma

PATHOLOGY

As with melanomas elsewhere, ciliary body melanomas can be amelanotic, pigmented or pseudopigmented (Figure 7.20).

PATTERNS OF TUMOUR GROWTH

a. Circumferential spread within the ciliary body to form a 'ring melanoma'.

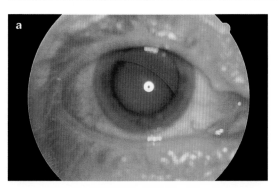

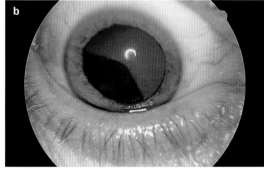

Figure 7.20 Ciliary body melanomas, which can be (**a**) amelanotic and (**b**) melantotic

b. Spread to the anterior chamber, with circumferential growth along the angle to cause eventual glaucoma (Figure 7.21).
c. Extraocular extension along a nerve or blood vessel, to form an episcleral pigmented nodule or an area of diffuse pigmentation (Figure 7.21).

SECONDARY CHANGES IN ADJACENT STRUCTURES

a. Lens complications, such as indentation, subluxation, and cataract formation (Figure 7.22).
b. Secondary glaucoma, caused by dispersion of melanomacrophages into the angle.
c. Dilatation of the overlying episcleral veins ('sentinel vessels') (Figures 7.21 and 7.23). Such vessels can occur with other types of tumour, benign or malignant.

SYMPTOMS

a. Blurred vision due to cataract or lenticular astigmatism, perhaps requiring a frequent change of spectacles.

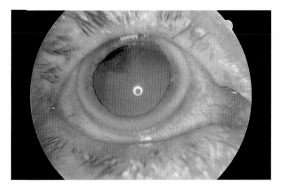

Figure 7.22 Cataract secondary to ciliary body melanoma

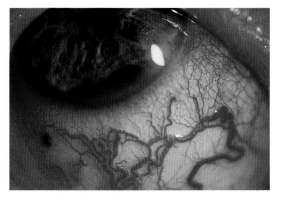

Figure 7.21 Ciliary body melanoma with anterior chamber invasion, extraocular extension and sentinel vessels

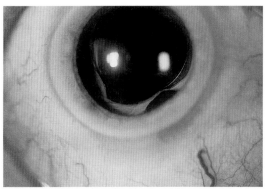

Figure 7.23 Sentinel vessel overlying ciliary body melanoma in a pseudophakic patient

b. Visual field loss due to exudative retinal detachment.
c. Red eye related to sentinel vessels.
d. Pain caused by secondary glaucoma

SIGNS

- Pigmented or amelanotic tumour involving the ciliary body or iris.
- Cataract or lens subluxation.
- Exudative retinal detachment.
- Invasion of the anterior chamber, with annular spread and secondary glaucoma.
- Extraocular extension.
- Sentinel vessels.

DIFFERENTIAL DIAGNOSIS

a. **Adenoma and adenocarcinoma** (Chapter 17).
b. **Uveal effusion** is lobulated (Figure 7.24**a**). It transilluminates brightly and appears cystic on ultrasonography (Figure 7.24**b**) or MRI (Figure 7.24**c**).
c. **Other amelanotic, benign tumours** (e.g. Schwannoma) may resemble a pigmented melanoma because of the overlying pigment epithelium. Transillumination with the light beam of the slitlamp reveals the amelanotic nature of the tumour.
d. **Benign cyst** may be falsely diagnosed if a melanoma is cystic (Figure 7.25).
f. **Sentinel vessels** are sometimes mistaken for episcleritis, which can sometimes occur over a melanoma (Figure 7.26)
g. **Staphyloma** in a patient with necrotizing scleritis may mimic extrascleral extension (Figure 7.27), but transilluminates brightly.

Iris melanoma

PATHOLOGY

Iris melanomas can be circumscribed or diffuse and may show varying degrees of pigmentation and vascularity.

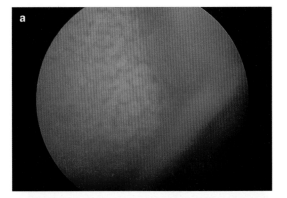

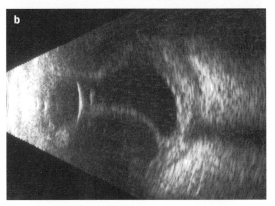

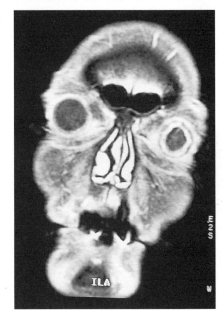

Figure 7.24 Uveal effusion syndrome: (**a**) colour photograph, (**b**) B-scan ultrasonogram and (**c**) MRI scan (coronal section)

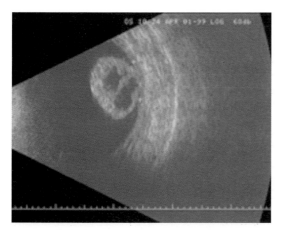

Figure 7.25 Ciliochoroidal melanoma with cystic spaces on ultrasonography

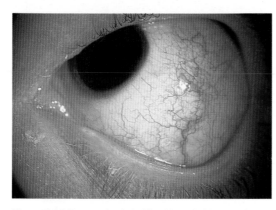

Figure 7.26 Temporal episcleritis with underlying uveal melanoma

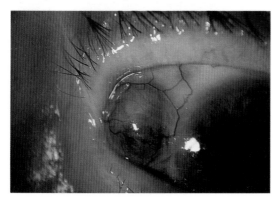

Figure 7.27 Scleral staphyloma mimicking extraocular extension. The staphyloma transilluminates brightly

SYMPTOMS

Patients usually present with a cosmetic blemish unless advanced disease causes cataract or secondary glaucoma.

SIGNS

- White, yellow, pink, brown or black colour, depending on vascularity and pigmentation (Figure 7.28).
- Smooth or irregular surface.
- Inferior location in most patients.

COMPLICATIONS

- Ectropion uveae, which may also occur with naevi.
- Circumferential spread around the angle, to cause secondary glaucoma.
- Posterior spread, to the ciliary body.
- Pressure on the lens, causing localized lens opacities.
- Contact with the corneal endothelium, resulting in corneal oedema and localized band keratopathy (Figure 7.29).
- Pupil margin cyst, rarely.

A minority of iris melanomas are diffuse (Figure 7.30), with a rare variant forming multiple amelanotic nodules across the iris surface ('tapioca melanoma') (Figure 7.31) (Hassenstein *et al.*, 1999).

DIFFERENTIAL DIAGNOSIS

a. **Naevus**. This is often difficult to distinguish from melanoma, both clinically and histologically. It has been suggested that many lesions diagnosed as iris melanomas are benign (Jakobiec and Silbert, 1981) (Chapter 5).
b. **Metastasis** (Chapter 19).
c. **Iris epithelial cyst** (Chapter 16).
d. **Leiomyoma** is very rare and can be differentiated from amelanotic melanoma only histologically.
e. **Haemangioma** is exceedingly rare.
f. **Heterochromia**.
g. **Foreign body** can mimic melanoma if rusty.

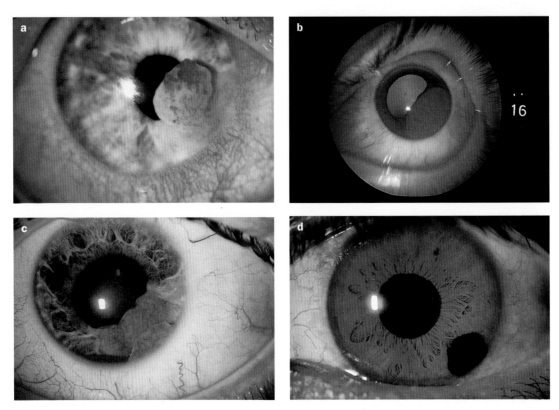

Figure 7.28 Iris melanomas, which can be (**a**) white, (**b**) pink (Courtesy of W.S. Foulds, Glasgow, UK), (**c**) grey or (**d**) brown

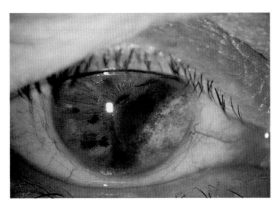

Figure 7.29 Band keratopathy over an iris melanoma

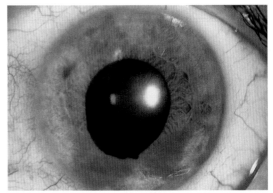

Figure 7.30 Diffuse iris melanoma (histologically confirmed)

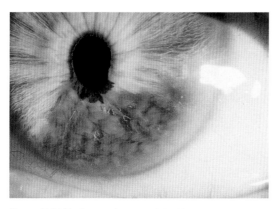

Figure 7.31 Tapioca melanoma of the iris

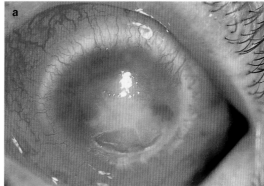

Advanced disease

If untreated, advanced uveal melanomas can result in the following conditions:

a. A painful, phthisical eye (Figure 7.32**a**).
b. Pseudo-cellulitis (Figure 7.32**b**).
c. Extraocular extension and proptosis (Figure 7.32 **c**).

INVESTIGATION OF THE PRIMARY TUMOUR

VISUAL FIELD EXAMINATION

Although choroidal melanomas tend to cause more severe visual field loss than naevi, this examination does not differentiate the two conditions.

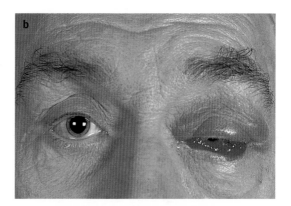

TRANSILLUMINATION

Transillumination is not of diagnostic value and gives only an approximate indication of tumour extent (Chapter 1).

FLUORESCEIN ANGIOGRAPHY

Choroidal melanomas usually show hyperfluorescence due to secondary RPE changes (Damato, 1992) (Figure 7.33) with a 'dual circulation' where the RPE is absent (Figure 7.34). Hypofluorescence can occur if the RPE over a pigmented melanoma is either absent, or normal

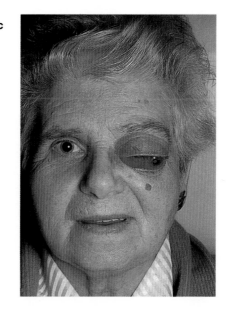

Figure 7.32 End-stage melanomas, giving rise to (**a**) phthisis, (**b**) cellulitis and (**c**) proptosis

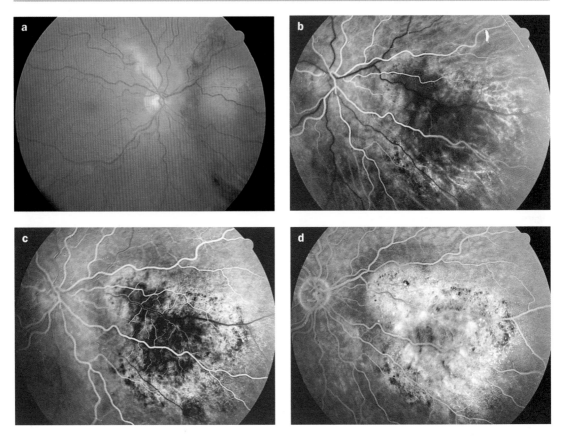

Figure 7.33 Fluorescein angiogram of a sub-RPE melanoma: (**a**) colour photograph, (**b**) 12 seconds, hypofluorescence corresponding to tumour pigment, with exposure of choroidal vessels, (**c**) 16 seconds, showing drusen in abnormal RPE and hypofluorescence at posterior tumour margin, corresponding to lateral tumour spread beneath normal RPE and (**d**) late hyperfluorescence due to fluid leakage under the retina

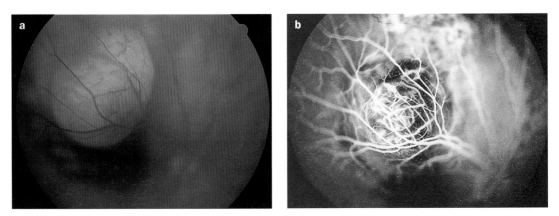

Figure 7.34 Fluorescein angiogram of a collar-stud melanoma, showing a 'dual circulation'

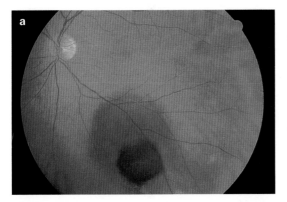 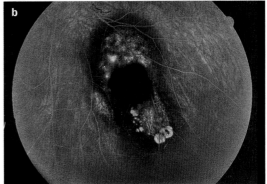

Figure 7.35 Deeply pigmented choroidal melanoma perforating retina. The tumour is hypofluorescent in exposed area and near margins, where overlying RPE is normal. Hyperfluorescent areas represent abnormalities in RPE and exposed sclera. (From Damato, B.E. (1990) Tumour-associated retinal pigment epitheliopathy. *Eye*, **4**, 382–7)

(Figure 7.35). Hypofluorescence is induced by photocoagulation, which destroys the choriocapillaris (see Figure 1.6).

Because none of the angiographic features of melanoma is pathognomonic, fluorescein angiography is of limited diagnostic value.

INDOCYANINE GREEN ANGIOGRAPHY

The infra-red light of indocyanine green angiography (IGA) penetrates deeper than the blue light of fluorescein angiography so that there is enhanced visualization of tumour and choroidal vessels and better definition of the tumour margins (in the case of pigmented tumours only) (Figure 7.36). Orange pigment is autofluorescent (Figure 7.36**b**).

ULTRASONOGRAPHY

Ultrasonography is useful for detecting a uveal melanoma, defining its extent, measuring its dimensions, and providing clues to diagnosis.

If the tumour has ruptured Bruch's membrane, there is a collar-stud configuration, which is almost pathognomonic of choroidal melanoma (Figure 7.37). Loss of internal acoustic reflectivity occurs towards the sclera. On A-scan ultrasonography, this produces a high initial spike with a descending slope (Figure 7.38). On B-scan ultrasonography, this contributes to the appearance of 'choroidal excavation' (Figure 7.38), which can

also be explained by tumour invasion of the sclera.

Computerized techniques for acoustic tissue characterization have been developed, which may be of diagnostic and prognostic value (Coleman *et al.*, 1991).

Ultrasonography is more likely to detect extraocular tumour extension than either computerized tomography or magnetic resonance imaging (Scott *et al.*, 1998). The extrascleral tumour is visible as a dark area adjacent to the eye (Figure 7.39).

High-frequency scans delineate ciliary body and iris tumours with good resolution (Figure 7.40).

COMPUTERIZED TOMOGRAPHY

This investigation is of limited diagnostic value but in some centres is routinely used for planning radiotherapy. Care must be taken to distinguish tumour from subretinal fluid (see Figure 1.14).

MAGNETIC RESONANCE IMAGING

Melanomas tend to have short T1 and T2 relaxation times, so that compared to vitreous they are hyper-intense on T1 weighted images and hypo-intense on T2 weighted images (De Potter *et al.*, 1995) (Figure 7.41). Gadolinium enhancement and fat suppression techniques improve image quality, demonstrating optic nerve and orbital invasion and facilitating differentiation from other types of tumour.

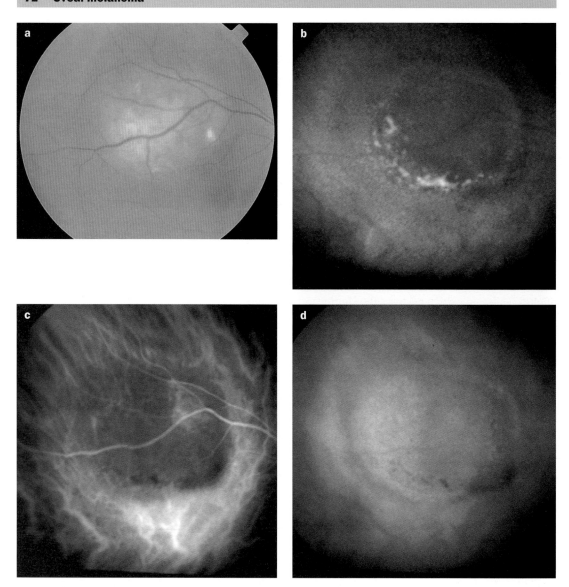

Figure 7.36 ICG features of a choroidal melanoma: (**a**) colour photograph, (**b**) autofluorescence of orange pigment, (**c**) early phase and (**d**) late phase. (Courtesy of B.A. Lafaut, Ghent, Belgium)

IMMUNOSCINTIGRAPHY

Radio-immunoscintigraphy using radio-labelled monoclonal antibodies is positive in more than 90% of uveal melanomas (Bomanji *et al.,* 1988), but does not distinguish small melanomas from large naevi (Bomanji *et al.,* 1988). This test is not widely used but may be helpful in special circumstances (Figure 7.42).

FINE NEEDLE ASPIRATION BIOPSY

Fine needle aspiration biopsy (FNAB) is performed if there is diagnostic uncertainty despite other investigations. If the sample is insufficient for immunohistochemistry, it may be difficult for the cytopathologist to differentiate an amelanotic melanoma from another malignant tumour.

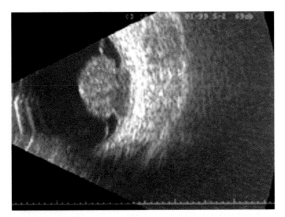

Figure 7.37 B-scan ultrasound of a collar-stud melanoma. Note that the internal acoustic reflectivity is greatest in the part of the tumour that has perforated Bruch's membrane

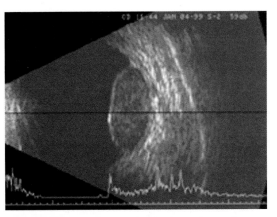

Figure 7.38 A- and B-scans showing internal acoustic reflectivity of a choroidal melanoma

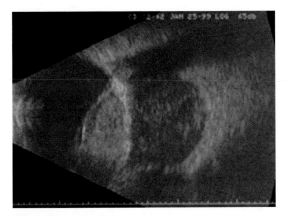

Figure 7.39 Juxtapapillary choroidal melanoma with large extraocular extension

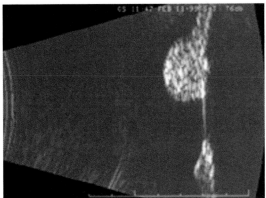

Figure 7.40 High-frequency scan of an iris melanoma

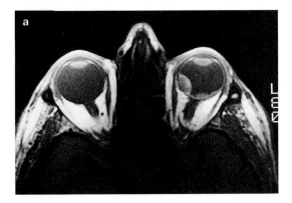

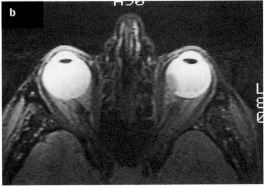

Figure 7.41 (**a**) T1 weighted and (**b**) T2 weighted MRI images of a choroidal melanoma. (Courtesy of P. De Potter, Brussels, Belgium)

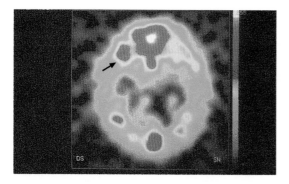

Figure 7.42 Radio-immunoscintigram of a temporal choroidal melanoma in the right eye of a 35-year-old male showing uptake in the tumour. (Courtesy of C. Mosci, Genoa, Italy)

INCISIONAL BIOPSY

Incisional biopsy is a more difficult surgical procedure than FNAB, but provides more tissue (Figure 7.43). Examination of frozen sections allows immediate diagnosis and treatment but preservation of cellular morphology is not as good as in fixed specimens, making it difficult to distinguish amelanotic melanoma from other tumours without the help of immunohistochemistry. To prevent

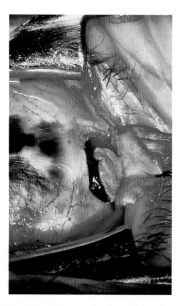

Figure 7.43 Incisional biopsy of a choroidal melanoma, performed under a lamellar scleral flap. (Courtesy of W.S. Foulds, Glasgow, UK)

possible spread of a melanoma through the scleral defect, plaque radiotherapy is commenced immediately if appropriate. Otherwise the scleral wound is sealed with tissue glue with subsequent enucleation or proton beam radiotherapy performed as soon as possible.

EXCISIONAL BIOPSY

Excision biopsy is difficult but in selected cases provides both a diagnosis and a cure if the surgeon is experienced in the technique.

SYSTEMIC INVESTIGATION

a. Any anaesthetic risks are identified by performing a full medical examination with serum biochemistry, haematology, electrocardiography, and, if necessary, chest radiography.

b. A search for an extraocular primary malignancy is indicated if the intraocular tumour may be a metastatic lesion. Investigations would include chest radiography, rectal examination, mammography in females and scrotal examination in males.

c. Metastatic spread of uveal melanoma to liver or lung is detected by liver ultrasonography and chest radiography. Such screening is usually restricted to patients with a high risk of metastasis (i.e., large tumour) or evidence of hepatic disease (i.e., palpable liver or abnormal liver enzymes). In other patients, routine liver ultrasonography may be counter-productive because detectable liver metastases are rare and outnumbered by innocuous cysts and angiomas, which may lead to FNAB and postponement of the ocular treatment.

TREATMENT OF THE PRIMARY TUMOUR

TREATMENT SELECTION

It is important to prioritize with each patient the following objectives:

a. Destruction of the primary tumour, in the hope that metastatic spread has not already occurred.

b. Prevention of a painful eye.

c. Conservation of central vision, particularly if there is poor vision in the fellow eye or a special need for stereopsis.

d. Conservation of peripheral vision, which may facilitate walking in crowded situations and driving.

e. Conservation of a cosmetically satisfactory eye, which to some patients is more important than vision.

NON-TREATMENT

Non-treatment is generally advocated mainly when trying to differentiate a large suspicious naevus from a small melanoma (Augsburger, 1993). In special cases, if treatment of a small melanoma in an only eye is likely to cause severe visual loss, it may be appropriate to delay treatment, especially if the patient is very elderly, because some tumours grow very slowly or remain stationary for many years. Special precautions should be taken to ensure that the patient is not lost to follow-up.

If treatment of a melanoma is withheld, it is advisable to obtain signed consent from the patient indicating an understanding of the risks involved.

PLAQUE RADIOTHERAPY (BRACHYTHERAPY)

In most centres, plaque radiotherapy is the first choice of treatment for choroidal melanoma because it is technically straightforward, inexpensive and effective.

Indications

a. Primary treatment of choroidal and ciliary body melanomas.

b. Primary treatment of selected, non-resectable iris melanomas (Shields *et al.*, 1995).

c. Adjunctive treatment after local resection or phototherapy, to prevent recurrent tumour.

d. Secondary treatment, for recurrent tumour after phototherapy or resection.

Contraindications

a. Tumour thickness more than 5 mm if a ruthenium-106 plaque is used, and more than 8–10 mm for an iodine-125 plaque.

b. Close proximity to the optic nerve head, unless a notched plaque is used.

The standard practice is to deliver a minimum apex dose of 80–100 Gy, although some also prescribe a minimum scleral surface dose of 400–700 Gy (Chapter 23).

Extraocular extension is either covered by the plaque or excised immediately before the plaque is positioned. Some surgeons recommend an unshielded iodine plaque, so as to irradiate the orbit.

Most tumours start to regress about 1 or 2 months after treatment, eventually forming a grey, slightly raised mass 2 or 3 years later (Figure 7.44).

The rate of tumour regression varies greatly, not only depending on the tumour cytology but also according to the type of plaque used. Regression is faster with ruthenium than with iodine plaques, presumably because the high basal dose causes radiation vasculopathy and tumour infarction.

Some tumours become almost completely replaced by fibrous tissue without any apparent regression. Other tumours may undergo rapid and complete regression. This marked response is associated with increased malignancy and a greater probability of metastatic death (Augsburger *et al.*, 1987).

Lightly pigmented tumours tend to become more pigmented as they regress, probably because of concentration of the same amount of melanin in melanomacrophages within a smaller tumour volume (Figure 7.45).

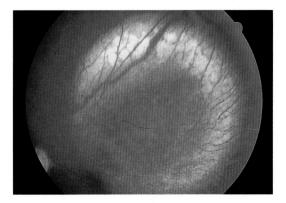

Figure 7.44 Radiational choroidal atrophy around a uveal melanoma 6 years after ruthenium plaque radiotherapy

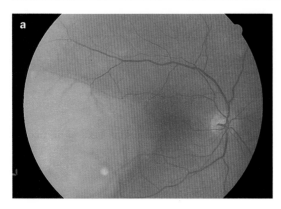
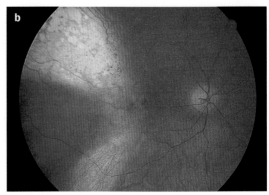

Figure 7.45 Choroidal melanoma (**a**) before ruthenium plaque radiotherapy and (**b**) 2 years later, when regression is associated with increased pigmentation

Radiational choroidal atrophy usually begins to appear about 2–6 months after treatment and tends to commence anteriorly before extending around the posterior tumour margin. Choroidal atrophy develops more rapidly and is more marked after ruthenium-106 than after iodine-125 plaque treatment.

Tumour destruction with retention of good vision is almost guaranteed with small peripheral tumours. Adverse factors are proximity to optic nerve head or fovea (i.e., <2 disc diameters), tumour thickness greater than 5 mm, indistinct tumour margins, retinal perforation and conditions such as diabetes predisposing to retinopathy (Packer *et al.*, 1992; Lommatzsch, 1993; Summanen *et al.*, 1995; Summanen *et al.*, 1996; Finger *et al.*, 1999).

Complications

a. Central tumour recurrence can be due to an inadequate dose of radiation or an unusually high degree of radio-resistance (Figure 7.46). This should only be diagnosed if increasing tumour thickness is demonstrable by sequential ultrasonography after taking into account the repeatability of this examination. This type of tumour recurrence may be mimicked by haemorrhage into a necrotic or fibrotic tumour, and prolapse of necrotic tumour through a defect in Bruch's membrane (Figure 7.47).

b. Marginal tumour recurrence is due to incorrect placement of the plaque (i.e., 'geographic miss') (Figure 7.48). This is recognized by

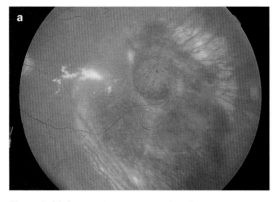
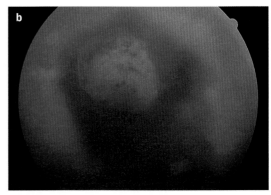

Figure 7.46 Choroidal melanoma in the left eye with progressive growth of a central tumour recurrence (**a**) 10 and (**b**) 12 years after cobalt plaque radiotherapy in 1973. (Courtesy of W.S. Foulds, Glasgow, UK)

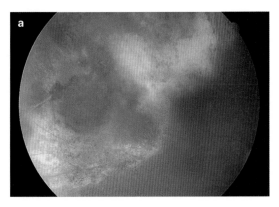

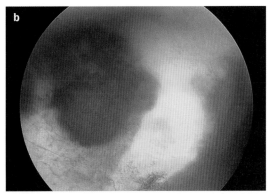

Figure 7.47 Collar-stud melanoma in the right eye showing progressive enlargement (**a**) 1 year and (**b**) 2 years after ruthenium plaque radiotherapy and photocoagulation. Endoresection of the tumour nodule showed only melanomacrophages

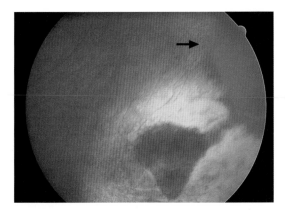

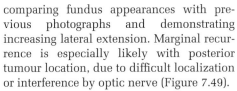

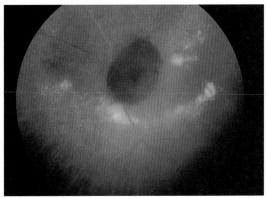

Figure 7.48 Marginal tumour recurrence after plaque radiotherapy peripheral to a wide zone of radiational atrophy after ruthenium plaque radiotherapy of a choroidal melanoma in the left eye

Figure 7.49 Marginal recurrence at disc in a patient with a juxtapapillary melanoma treated with an iodine plaque

comparing fundus appearances with previous photographs and demonstrating increasing lateral extension. Marginal recurrence is especially likely with posterior tumour location, due to difficult localization or interference by optic nerve (Figure 7.49).
c. Non-contiguous recurrence is rare (Duker *et al.*, 1989). It is presumably due to ocular micro-metastases already present at the time of treatment.
d. Recurrent vitreous haemorrhage from the tumour apex can occur if the tumour has ruptured the retina.
e. Non-specific radiational complications (Chapter 23).

To determine the safety of plaque radiotherapy, the Collaborative Ocular Melanoma Study (COMS) is performing a large, randomized prospective study evaluating patient survival after iodine plaque radiotherapy in comparison with enucleation (Schachat, 1994). Previous studies using historical controls have shown no significant difference in survival between enucleation and ruthenium plaque (Guthoff *et al.*, 1992) or cobalt plaque radiotherapy (Augsburger *et al.*, 1998).

CHARGED PARTICLE RADIOTHERAPY

In a few centres, highly focused radiotherapy can be delivered using charged particles, such as protons or helium ions (Gragoudas and Char, 1994).

The indications and contraindications vary from one centre to another.

Indications

a. Small choroidal melanoma that is difficult to treat with plaque radiotherapy because of posterior location or irregular shape.
b. Choroidal or ciliary body melanoma that is too thick for plaque radiotherapy, especially if the patient is highly motivated to retain the eye (e.g., if the other eye is blind).
c. Optic nerve involvement precluding plaque radiotherapy, if the patient is keen to retain the eye irrespective of vision.
d. Iris melanoma, as a means of avoiding a surgical coloboma and resultant photophobia (Figure 7.50).

Contraindications

a. High probability of success with plaque radiotherapy.
b. Inevitable blindness due to radiational optic neuropathy, if the cosmetic results of enucleation are likely to be acceptable to the patient.
c. Large tumour size, and hence, high risk of exudative retinal detachment and neovascular glaucoma, particularly if trans-scleral local resection is possible or if enucleation is acceptable to the patient.
d. Extensive diffuse melanomas, because the risk of local recurrence is high.

The dose of radiation generally administered for uveal melanoma varies between 50 and 70 Gy, delivered in four to eight fractions (Chapter 23).

Tumour regression tends to be slower than after plaque radiotherapy, except for the rare, highly malignant tumours, which regress dramatically (Glynn *et al.,* 1989) (Figure 7.51). Radiational choroidal atrophy is also less conspicuous and more gradual than with brachytherapy.

The best results occur with small tumours not extending close to optic nerve head or fovea and covered by an intact retina (Seddon *et al.,* 1986; Gragoudas *et al.,* 1987; Seddon *et al.,* 1987; Egan *et al.,* 1989; Char *et al.,* 1990; Bercher *et al.,* 1991; Guyer *et al.,* 1992; Char *et al.,* 1998) (Figure 7.52).

Complications

a. Central tumour recurrence, which is rare (i.e., <5%) (Bercher *et al.,* 1991). This must be differentiated from transient enlargement, which can occur during the first year after treatment, probably due to oedema.
b. Marginal tumour recurrence, which is most likely to occur if there is diffuse, sub-clinical tumour extension laterally, which has not been included in the treatment field. True marginal tumour growth needs to be differentiated from unmasking of hidden lateral tumour extensions as radiational choroidal atrophy develops (Figure 7.53).
c. Recurrent vitreous haemorrhage, which can be a problem if the tumour has perforated the retina.

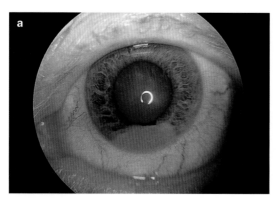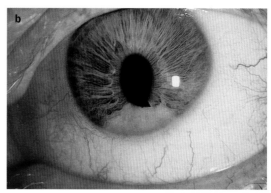

Figure 7.50 Iris melanoma (**a**) before and (**b**) 7 months after proton beam radiotherapy and lens extraction. The vision was 6/9 almost 3 years postoperatively

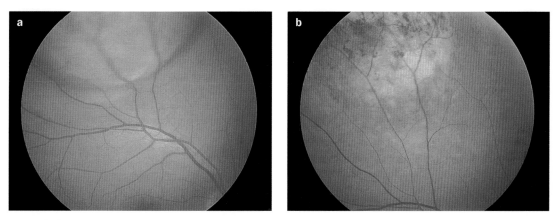

Figure 7.51 Choroidal melanoma (**a**) before and (**b**) 7 months after proton beam radiotherapy, showing rapid regression. The patient died of metastatic disease 9 months after treatment

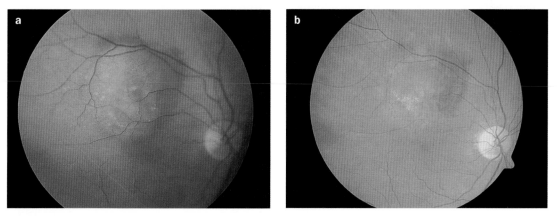

Figure 7.52 Juxtafoveal choroidal melanoma in the right eye (**a**) before and (**b**) 4.5 years after proton beam radiotherapy, when the visual acuity was still 6/9. Retention of such good acuity so long after high-dose macular irradiation is unusual

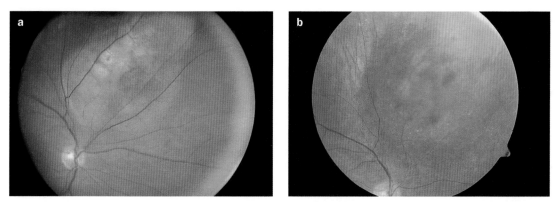

Figure 7.53 Choroidal melanoma (**a**) before proton beam radiotherapy and (**b**) almost 5 years later, when choroidal atrophy has unmasked previously hidden lateral tumour extensions, mimicking lateral growth

d. Persistent exudative retinal detachment, which occurs in about 40% of eyes if the tumour is 6–10 mm in thickness (Bercher *et al.,* 1991).

e. Neovascular glaucoma, which occurs in about 50% of eyes with persistent retinal detachment (Bercher *et al.,* 1991).

f. Non-specific complications (Chapter 23).

Survival after proton beam radiotherapy is not significantly different from that after enucleation (Seddon *et al.,* 1990). Some argue that longer follow-up is required before the safety of radiotherapy can be proven (Manschot and van Strik, 1992).

STEREOTACTIC RADIOTHERAPY

There is growing interest in stereotactic radiotherapy, which is described in Chapter 23. Further studies are required to evaluate the scope of this treatment (Marchini *et al.,* 1995; Zehetmayer *et al.,* 1997).

CHOROIDECTOMY

Choroidectomy and cyclochoroidectomy are difficult procedures and therefore performed only in selected cases as an alternative to enucleation if a tumour is deemed unsuitable for radiotherapy (Peyman and Gremillion, 1989; Shields *et al.,* 1991; Damato and Foulds, 1994).

Indications

a. Tumour thickness excessive for plaque radiotherapy.

b. High risk of persistent retinal detachment after proton beam radiotherapy.

c. Proximity of a large tumour to optic nerve, if conservation of vision is important.

d. Persistent exudative retinal detachment after proton beam radiotherapy.

e. Excision biopsy of a large tumour.

Contraindications

a. Tumour diameter greater than 16 mm, because the risk of local recurrence is high.

b. Diffuse melanoma because of poor localization.

c. Optic nerve head invasion; because complete excision is not possible.

d. Involvement of more than 2–3 clock hours of ciliary body or angle, because the chances of hypotony and phthisis are high.

e. Tumour extension to within 1–2 DD of optic nerve head or fovea if the increased risks of residual tumour and visual loss are unacceptable.

f. Posterior scleral perforation because of difficulty in suturing a full-thickness graft.

g. Retinal invasion or penetration if vitreoretinal surgery is not possible or undesirable.

h. Systemic conditions precluding hypotensive anaesthesia. Old age is not in itself a contraindication.

The surgical methods are described in Chapter 24. The best visual results occur after the resection of nasal choroidal melanomas not extending to within 2 DD of the optic nerve head or fovea (Damato *et al.,* 1993) (Figure 7.54).

Complications

a. Visible residual tumour at the end of the operation. This is most likely to occur with tumours extending to within 1or 2 DD of the optic nerve head and with tumours having a tapering edge (Damato *et al.,* 1996b) (Figure 7.55).

b. Tumour recurrence from microscopic deposits, developing after a delay of months or years (Figures 7.56–7.58) (Damato *et al.,* 1996b). Extraocular tumour recurrence is rare (Figure 7.59). Recurrence must be differentiated from reactive hyperplasia of the RPE (Figure 7.60) and organized haematoma (Figure 7.61) (Lee, 1987). Recurrence has become less common with the introduction of adjunctive plaque radiotherapy.

c. Non-specific complications (Chapter 24).

IRIDOCYCLECTOMY

Indications

Iridocyclectomy is indicated for iris tumours involving the angle and for ciliary body tumours (Naumann and Rummelt, 1996).

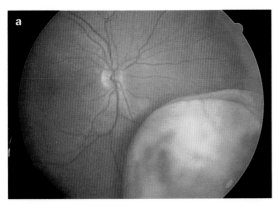

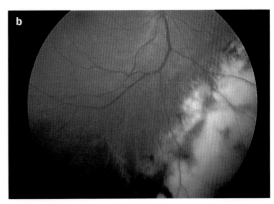

Figure 7.54 Choroidal melanoma having a thickness of 7 mm (**a**) before trans-scleral local resection and (**b**) 8 years later, when the vision was still 6/5

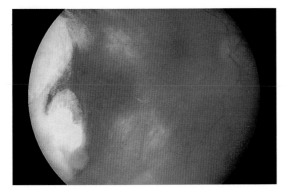

Figure 7.55 Residual tumour at the posterior margin of the surgical coloboma after trans-scleral local resection and adjunctive plaque radiotherapy. Two years postoperatively, the vision was 6/12

Contraindications

Iridocyclectomy is contraindicated if the tumour involves more than 2–3 clock hours of the ciliary body or angle.

The surgical technique is described in Chapter 24. As with iridectomy, the visual prognosis is good, but the iris defect causes photophobia.

Complications

Local tumour recurrence is rare if the procedure is performed by an experienced surgeon. It tends to develop at the margins of the surgical scar and can be pigmented or amelanotic. Some surgeons

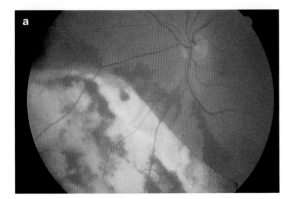

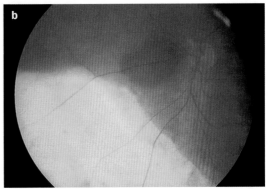

Figure 7.56 Surgical coloboma (**a**) soon after local resection, suggesting complete tumour excision and (**b**) after local tumour recurrence from microscopic deposits

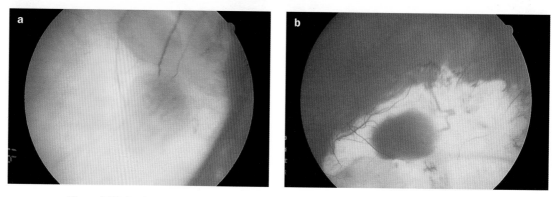

Figure 7.57 Surgical colobomas with (**a**) amelanotic and (**b**) pigmented local tumour recurrences

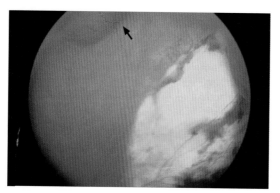

Figure 7.58 Local tumour recurrence distant from the site of the primary tumour

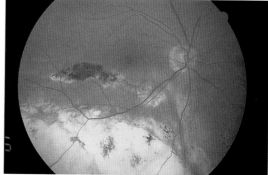

Figure 7.60 Reactive pigment epithelial hyperplasia

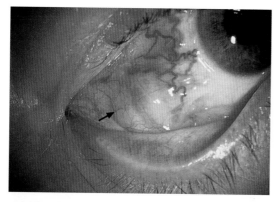

Figure 7.59 Extraocular recurrence 7 years after local resection of a choroidal melanoma

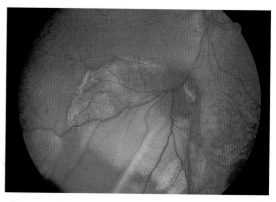

Figure 7.61 Organized subretinal haematoma

recommend full-thickness scleral resection because of fears of local tumour recurrence within a lamellar scleral flap (Naumann and Rummelt, 1996), but this is not reported to be a significant problem by those preferring the lamellar resection technique (Damato and Foulds, 1994).

Other problems, which are more likely after extensive procedures (i.e. >2 clock hours), include cataract, lens subluxation, bullous keratopathy and ocular hypotony. Retinal detachment should not occur if the dissection does not extend posterior to the ora serrata.

IRIDECTOMY

Iridectomy is indicated for discrete iris melanomas not involving the angle or ciliary body. It is contra-indicated if the tumour has a significant diffuse element. The surgical technique is described in Chapter 24.

The visual prognosis is good if the tumour is small, but the iris defect can cause problematic photophobia. This can be treated with a painted contact lens or, in pseudophakic patients, an artificial iris (Figure 7.62).

The most serious complication is tumour recur-

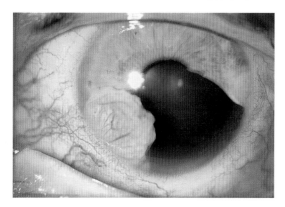

Figure 7.63 Local tumour recurrence of an amelanotic iris melanoma 3 years after iridocyclectomy. (Courtesy of W.S. Foulds, Glasgow, UK)

rence, which is most likely to occur if the tumour has a diffuse component, especially if it is amelanotic (Figure 7.63).

PHOTOCOAGULATION

Photocoagulation can give good results with small, posterior tumours (Figure 7.64) but is rarely selected as a primary form of treatment for uveal melanomas because it has been superseded by methods such as transpupillary thermotherapy, which are more reliable and less labour-intensive.

Indications

a. Treatment of a small recurrence or suspicious pigmentation within or at the margin of a surgical scar after local resection (Figure 7.65).
b. Treatment of the posterior tumour margin after a plaque has deliberately been placed eccentrically to avoid radiational maculopathy or optic neuropathy (Figure 7.66).
c. In some centres, treatment of the tumour apex if the tumour thickness is too great for plaque radiotherapy alone.

Contraindications

a. Poor tumour visualization, because of peripheral location or media opacities.

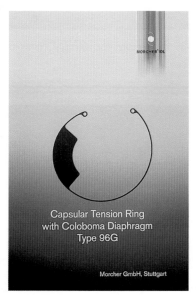

Figure 7.62 Artificial iris. (Courtesy of Morcher GmbH, Stuttgart, Germany)

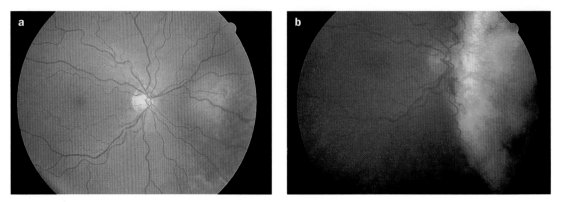

Figure 7.64 Choroidal melanoma (**a**) before treatment and (**b**) after photocoagulation. Ten years after treatment the eye had no evidence of active tumour and the vision was 6/5

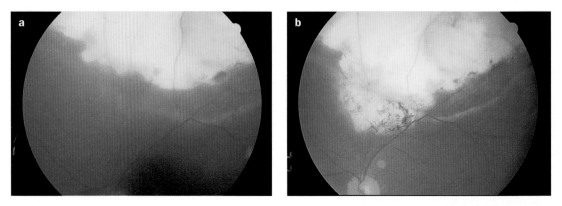

Figure 7.65 Photocoagulation of local tumour recurrence after trans-scleral resection of a choroidal melanoma

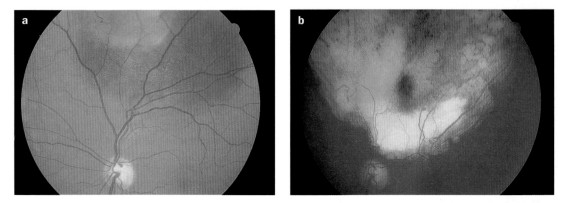

Figure 7.66 Superior choroidal melanoma in the left eye (**a**) before treatment and (**b**) after ruthenium plaque radiotherapy with adjunctive photocoagulation applied to the posterior part of the tumour

b. Tumour thickness exceeding 3 mm.

c. Involvement of more than a third of the optic nerve head.

The methods are described in Chapter 25. Photocoagulation is effective in carefully selected cases if administered by an experienced practitioner (Foulds and Damato, 1986; Bornfeld and Wessing, 1994).

Complications

a. Central recurrence because residual tumour has been mistaken for scar tissue. Non-fluorescence on angiography should not be misinterpreted as tumour destruction (Damato, 1991).

b. Marginal recurrence, which is most likely to occur with amelanotic melanomas (Figure 7.67).

c. Extraocular recurrence if the photocoagulation has not penetrated deeply enough.

d. Non-specific complications, described in Chapter 25.

TRANSPUPILLARY THERMOTHERAPY (TTT)

This has been developed as a primary treatment for small, juxtapapillary tumours to avoid radiational optic neuropathy (Oosterhuis *et al.,* 1995). The indications and contraindications are similar to photocoagulation. The methods are described in Chapter 25.

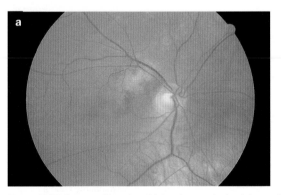
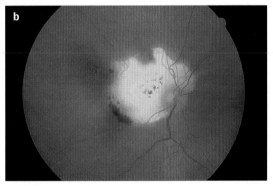

Figure 7.67 Juxtapapillary choroidal melanoma in the right eye (**a**) before photocoagulation and (**b**) 3 years later, when marginal recurrences developed

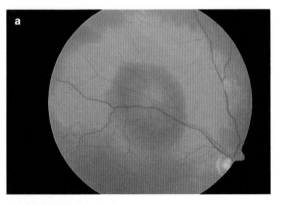
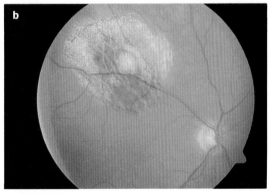

Figure 7.68 Superior choroidal melanoma in the right eye of a 69 year old diabetic man (**a**) before transpupillary thermotherapy, when the tumour was 2 mm thick, reducing the acuity to 6/9 and (**b**) 3 months later, showing complete regression, with improvement of vision to 6/5

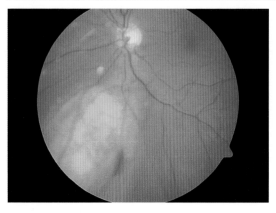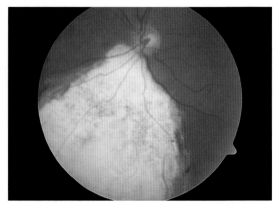

Figure 7.69 Juxtapapillary choroidal melanoma in the left eye (**a**) before endoresection and (**b**) a year later, when the vision was 6/5

A single treatment session is effective for tumours up to 4 mm in thickness. After treatment, the tumour regresses gradually over several months (Figure 7.68). (Robertson *et al.,* 1999)

The need for adjunctive radiotherapy is disputed (Oosterhuis *et al.,* 1995; Shields *et al.,* 1998).

Early results are encouraging (Oosterhuis *et al.,* 1998; Shields *et al.,* 1998), but long term studies are required to establish whether TTT is superior to photocoagulation.

PHOTODYNAMIC THERAPY

A small number of patients have been treated with photodynamic therapy using haematoporphyrin derivatives (HPD) (Bruce Jr., 1984). This preparation causes severe and prolonged photosensitivity and has therefore been superseded by phthalocyanines and other agents (Young *et al.,* 1996) (Chapter 25).

ENDORESECTION

This operation is performed in a few centres, but is still controversial (Lee *et al.,* 1993; Damato *et al.,* 1998). The indications and contraindications should therefore be regarded as tentative.

Indications

a. Tumour extension to within a disc diameter

of the optic disc, to avoid radiational optic neuropathy.

b. Residual tumour after other forms of conservative treatment.

Contraindications

a. Tumour size and location more suitable for plaque or proton beam radiotherapy.

b. Diffuse melanoma, because of the difficulties in defining the tumour margins.

c. Optic disc involvement greater than 3 clock hours, because conservation of useful vision is unlikely.

d. Tumour diameter greater than 10–12 mm, because of the increased risk of (a) recurrence, unless adjunctive plaque radiotherapy is administered, and (b) hypotony, unless the procedure is performed under a retinal flap.

The techniques are described in Chapter 24. With nasal tumours, retention of good acuity is possible (Figure 7.69), but with macular tumours, the main objective is to conserve the temporal visual field.

Complications

The commonest complications are those of vitrectomy, and are mostly entry site retinal tears, rhegmatogenous retinal detachment and cataract. Although the efficacy of tumour control seems comparable to other forms of conservative treatment, further studies are required.

CRYOTHERAPY

A few small choroidal melanomas have been treated successfully with cryotherapy (Wilson and Klein, 1999) although this method is not widely used.

ENUCLEATION

Enucleation is increasingly being replaced by treatment aimed at conserving the eye with as much vision as possible.

Indications

a. Tumour diameter greater than 16 mm.
b. Optic nerve invasion.
c. Tumour involvement of more than 2–3 hours of the ciliary body or angle.
d. Vitreous seeding.
e. Extensive diffuse melanoma.
f. Large extraocular tumour extension.
g. Secondary glaucoma due to tumour invasion of angle.
h. Lack of motivation to keep the eye or to attend for life-long follow up.
i. Fear of residual or recurrent tumour after conservative treatment.
j. Local tumour recurrence after conservative treatment that cannot adequately be treated by further eye salvaging therapy.
k. After conservative treatment, inability to monitor the posterior segment by ophthalmoscopy because of untreatable media opacities, such as retinal detachment.
l. Uncontrollable inflammation after conservative therapy, because of the risk of sympathetic ophthalmitis (Fries et al., 1987).

Contraindications

a. Significant diagnostic uncertainty, unless biopsy is impractical or undesirable.
b. Limited life expectancy if the tumour is small and unlikely to cause pain or metastasis, particularly if the patient can be monitored adequately.

Informed consent for enucleation implies that the patient has been given the chance to consider the alternatives.

Enucleation is performed in the standard fashion (Chapter 24), with an orbital implant.

If extraocular tumour extension is present, the risk of orbital recurrence after enucleation is between 8% and 18% (Starr and Zimmerman, 1962; Jensen, 1982). The choice of management in patients with extraocular extension is therefore between:

a. External beam radiotherapy to the orbit immediately after enucleation, which virtually eliminates any chance of local recurrence, but which causes cosmetic deformity and discomfort.
b. Observation, with local excision and external beam radiotherapy if any recurrences occur.

Pre-enucleation radiotherapy does not prevent metastasis (Char and Phillips, 1985; Collaborative Ocular Melanoma Study Group, 1998).

EXENTERATION

Exenteration for extraocular tumour extension does not improve survival (Kersten et al., 1985) and is now reserved for disease that cannot be controlled with less radical methods.

Metastatic disease

Most patients with metastatic disease from uveal melanoma die from hepatic metastasis. Less common sites of metastasis are lung, skin, bone and brain (Albert et al., 1996; Lorigan et al., 1991).

PROGNOSTICATION

At the time of the treatment of the primary tumour the overall 10-year survival is about 50% (Jensen, 1982), this statistic is unduly pessimistic for many patients. It is therefore preferable to estimate the prognosis for survival more precisely by using a predictive model (see below).

Factors related to an increased probability of metastatic death are:

CLINICAL FEATURES

a. Rapid tumour growth before treatment.
b. Anterior extension of choroidal melanomas, especially with ciliary body involvement.
c. Large tumour size (Diener-West *et al.*, 1992).
d. Extraocular tumour extension (Affeldt *et al.*, 1980; Pach *et al.*, 1986).
e. Old age at treatment (Damato *et al.*, 1996a).
f. Nulliparity in women (Egan *et al.*, 1999).
g. Blue or grey iris (Regan *et al.*, 1999).

PATHOLOGICAL FEATURES

a. Epithelioid cells (Seddon *et al.*, 1983).
b. Chromosomal monosomy 3 and trisomy 8 (Prescher *et al.*, 1996).
c. Presence of closed microvascular loops and networks (Folberg *et al.*, 1993; Mäkitie *et al.*, 1999a) and high microvascular density (Mäkitie *et al.*, 1999b).
d. Hypodiploidy (Toti *et al.*, 1998).
e. Large mean nucleolar diameter (McCurdy *et al.*, 1991).
f. Short cell cycling times, as demonstrated by immunohistochemical markers (e.g., PC-10) (Seregard *et al.*, 1998).
g. Significant lymphocytic infiltration (de la Cruz Jr. *et al.*, 1990).
h. Human leukocyte antigen (HLA) class 1 expression (Blom *et al.*, 1997).

i. Weak expression of the intercellular cell adhesion molecule-1 (ICAM-1) (Anastassiou *et al.*, 2000).

TUMOUR BEHAVIOUR AFTER TREATMENT

a. Rapid tumour regression after radiotherapy (Augsburger *et al.*, 1987).
b. Local tumour recurrence after plaque radiotherapy (Karlsson *et al.*, 1989) or proton beam radiotherapy (Egan *et al.*, 1998), and large recurrence after local resection (Damato *et al.*, 1996a). It is not known whether the recurrence is the cause of the metastasis or merely an indicator of aggressive disease.

Most of these predictive factors are interrelated. For example, extraocular tumour extension is more likely with large tumours containing epithelioid cells, which would also be expected to show nucleolar variation, rapid growth, closed vascular loops and chromosomal abnormalities.

The prognosis can be estimated using predictive models based on the number of independent prognostic factors, each identified by Cox multivariate analysis (Figure 7.70) (Damato *et al.*, unpublished data).

Iris melanomas have a relatively good prognosis. It is not known whether this is due to their small size and favourable histology, or whether early detection gives a false impression of improved prognosis (i.e., 'lead time bias').

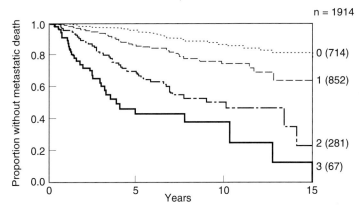

Figure 7.70 Kaplan–Meier survival curves showing survival after enucleation or local resection of uveal melanoma according to the number of risk factors (i.e., tumour diameter >15 mm, epithelioid cells, ciliary body involvement)

FEATURES OF HEPATIC METASTASIS

a. Symptoms such as anorexia, weight loss, localized tenderness, vague 'dyspepsia', abdominal swelling and discomfort, weight gain in the presence of ascites, jaundice, nausea and vomiting.
b. Clinical signs, which include a palpable liver, ascites, right hypochondrial tenderness and jaundice.
c. Abnormal biochemical test results, mainly serum lactate dehydrogenase, alkaline phosphatase and bilirubin.
d. Positive scanning, by ultrasonography, computerized tomography or magnetic resonance imaging. These tend to detect tumour nodules but not micro-metastases.

The scope of screening for metastatic disease is controversial. It would depend on (1) whether or not some form of curative treatment would be considered in the event of tumour spread, and (2) the probability of developing metastatic disease. It is estimated that liver function tests and ultrasonography would detect about 60% of patients with metastasis at an asymptomatic stage if performed once a year, with this percentage increasing to more than 90% if screening is performed every 6 months (Eskelin et al., 1999).

Without treatment, the median survival of patients with hepatic metastatic disease is about 5–7 months (Bedikian et al., 1995). Survival tends to be better in patients with pulmonary or subcutaneous metastatic disease without clinical hepatic metastasis (Rajpal et al., 1983; Kath et al., 1993).

ADJUNCTIVE THERAPY FOR THE PREVENTION OF METASTATIC DISEASE

A variety of adjuvant treatments are being investigated in patients with cutaneous melanoma, which might be applicable to patients with a high risk of metastatic uveal melanoma. These include:

a. High dose interferon-alpha-2b (Kirkwood, 1994).
b. Immunotherapy using a variety of vaccines (Barth et al., 1994; Livingston et al., 1994).
c. Chemotherapy (Retsas et al., 1994).

TREATMENT OF METASTATIC DISEASE

Before treatment is started, the diagnosis should be confirmed by biopsy to differentiate metastatic melanoma from another malignancy, which may be more treatable. The following therapies have been developed for metastatic melanoma:

a. Systemic chemotherapy, such as the BOLD protocol, consisting of recombinant alpha-2b-interferon with vincristine, bleomycin, lomustine and dacarbazine (Fiedler et al., 1992).
b. Intra-arterial hepatic infusion of fotemustine, a third generation nitrosourea, which is administered using an indwelling cannula (Leyvraz et al., 1997).
c. Resection of isolated liver metastases (Gündüz et al., 1998), with or without adjuvant chemotherapy.
d. Palliative radiotherapy to painful metastases in bone, brain and liver.
e. Vaccination with synthetic peptides, such as, g209-GM, delivered with Freund's adjuvant and interleukin-2 (Rosenberg et al., 1998).
f. Vaccination with dendritic cells pulsed in vitro with melanoma lysates or peptides (Nestle et al., 1998).

It is important to address the fear and grief that affect patients with terminal illness and their families (Parkes, 1998).

REFERENCES

Affeldt, J.C., Minckler, D.S., Azen, S.P. and Yeh, L. (1980) Prognosis in uveal melanoma with extrascleral extension. Arch. Ophthalmol., **98**, 1975–9.

Albert, D.M., Ryan, L.M. and Borden, E.C. (1996) Metastatic ocular and cutaneous melanoma: a comparison of patient characteristics and prognosis. Arch. Ophthalmol., **114**, 107–8.

Anastassiou, G., Schilling, H., Stang, A., Djakovic, S., Heilinghaus, A. and Bornfeld, N. (2000) Expression of the cell adhesion molecules ICAM-1, VCAM-1 and NCAM in uveal melanoma: a clinicopathological study. Oncology, **58**, 83–8.

Augsburger, J.J. (1993) Is observation really appropriate for small choroidal melanomas? Trans. Am. Ophthalmol. Soc., **91**, 147–68.

Augsburger, J.J., Corrêa, Z.M., Freire, J. and Brady, L.W. (1998) Long-term survival in choroidal and ciliary body melanoma after enucleation versus plaque radiation therapy. Ophthalmology, 105, 1670–8.

Augsburger, J.J., Gamel, J.W., Shields, J.A., Markoe, A.M. and Brady, L.W. (1987) Post-irradiation regression of choroidal melanomas as a risk factor for death from metastatic disease. *Ophthalmology*, **94**, 1173–7.

Barth, A., Hoon, D.S.B., Foshag, L.J., Nizze, J.A., Famatiga, E., Okun, E. and Morton, D.L. (1994) Polyvalent melanoma cell vaccine induces delayed-type hypersensitivity and *in vitro* cellular immune response. *Cancer Res.*, **54**, 3342–5.

Bataille, V., Sasieni, P., Cuzick, J., Hungerford, J.L., Swerdlow, A. and Bishop, J.A. (1995) Risk of ocular melanoma in relation to cutaneous and iris naevi. *Int. J. Cancer*, **60**, 622–6.

Bedikian, A.Y., Legha, S.S., Mavligit, G., Carrasco, C.H., Khorana, S., Plager, C., Papadopoulos, N. and Benjamin, R.S. (1995) Treatment of uveal melanoma metastatic to the liver: a review of the M.D. Anderson Cancer Center experience and prognostic factors. *Cancer*, **76**, 1665–70.

Bercher, L., Zografos, L., Chamot, L., Egger, E., Perret, C., Uffer, S. and Gailloud, C. (1991) Functional results of 450 cases of uveal melanoma treated with proton beam. In: N. Bornfeld, E.S. Gragoudas, W. Höpping, P.K. Lommatzsch, A. Wessing and L. Zografos (eds), *Tumors of the Eye*. Amsterdam: Kugler, pp. 507–10.

Blom, D-J.R., Luyten, G.P.M., Mooy, C., Kerkvliet, S., Zwinderman, A.H. and Jager, M.J. (1997) Human leukocyte antigen class I expression. Marker of poor prognosis in uveal melanoma. *Invest. Ophthalmol. Vis. Sci.*, **38**, 1865–72.

Bomanji, J., Hungerford, J.L., Granowska, M. and Britton, K.E. (1988) Uptake of ^{99m}Tc labelled (Fab$'$)$_2$ fragments of monoclonal antibody 225.28S by a benign ocular naevus. *Eur. J. Nucl. Med.*, **14**, 165–6.

Bomanji, J., Nimmon, C.C., Hungerford, J.L., Solanki, K., Granowska, M. and Britton, K.E. (1988) Ocular radioimmunoscintigraphy: sensitivity and practical considerations. *J. Nucl. Med.*, **29**, 1038–44.

Bornfeld, N. and Wessing, A. (1994) Photocoagulation of choroidal melanoma. In: S.J. Ryan (ed.), *Retina*. St Louis: Mosby, Vol. 1, Ch. 49, pp. 815–23.

Bruce, R.A., Jr (1984) Evaluation of hematoporphyrin photoradiation therapy to treat choroidal melanomas. *Lasers. Surg. Med.*, **4**, 59–64.

Char, D.H., Castro, J.R., Kroll, S.M., Irvine, A.R., Quivey, J.M. and Stone, R.D. (1990) Five-year follow-up of helium ion therapy for uveal melanoma. *Arch. Ophthalmol.*, **108**, 209–14.

Char, D.H., Kroll, S.M. and Castro, J. (1998) Ten-year follow-up of helium ion therapy for uveal melanoma. *Am. J. Ophthalmol.*, **125**, 81–9.

Char, D.H. and Phillips, T.L. (1985) Pre-enucleation irradiation of uveal melanoma. *Br. J. Ophthalmol.*, **69**, 177–9.

Coleman, D.J., Silverman, R.H., Rondeau, M.J., Coleman, J.A., Rosberger, D., Ellsworth, R.M. and Lizzi, F.L. (1991) Ultrasonic tissue characterization of uveal melanoma and prediction of patient survival after enucleation and brachytherapy. *Am. J. Ophthalmol.*, **112**, 682–8.

Collaborative Ocular Melanoma Study Group (1998) The Collaborative Ocular Melanoma Study (COMS) randomized trial of pre-enucleation radiation of large choroidal melanoma, II. Initial mortality findings. *Am. J. Ophthalmol.*, **125**, 779–96.

Damato, B.E. (1991) Why do choroidal melanomas fluoresce on angiography? In: N. Bornfeld, E.S. Gragoudas, W. Höpping, P.K. Lommatzsch, A. Wessing and L. Zografos (eds), *Tumors of the Eye*. Amsterdam: Kugler, pp. 223–30.

Damato, B.E. (1992) Tumour fluorescence and tumour-associated fluorescence of choroidal melanomas. *Eye*, **6**, 587–93.

Damato, B.E. and Foulds, W.S. (1990) Tumour-associated retinal pigment epitheliopathy. *Eye*, **4**, 382–7.

Damato, B.E. and Foulds, W.S. (1994) Surgical resection of choroidal melanomas. In: S.J. Ryan (ed.), *Retina*. St Louis: Mosby, Vol. 1, Ch. 47, pp. 795–807.

Damato, B.E., Paul, J. and Foulds, W.S. (1993) Predictive factors of visual outcome after local resection of choroidal melanoma. *Br. J. Ophthalmol.*, **77**, 616–23.

Damato, B., Groenewald, C., McGalliard, J. and Wong, D. (1998) Endoresection of choroidal melanoma. *Br. J. Ophthalmol.* **82**, 213–18.

Damato, B.E., Paul, J. and Foulds, W.S. (1996a) Risk factors for metastatic uveal melanoma after trans-scleral local resection. *Br. J. Ophthalmol.*, **80**, 109–16.

Damato, B.E., Paul, J. and Foulds, W.S. (1996b) Risk factors for residual and recurrent uveal melanoma after trans-scleral local resection. *Br. J. Ophthalmol.*, **80**, 102–8.

de la Cruz, P.O., Jr., Specht, C.S. and McLean, I.W. (1990) Lymphocytic infiltration in uveal malignant melanoma. *Cancer*, **65**, 112–15.

De Potter, P., Shields, J.A. and Shields, C.L. (1995) *MRI of the Eye and Orbit*. Philadelphia: J.B. Lippincott.

Diener-West, M., Hawkins, B.S., Markowitz, J.A. and Schachat, A.P. (1992) A review of mortality from choroidal melanoma. II. A meta-analysis of 5-year mortality rates following enucleation, 1966 through 1988. *Arch. Ophthalmol.*, **110**, 245–50.

Duker, J.S., Augsburger, J.J. and Shields, J.A. (1989) Noncontiguous local recurrence of posterior uveal melanoma after Cobalt 60 episcleral plaque therapy. *Arch. Ophthalmol.*, **107**, 1019–22.

Dunn, W.U., Lambert, H.M., Kincaid, M.C., Dieckert, J.P. and Shore, J.W. (1988) Choroidal malignant melanoma with early vitreous seeding. *Retina*, **8**, 188–92.

Egan, K.M., Gragoudas, E.S., Seddon, J.M., Glynn, R.J., Munzenreider, J.E., Goitein, M., Verhey, L., Urie, M. and Koehler, A. (1989) The risk of enucleation after proton beam irradiation of uveal melanoma. *Ophthalmology*, **96**, 1377–82.

Egan, K.M., Ryan, L.M. and Gragoudas, E.S. (1998) Survival implications of enucleation after definitive radiotherapy for choroidal melanoma: an example of regression on time-dependent covariates. *Arch. Ophthalmol.*, **116**, 366–70.

Egan, K.M., Seddon, J.M., Glynn, R.J., Gragoudas, E.S. and Albert, D.M. (1988) Epidemiologic aspects of uveal melanoma. *Surv. Ophthalmol.*, **32**, 239–51.

Eskelin, S., Pyrhönen, S., Summanen, P., Prause, J.U. and Kivelä, T. (1999) Screening for metastatic malignant melanoma of the uvea revisited. *Cancer*, **85**, 1151–9.

Fiedler, W., Jasmin, C., De Mulder, P.H.M., Pyrhönen, S., Palmer, P.A., Franks, C.R., Oskam, R. and Hossfeld, D.K. (1992) A phase II study of sequential recombinant interleukin-2 followed by dacarbazine in metastatic melanoma. *Eur. J. Cancer*, **28**, 443–6.

Finger, P.T., Berson, A. and Szechter, A. (1999) Palladium-103 plaque radiotherapy for choroidal melanoma. Results of a seven year study. *Ophthalmology*, **106**, 606–13.

Folberg, R., Rummelt, V., Parys-Van Ginderdeuren, R., Hwang, T., Woolson, R.F., Pe'er, J. and Gruman, L.M. (1993) The prognostic value of tumor blood vessel morphology in primary uveal melanoma. *Ophthalmology*, **100**, 1389–98.

Foulds, W.S. and Damato, B.E. (1986) Low-energy long-exposure laser therapy in the management of choroidal melanoma. *Graefes Arch. Clin. Exp. Ophthalmol.*, **224**, 26–31.

Friedman, S.M. and Margo, C.E. (1998) Choroidal melanoma and neurofibromatosis type 1. *Arch. Ophthalmol.*, **116**, 694–5.

Fries, P.D., Char, D.H., Crawford, J.B. and Waterhouse, W. (1987) Sympathetic ophthalmia complicating helium ion irradiation of a choroidal melanoma. *Arch. Ophthalmol.*, **105**, 1561–4.

Glynn, R.J., Seddon, J.M., Gragoudas, E.S., Egan, K.M. and Hart, L.J. (1989) Evaluation of tumor regression and other prognostic factors for early and late metastasis after proton irradiation of uveal melanoma. *Ophthalmology*, **96**, 1566–73.

Gragoudas, E.S. and Char, D.H. (1994) Charged particle irradiation of uveal melanomas. In: D.M. Albert and F.A. Jakobiec (eds), *Principles and Practice of Ophthalmology*. Philadelphia: W.B. Saunders, Vol. 5, Ch. 262, pp. 3233–44.

Gragoudas, E.S., Seddon, J.M., Egan, K., Glynn, R., Munzenrider, J., Austin-Seymour, M., Goitein, M., Verhey, L., Urie, M. and Koehler, A. (1987) Long-term results of proton beam irradiated uveal melanomas. *Ophthalmology*, **94**, 349–53.

Gündüz, K., Shields, J.A., Shields, C.L., Sato, T. and Mastrangelo, M.J. (1998) Surgical removal of solitary hepatic metastasis from choroidal melanoma. *Am. J. Ophthalmol.*, **125**, 407–9.

Guthoff, R., Frischmuth, J., Jensen, O.A., Bjerrum, K. and Prause, J.U. (1992) Das Aderhautmelanom. Eine retrospektive randomisierte Vergleichsstudie Ruthenium-Bestrahlung vs Enukleation. *Klin. Monatsbl. Augenheilkd.*, **200**, 257–61.

Guyer, D.R., Mukai, S., Egan, K.M., Seddon, J.M., Walsh, S.M. and Gragoudas, E.S. (1992) Radiation maculopathy after proton beam irradiation for choroidal melanoma. *Ophthalmology*, **99**, 1278–85.

Hassenstein, A., Bialasiewicz, A.A., von Domarus, D., Schäfer, H. and Richard, G. (1999) Tapioca melanomas of the iris: immunohistology and report on two cases. *Graefes Arch Clin Exp. Ophthalmol.*, **237**, 424–8.

Haut, J., Sobel-Martin, A., Dureuil, J., Larricart, P. and Sarnikowski, C. (1984) Atrophies 'like flows' of the retinal pigment epithelium: a neuroepithelium-draining method of the posterior pole. *Ophthalmologica*, **189**, 121–7.

Holly, E., Aston, D.A., Ahn, D.K., Kristiansen, J.J. and Char, D.H. (1991) No excess prior cancer in patients with uveal melanoma. *Ophthalmology*, **98**, 608–11.

Jakobiec, F.A. and Silbert, G. (1981) Are most iris "melanomas" really nevi? A clinicopathologic study of 189 lesions. *Arch. Ophthalmol.*, **99**, 2117–32.

Jensen, O.A. (1982) Malignant melanomas of the human uvea: a 25-year follow-up of cases in Denmark, 1943–1952. *Acta Ophthalmol. (Copenh.)*, **60**, 161–82.

Karlsson, U.L., Augsburger, J.J., Shields, J.A., Markoe, A.M., Brady, L.W. and Woodleigh, R. (1989) Recurrence of posterior uveal melanoma after ^{60}Co episcleral plaque therapy. *Ophthalmology*, **96**, 382–8.

Kath, R., Hayungs, J., Bornfeld, N., Sauerwein, W., Höffken, K. and Seeber, S. (1993) Prognosis and treatment of disseminated uveal melanoma. *Cancer*, **72**, 2219–23.

Kersten, R.C., Tse, D.T. Anderson, R.L. and Blodi, F.C. (1985) The role of orbital exenteration in choroidal melanoma with extrascleral extension. *Ophthalmology*, **92**, 436–43.

Kirkwood, J.M. (1994) The role of interferons in the therapy of melanoma. *Immunol. Ser.*, **61**, 239–50.

Kivelä, T. (1995) Immunohistochemical staining followed by bleaching of melanin: a practical method for ophthalmic pathology. *Br. J. Ophthalmol.*, **52**, 325–6.

Kivelä, T. and Summanen, P. (1997) Retinoinvasive malignant melanoma of the uvea. *Br. J. Ophthalmol.*, **81**, 691–7.

Lee, K.J., Peyman, G.A. and Raichand, S. (1993) Internal eye wall resection for posterior uveal melanoma. *Jpn J. Ophthalmol.*, **37**, 287–92.

Lee, W.R. (1987) Pseudomelanomas after conservative management of uveal melanoma. *Eye*, **1**, 668–75.

Leyvraz, S., Spataro, V., Bauer, J., Pampallona, S., Salmon, R., Dorval, T., Meuli, R., Gillet, M., Lejeune, F. and Zografos, L. (1997) Treatment of ocular melanoma metastatic to the liver by hepatic arterial chemotherapy. *J. Clin. Oncol.*, **15**, 2589–95.

Livingston, P.O., Wong, G.Y., Adluri, S., Tao, Y., Padavan, M., Parente, R., Hanlon, C., Calves, M.J.,

Helling, F., Ritter, G. *et al.* (1994) Improved survival in stage III melanoma patients with GM2 antibodies: a randomized trial of adjuvant vaccination with GM2 ganglioside. *J. Clin. Oncol.*, **12**, 1036–44.

Lommatzsch, P.K. (1993) Treatment of choroidal melanomas with ^{106}Ru/^{106}Rh beta ray applications. In: W.E. Alberti and R.H. Sagerman (eds), *Radiotherapy of Intraocular and Orbital Tumors*. Berlin: Springer-Verlag, Ch. 4, pp. 23–30.

Lorigan, J. G., Wallace, S. and Mavligit, G. M. (1991) The prevalence and location of metastases from ocular melanoma: imaging study in 110 patients. *Am. J. Roentgenol.*, **157**, 1279–81.

Mäkitie, T., Summanen, P., Tarkkanen, A. and Kivelä, T. (1999a) Microvascular loops and networks as prognostic indicators in choroidal and ciliary body melanomas. *J. Natl Cancer Inst.*, **91**, 359–67.

Mäkitie, T., Summanen, P., Tarkkanen, A. and Kivelä, T. (1999b) Microvascular density in predicting survival in patients with choroidal and ciliary body melanoma. *Invest. Ophthalmol. Vis. Sci.*, **40**, 2471–80.

Manschot, W.A. and van Strik, R. (1992) Uveal melanoma: therapeutic consequences of doubling times and irradiation results: a review. *Int. Ophthalmol.*, **16**, 91–9.

Marchini, G., Babighian, S., Tomazzoli, L., Gerosa, M.A., Nicolato, A., Bricolo, A., Piovan, E., Zampieri, P.G., Alessandrini, F., Benati, A. *et al.* (1995) Stereotactic radiosurgery of uveal melanomas: preliminary results with Gamma Knife treatment. *Stereotact. Funct. Neurosurg.*, **64** (Suppl 1), 72–9.

Margo, C.E., Mulla, Z. and Billiris, K. (1998) Incidence of surgically treated uveal melanoma by race and ethnicity. *Ophthalmology*, **105**, 1087–90.

McCurdy, J., Gamel, J. and McLean, I. (1991) A simple, efficient and reproducible method for estimating the malignant potential of uveal melanoma from routine H & E slides. *Pathol. Res. Pract.*, **187**, 1025–7.

McLean, I.W., Foster, W.D., Zimmerman, L.E. and Gamel, J.W. (1983) Modifications of Callender's classification of uveal melanoma at the Armed Forces Institute of Pathology. *Am. J. Ophthalmol.*, **96**, 502–9.

Naumann, G.O.H. and Rummelt, V. (1996) Block excision of tumors of the anterior uvea. *Ophthalmology*, **103**, 2017–28.

Nestle, F.O., Alijagic, S., Gilliet, M., Sun, Y., Grabbe, S., Dummer, R., Burg, G. and Schadedorf, D. (1998) Vaccination of melanoma patients with peptide- or tumor lysate-pulsed dendritic cells. *Nature Med.*, **4**, 328–32.

Oosterhuis, J.A., Journée-de Korver, H.G., Kakebeeke-Kemme, H.M. and Bleeker, J.C. (1995) Transpupillary thermotherapy in choroidal melanomas. *Arch. Ophthalmol.*, **113**, 315–21.

Oosterhuis, J.A., Journée de Korver, H.G. and Keunen, J.E.E. (1998) Transpupillary thermotherapy: results in 50 patients with choroidal melanoma. *Arch. Ophthalmol.*, **116**, 157–62.

Pach, J.M., Robertson, D.M., Taney, B.S., Martin, J.A., Campbell, R.J. and O'Brien, P.C. (1986) Prognostic factors in choroidal and ciliary body melanomas with extrascleral extension. *Am. J. Ophthalmol.*, **101**, 325–31.

Packer, S., Stoller, S., Lesser, M.L., Mandel, F.S. and Finger, P.T. (1992) Long-term results of iodine 125 irradiation of uveal melanoma. *Ophthalmology*, **99**, 767–74.

Parkes, C.M. (1998) Coping with loss. The dying adult. *Br. Med. J.*, **316**, 1313–15.

Peyman, G.A. and Gremillion, C.M. (1989) Eye wall resection in the management of uveal neoplasms. *Jpn J. Ophthalmol.*, **33**, 458–71.

Prescher, G., Bornfeld, N., Hirche, H., Horsthemke, B., Jöckel, K-H. and Becher, R. (1996) Prognostic implications of monosomy 3 in uveal melanoma. *Lancet*, **347**, 1222–5.

Rajpal, S., Moore, R. and Karakousis, C.P. (1983) Survival in metastatic ocular melanoma. *Cancer*, **52**, 334–6.

Regan, S., Judge, H.E., Gragoudas, E.S. and Egan, K.M. (1999) Iris color, as a prognostic factor in ocular melanoma. *Arch. Ophthalmol.*, **117**, 811–14.

Retsas, S., Quigley, M., Pectasides, D., Macrae, K. and Henry, K. (1994) Clinical and histologic involvement of regional lymph nodes in malignant melanoma. Adjuvant vindesine improves survival. *Cancer*, **73**, 2119–30.

Robertson, D.M., Buettner, H. and Bennett, S.R. (1999) Transpupillary thermotherapy as primary treatment for small choroidal melanomas. *Arch. Ophthalmol.*, **117**, 1512–19.

Rosenberg, S.A., Yang, J.C., Schwartzentruber, D.J., Hwu, P., Marinocola, F.M., Topalian, S.L., Restifo, N.P., Dudley, M.E., Schwarz, S.L., Spiess, P.J., Wunderlich, J.R., Parkhurst, M.R., Kawakami, Y., Seipp, C.A., Einhorn, J.H. and White, D.E. (1998) Immunologic and therapeutic evaluation of a synthetic peptide vaccine for the treatment of patients with metastatic melanoma. *Nature Med.*, **4**, 321–7.

Rummelt, V., Folberg, R., Rummelt, C., Gruman, L.M., Hwang, T., Woolson, R.F., Yi, H. and Naumann, G.O.H. (1994) Microcirculation architecture of melanocytic nevi and malignant melanomas of the ciliary body and choroid. A comparative histopathologic and ultrastructural study. *Ophthalmology*, **101**, 718–27.

Sarvananthan, N., Wiselka, M. and Bibby, K. (1998) Intraocular tuberculosis without detectable systemic infection. *Arch. Ophthalmol.*, **116**, 1386–8.

Schachat, A.P. (1994) Collaborative ocular melanoma study. In: S.J. Ryan (ed.), *Retina*. St Louis: Mosby, Vol. 1, Ch. 51, pp. 828–31.

Scott, I.U., Murray, T.G. and Hughes, J.R. (1998) Evaluation of imaging techniques for detection of extraocular extension of choroidal melanoma. *Arch. Ophthalmol.*, **116**, 897–9.

Scotto, J., Fraumeni, J.F., Jr. and Lee, J.A.H. (1976) Melanomas of the eye and other noncutaneous sites: epidemiologic aspects. *J. Natl. Cancer Inst.*, **56**, 489–91.

Seddon, J.M., Albert, D.M., Lavin, P.T. and Robinson, N. (1983) A prognostic factor study of disease-free interval and survival following enucleation for uveal melanoma. *Arch. Ophthalmol.*, **101**, 1894–9.

Seddon, J.M. and Egan, K. (1993) Application of epidemiological methods to the study of eye disease: uveal melanoma. In: D.M. Albert and F.A. Jakobiec (eds), *Principles and Practice of Ophthalmology. Basic Sciences.* Philadelphia: W.B. Saunders, Ch. 106, pp. 1245–9.

Seddon, J.M., Gragoudas, E.S., Egan, K.M., Glynn, R.J., Howard, S., Fante, R.G. and Albert, D.M. (1990) Relative survival rates after alternative therapies for uveal melanoma. *Ophthalmology*, **97**, 769–77.

Seddon, J.M., Gragoudas, E.S., Polivogianis, L., Hsieh, C-C., Egan, K.M., Goitein, M., Verhey, L., Munzenrider, J., Austin-Seymour, M., Urie, M. *et al.* (1986) Visual outcome after proton beam irradiation of uveal melanoma. *Ophthalmology*, **93**, 666–74.

Seddon, J.M., Polivogianis, L., Hsieh, C-C., Albert, D.M., Gamel, J.W. and Gragoudas, E.S. (1987) Death from uveal melanoma. Number of epithelioid cells and inverse SD of nucleolar area as prognostic factors. *Arch. Ophthalmol.*, **105**, 801–6.

Seregard, S., Oskarsson, M. and Spångberg, B. (1996) PC-10 as a predictor of prognosis after antigen retrieval in posterior uveal melanoma. *Invest. Ophthalmol. Vis. Sci.*, **37**, 1451–8.

Seregard, S., Spångberg, B., Juul, C. and Oskarsson, M. (1998) Prognostic accuracy of the mean of the largest nucleoli, vascular patterns, and PC-10 in posterior uveal melanoma. *Ophthalmology*, **105**, 485–91.

Shields, C.L., Shields, J.A., Cater, J., Lois, N., Edelstein, C., Gündüz, K. and Mercado, G. (1998) Transpupillary thermotherapy for choroidal melanoma: tumor control and visual results in 100 consecutive cases. *Ophthalmology*, **105**, 581–90.

Shields, C.L., Shields, J.A., De Potter, P., Cater, J., Tardio, D. and Barrett, J. (1996) Diffuse choroidal melanoma. Clinical features predictive of metastasis. *Arch. Ophthalmol.*, **114**, 956–63.

Shields, C.L., Shields, J.A., De Potter, P., Singh, A.D., Hernandez, C. and Brady, L.W. (1995) Treatment of non-resectable malignant iris tumours with custom designed plaque radiotherapy. *Br. J. Ophthalmol.*, **79**, 306–12.

Shields, C.L., Shields, J.A., Yarian, D.L. and Augsburger, J.J. (1987) Intracranial extension of choroidal melanoma via the optic nerve. *Br. J. Ophthalmol.*, **71**, 172–6.

Shields, J.A., Shields, C.L., Shah, P. and Sivalingam, V. (1991) Partial lamellar sclerouvectomy for ciliary body and choroidal tumors. *Ophthalmology*, **98**, 971–83.

Simpson, E.R. (1999) Personal communication: International Congress of Ocular Oncology, Philadelphia.

Singh, A.D., De Potter, P., Fijal, B.A., Shields, C.L., Shields, J.A. and Elston, R.C. (1998) Lifetime prevalence of uveal melanoma in white patients with oculo (dermal) melanocytosis. *Ophthalmology*, **105**, 195–8.

Singh, A.D., Shields, C.L., De Potter, P., Shields, J.A., Trock, B., Cater, J. and Pastore, D. (1996) Familial uveal melanoma. Clinical observations on 56 patients. *Arch. Ophthalmol.*, **114**, 392–9.

Spencer, W.H. (1975) Optic nerve extension of intraocular neoplasms. *Am. J. Ophthalmol.*, **80**, 465–71.

Starr, H.J. and Zimmerman, L.E. (1962) Extrascleral extension and orbital recurrence of malignant melanomas of the choroid and ciliary body. *Int. Ophthalmol. Clin.* 369–85.

Summanen, P., Immonen, I., Kivelä, T., Tommila, P., Heikkonen, J. and Tarkkanen, A. (1995) Visual outcome of eyes with malignant melanoma of the uvea after ruthenium plaque radiotherapy. *Ophthalmic Surg.*, **26**, 449–60.

Summanen, P., Immonen, I., Kivelä, T., Tommila, P., Heikkonen, J. and Tarkkanen, A. (1996) Radiation related complications after ruthenium plaque radiotherapy of uveal melanoma. *Br. J. Ophthalmol.*, **80**, 732–9.

Toti, P., Greco, G., Mangiavacchi, P., Bruni, A., Palmeri, M.L.D. and Luzi, P. (1998) DNA ploidy pattern in choroidal melanoma: correlation with survival. A flow cytometry study on archival material. *Br. J. Ophthalmol.*, **82**, 1433–7.

Wilson, D. and Klein, M. (1999) Personal communication; International Congress of Ocular Oncology, Philadelphia.

Wiznia, R.A., Freedman, J.K., Mancini, A.D. and Shields, J.A. (1978) Malignant melanoma of the choroid in neurofibromatosis. *Am. J. Ophthalmol.*, **86**, 684–7.

Young, L.H., Howard, M.A., Hu, L.K., Kim, R.Y. and Gragoudas, E.S. (1996) Photodynamic therapy of pigmented choroidal melanomas using a liposomal preparation of benzoporphyrin derivative. *Arch. Ophthalmol.*, **114**, 186–92.

Zehetmayer, M., Menapace, R., Kitz, K., Ertl, A., Strenn, K. and Ruhswurm, I. (1997) Stereotactic irradiation of uveal melanoma with the Leksell Gamma Unit. In: T. Wiegel, N. Bornfeld, M.H. Foerster and W. Hinkelbein (eds), *Radiotherapy of Ocular Disease.* Basle: Karger, Vol. 30, pp. 47–55.

Chapter 8

Choroidal haemangioma

Choroidal haemangiomas are relatively rare. The incidence of asymptomatic lesions is probably underestimated. Clinically, they may be circumscribed or diffuse.

Diffuse choroidal haemangiomas are associated with the Sturge–Weber syndrome, which tends to develop sporadically.

PATHOLOGY

Choroidal haemangiomas are vascular hamartomas. Most are of the cavernous or mixed variety (i.e., cavernous–capillary) (Witschel and Font, 1976) (Figure 8.1)

The RPE overlying the haemangioma degenerates, accumulating lipofuscin pigment and occasionally developing fibrous or osseous metaplasia.

The overlying retina becomes cystic and there is typically a serous retinal detachment. This may become total to cause painful, neovascular glaucoma.

PRESENTATION

Circumscribed choroidal haemangiomas (Anand *et al.,* 1989) are not associated with any systemic disease. They are usually detected in adulthood,

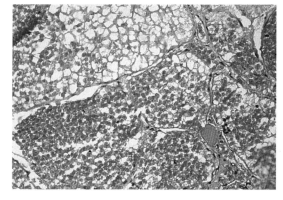

Figure 8.1 Light micrograph of a choroidal haemangioma

either because of visual symptoms or on routine examination.

Diffuse choroidal haemangiomas tend to cause symptoms in childhood.

SYMPTOMS

- Blurred vision, metamorphopsia and micropsia due to serous retinal detachment affecting the fovea.
- Hypermetropia, if the retina is elevated by tumour or fluid.

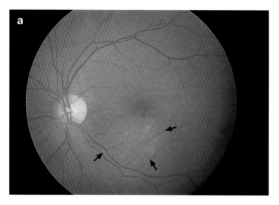
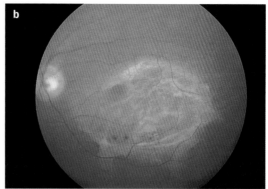

Figure 8.2 Clinical photographs of localized choroidal haemangiomas (**a**) without and (**b**) with subretinal fibrosis

Many patients are asymptomatic with normal visual acuity.

SIGNS

CIRCUMSCRIBED CHOROIDAL HAEMANGIOMA

- Red or pink tumour (Figure 8.2**a**), perhaps with a network of subretinal fibrosis (Figure 8.2**b**), dusting of orange pigment and black clumps of RPE cells.
- Round or oval shape, with smooth surface and indistinct margins.
- Post-equatorial location, usually extending to within 2 DD of optic disc or fovea.
- Small size, usually less than 10 mm in diameter and less than 5 mm in thickness, although tumours up to 18 mm in diameter and 7 mm in thickness have been recorded.

DIFFUSE CHOROIDAL HAEMANGIOMA

- Bright red pupillary reflex ('tomato ketchup fundus')
- Diffuse red–orange choroidal thickening with indistinct margins and sometimes involving the entire fundus.
- RPE stippling, which can mimic retinitis pigmentosa.
- Dilated, tortuous retinal vessels overlying the haemangioma (Figure 8.3)

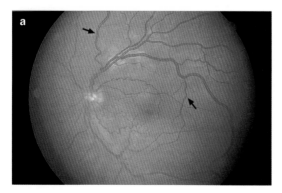
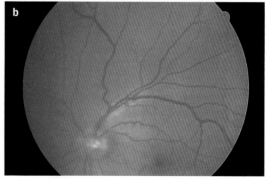

Figure 8.3 Diffuse choroidal haemangioma in the superior part of the left eye: (**a**) at presentation, showing dilated and tortuous retinal veins over the lesion and (**b**) 5 months after external beam radiotherapy, showing that the retinal vessels have returned to normal

COMPLICATIONS

- Macular hard exudates and macular pucker.
- Cystic degeneration of overlying retina and exudative retinal detachment, which may become total.
- Neovascular glaucoma secondary to retinal detachment.
- Secondary cataract, with leukocoria and band keratopathy in cases with total retinal detachment.

OTHER MANIFESTATIONS OF STURGE–WEBER SYNDROME

- Naevus flammeus ('port wine stain') affecting the face, on the same side as the ocular haemangioma (Figure 8.4).
- Leptomeningeal disease, which can affect the parietal and occipital cortex to cause seizures, intellectual deficit and visual field loss.
- Glaucoma, due to abnormal development of the anterior chamber angle or raised episcleral venous pressure, which can lead to buphthalmos in young children (i.e., before the age of three years).
- Iris heterochromia, with increased ipsilateral pigmentation.

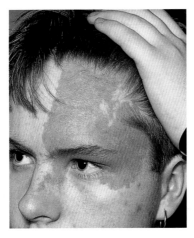

Figure 8.4 Cutaneous manifestations of Sturge–Weber syndrome

- Conjunctival and episcleral telangiectasia.
- Ocular melanosis and naevus of Ota, rarely.

INVESTIGATIONS

VISUAL FIELD EXAMINATION

Causes of visual field loss include:

- Leptomeningeal disease, which causes homonymous defects.
- Macular oedema, causing a central scotoma.
- Retinal detachment.
- Glaucoma.

FLUORESCEIN ANGIOGRAPHY

There is rapid hyperfluorescence, usually preceding retinal arteriolar filling, with diffuse leakage in the later stages (Figure 8.5). These appearances are typical of haemangioma but not pathognomonic, as they can occur with melanoma.

INDOCYANINE GREEN ANGIOGRAPHY

Angiomas rapidly develop a lacy hyperfluorescence, followed by a 'washout' of dye after about 15–20 minutes, so that they become iso- or hypofluorescent relative to surrounding choroid (Sallet *et al.*, 1995; Shields *et al.*, 1995) (Figure 8.6).

ULTRASONOGRAPHY

A- and B-scan ultrasonography show high internal reflectivity without acoustic hollowness (Figure 8.7). Osseous fibroplasia, if present, has a highly reflective surface, with orbital shadowing. A collar-stud configuration does not occur.

Colour Doppler imaging shows a high maximum systolic Doppler shift, which can also occur with melanoma.

COMPUTERIZED TOMOGRAPHY

There is moderate enhancement with contrast material. Calcification is evident if there is any osseous fibroplasia.

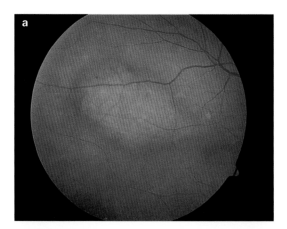

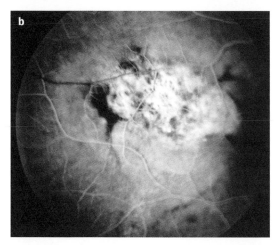

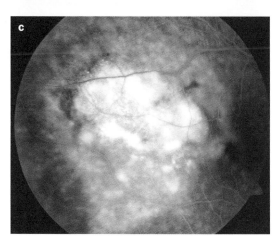

Figure 8.5 Fluorescein angiogram of a choroidal haemangioma showing (**a**) colour photograph; (**b**) rapid filling and (**c**) late diffuse hyperfluorescence

MAGNETIC RESONANCE IMAGING

Haemangiomas are iso- or hyper-intense to vitreous in T1 weighted images and iso-intense to vitreous in T2 weighted images (De Potter *et al.*, 1995) (Figure 8.8). There is marked enhancement with gadolinium, which aids differentiation from surrounding retinal detachment.

DIFFERENTIAL DIAGNOSIS

1. **Amelanotic melanoma** (Chapter 7).
2. **Metastasis** (Chapter 19).
3. **Choroidal osteoma** (Chapter 9).
4. **Posterior scleritis** (Calthorpe *et al.*, 1988; Benson, 1988). This may be associated with massive scleral thickening (Finger *et al.*, 1990), inflammatory signs, pain, disc swelling and exudative retinal detachment. Other features that may be present include choroidal folds, calcification, ciliochoroidal detachment, limited eye movements, proptosis and lower lid retraction on attempted elevation of the eye (Figure 8.9).
5. **RPE detachment.** This shows uniform hyperfluorescence on angiography and is acoustically hollow on ultrasonography.

MANAGEMENT

OBSERVATION

Asymptomatic lesions not threatening vision can be observed without treatment.

EXTERNAL BEAM RADIOTHERAPY

Radiotherapy has become the first choice of treatment in many centres. A total dose of 12.5–20 Gy is delivered in six to ten divided fractions, using a lateral, lens-sparing technique (Schilling *et al.*, 1997) (see Figure 8.3**b**) or stereotactic radiotherapy (Chapter 23).

PLAQUE RADIOTHERAPY (BRACHYTHERAPY)

Plaque radiotherapy may be preferred for circumscribed haemangiomas not extending close to optic disc or fovea (Zografos *et al.*, 1996).

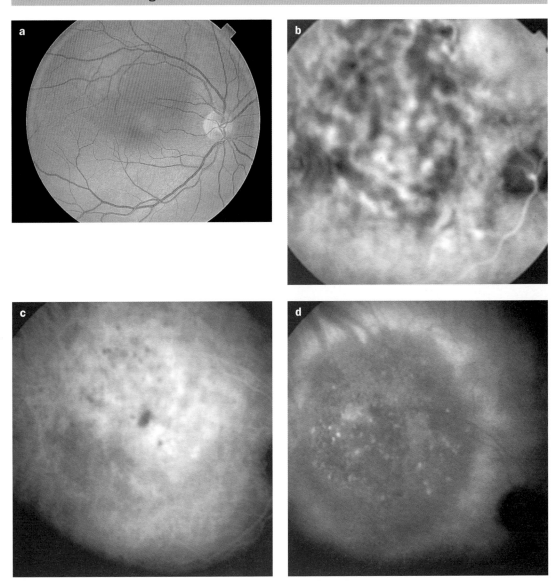

Figure 8.6 Indocyanine green angiogram of a superior choroidal haemangioma in the right eye: (**a**) colour photograph showing smooth pink tumour, (**b**) 20 seconds, showing patchy hyperfluorescence, (**c**) 5 minutes, showing diffuse hyperfluorescence and (**d**) 40 minutes, with generalized hypofluorescence and pinpoint hyperfluorescence. (Courtesy of B.A. Lafaut, Ghent, Belgium)

Advocates of plaque radiotherapy believe that this approach induces more tumour regression and therefore a better final visual acuity than external beam radiotherapy (Madreperla *et al.*, 1997). Approximately 45 Gy is delivered to the tumour apex (Chapter 23).

PROTON BEAM RADIOTHERAPY

Proton beam radiotherapy is relatively expensive, requires insertion of tantalum markers and is not widely available. Advocates of this technique consider it to be superior to brachytherapy because it

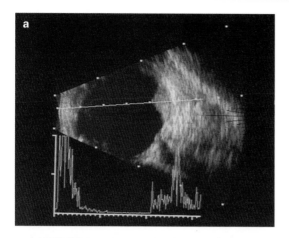

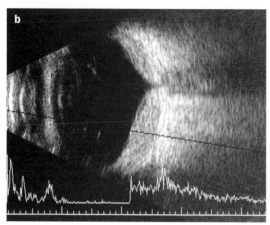

Figure 8.7 Ultrasonography of (**a**) circumscribed and (**b**) diffuse choroidal haemangiomas showing high intensity echoes on A-scan and bright reflectivity throughout lesion

provides a homogenous dose of radiation to the entire tumour while sparing surrounding tissues (Hannouche *et al.*, 1997; Zografos *et al.*, 1998). A total dose of approximately 18 Gy is delivered in four daily fractions (Chapter 23).

PHOTOTHERAPY

Photocoagulation is applied by delivering light, non-confluent, 200–500 µm burns to the tumour surface over two or three sessions (Chapter 25). The objective is not to destroy the tumour but to achieve chorioretinal adhesion. Excessive subretinal fluid can be drained by posterior sclerotomy,

replacing the intraocular volume with intravitreal gas or fluid (Shields and Shields, 1992). It is often necessary to repeat the treatment, because of persistent or recurrent retinal detachment (Sanborn *et al.*, 1982). Treatment of sub-macular tumour is not possible without loss of central vision.

Transpupillary thermotherapy, delivering long applications, can induce tumour regression and resolution of the retinal detachment (Othmane *et al.*, 1999) (Chapter 25).

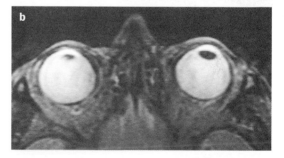

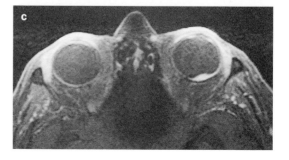

Figure 8.8 MRI scan showing (**a**) T1 weighted image, (**b**) T2 weighted image and (**c**) post-contrast T1 weighted image with fat suppression technique. (Courtesy of P. De Potter, Brussels, Belgium)

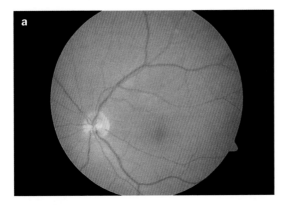

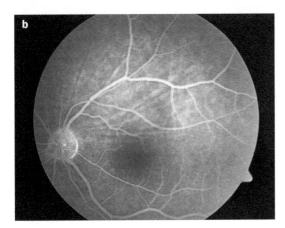

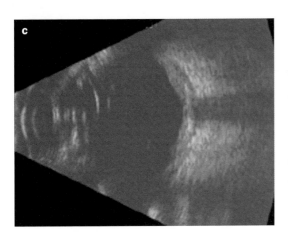

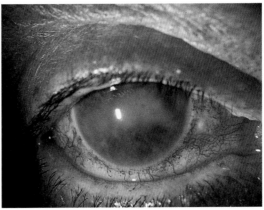

ENUCLEATION

If there is total, intractable retinal detachment with neovascular glaucoma, enucleation may be the only treatment that can prevent pain.

PROGNOSIS

The prognosis in asymptomatic cases is not known. If a choroidal haemangioma causes persistent and total retinal detachment, the eye is likely to develop neovascular glaucoma, cataract and band keratopathy (Figure 8.10).

After radiotherapy, tumour regression is more likely to occur with diffuse haemangiomas and with higher doses of radiotherapy. Retinal detachment tends to resolve even if the tumour does not regress.

After successful resolution of the retinal detachment, there may be permanent distortion of vision if the tumour remains elevated.

Vision is unlikely to improve if the tumour is subfoveal or if prolonged retinal detachment has resulted in irreversible macular changes. Years after initial improvement, vision may deteriorate because of subretinal fibrosis.

The visual outcome may be poor in patients with the Sturge–Weber syndrome despite successful treatment of the angioma because of other problems, such as glaucoma.

Figure 8.9 Posterior scleritis of left eye showing (**a**) choroidal folds, (**b**) lack of hyperfluorescence on fluorescein angiography and (**c**) scleral thickening with the typical T-sign of extraocular oedema around the optic nerve head on B-scan ultrasonography

Figure 8.10 End-stage eye in a patient with Sturge–Weber syndrome, with total retinal detachment, cataract and band keratopathy

REFERENCES

Anand, R., Augsburger, J.J. and Shields, J.A. (1989) Circumscribed choroidal hemangiomas. *Arch. Ophthalmol.*, **107**, 1338–42.

Benson, W.E. (1988) Posterior scleritis. *Surv. Ophthalmol.*, **32**, 297–316.

Calthorpe, C.M., Watson, P.G. and McCartney, A.C. (1988) Posterior scleritis: a clinical and histological survey. *Eye*, **2**, 267–77.

De Potter, P., Shields, J.A. and Shields, C.L. (1995) *MRI of the Eye and Orbit*. Philadelphia: J.B. Lippincott, Ch. 6, p. 60.

Finger, P.T., Perry, H.D., Packer, S., Erdey, R.A., Weisman, G.D. and Sibony, P.A. (1990) Posterior scleritis as an intraocular tumour. *Br. J. Ophthalmol.*, **74**, 121–2.

Hannouche, D., Frau, E., Desjardins, L., Cassoux, N., Habrand, J-L. and Offret, H. (1997) Efficacy of proton therapy in circumscribed choroidal hemangiomas associated with serous retinal detachment. *Ophthalmology*, **104**, 1780–4.

Madreperla, S.A., Hungerford, J.L., Plowman, P.N., Laganowski, H.C. and Gregory, P.T.S. (1997) Choroidal haemangiomas: treatment by photocoagulation or radiotherapy. *Ophthalmology*, **104**, 1773–9.

Othmane, I.S., Shields, C.L., Shields, J.A., Gündüz, K. and Mercado, G. (1999) Circumscribed choroidal hemangioma managed by transpupillary thermotherapy. *Arch. Ophthalmol.*, **117**, 136–7.

Sallet, G., Amoaku, W.M., Lafaut, B.A., Brabant, P. and De Laey, J.J. (1995) Indocyanine green angiography of choroidal tumors. *Graefes Arch. Clin. Exp. Ophthalmol.*, **233**, 677–89.

Sanborn, G.E., Augsburger, J.J. and Shields, J.A. (1982) Treatment of circumscribed choroidal hemangiomas. *Ophthalmology*, **89**, 1374–80.

Schilling, H., Sauerwein, W., Lommatzsch, A., Friedrichs, W., Brylak, S., Bornfeld, N. and Wessing, A. (1997) Long term results after low dose ocular irradiation for choroidal haemangiomas. *Br. J. Ophthalmol.*, **81**, 267–73.

Shields, C.L., Shields, J.A. and De Potter, P. (1995) Patterns of indocyanine green videoangiography of choroidal tumours. *Br. J. Ophthalmol.*, **79**, 237–45.

Shields, J.A. and Shields, C.L. (1992) *Intraocular Tumors. A Text and Atlas*. Philadelphia: W.B. Saunders, Ch. 13, pp. 249–51.

Witschel, H. and Font, R.L. (1976) Hemangioma of the choroid. A clinicopathologic study of 71 cases and a review of the literature. *Surv. Ophthalmol.*, **20**, 415–31.

Zografos, L., Bercher, L., Chamot, L., Gailloud, C., Raimondi, S. and Egger, E. (1996) Cobalt-60 treatment of choroidal hemangiomas. *Am. J. Ophthalmol.*, **121**, 190–9.

Zografos, L., Egger, E., Bercher, L., Chamot, L. and Munkel, G. (1998) Proton beam irradiation of choroidal hemangiomas. *Am. J. Ophthalmol.*, **126**, 261–8.

Chapter 9

Choroidal osteoma

Choroidal osteoma is a very rare tumour. It is usually detected in early adulthood, but can occur in children (Fava *et al.*, 1980). Most patients are female. Familial cases have been reported (Noble, 1990; Eting and Savir, 1992).

PATHOLOGY

Choroidal osteoma consists of mature, cancellous bone (Williams *et al.*, 1978). The overlying RPE is atrophic. Choroidal neovascularization tends to develop to cause visual loss.

The cause is unknown. Some workers have suggested that the lesion is a choristoma. Osteomas have been observed to develop at sites of previous inflammation (Trimble and Schatz, 1983), in siblings (Aylward *et al.*, 1998) and in a family with autosomal dominant limbal dermoids (Magli *et al.*, 1999). Intrascleral ossification can arise in association with the naevus sebaceus of Jadassohn (Traboulsi *et al.*, 1999).

Slow growth can occur, either by generalized enlargement or by the formation of finger-like projections. Spontaneous decalcification has been reported (Trimble *et al.*, 1998).

SYMPTOMS

This condition is asymptomatic unless the fovea is involved by tumour, associated neovascularization or exudative retinal detachment.

SIGNS

- White, yellow or orange colour, perhaps with visible, pink, vascular tufts on the surface.
- Wavy margins, which are well defined.
- Flat or irregularly undulating surface.
- Posterior location, usually adjacent to or surrounding disc and often involving macula (Figure 9.1).
- Bilateral in about 25% of cases.

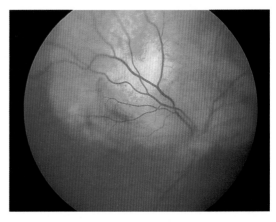

Figure 9.1 Superior juxtapapillary choroidal osteoma in the right eye, with well-defined wavy margins and an early neovascular membrane

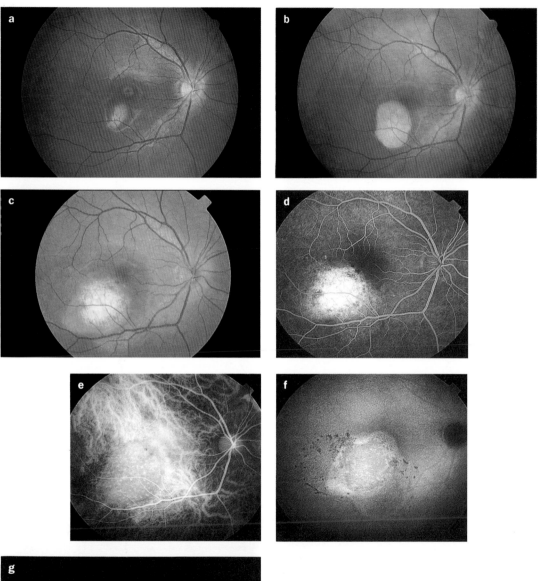

Figure 9.2 Inferotemporal choroidal osteoma in the right eye: (**a**) at presentation, (**b**) 3 years later, (**c**) 7 years later, (**d**) fluorescein angiogram showing diffuse hyperfluorescence, (**e**) early ICG angiogram showing early hypofluorescence with hyperfluorescent spots, (**f**) late ICG angiogram showing diffuse hyperfluorescence with abnormality in ophthalmoscopically normal choroid and (**g**) B-scan ultrasonograph, showing high surface reflectivity and orbital shadowing. (Courtesy of G. Modorati, Milan, Italy)

- Diameter varying between 2 DD to more than 20 mm.
- Thickness less than 5 mm.
- Growth in about 50% of cases, which is usually slow (Figure 9.2**a–c**).

INVESTIGATIONS

FLUORESCEIN ANGIOGRAPHY

There is irregular, diffuse hyperfluorescence, with highlighting of vascular tufts and masking by residual pigment on the tumour surface (Figure 9.2**d**). A neovascular membrane may be evident.

INDOCYANINE GREEN ANGIOGRAPHY

ICG angiography shows early hypofluorescence with late staining, also revealing abnormality in ophthalmoscopically normal choroid (Yuzawa *et al.,* 1994) (Figure 9.2**e–f**).

ULTRASONOGRAPHY

Osteomas have a highly reflective anterior surface and cast a shadow into the orbit (Figure 9.2**g**).

COMPUTERIZED TOMOGRAPHY

The radiographic features are the same as bone (Figure 9.3).

MAGNETIC RESONANCE IMAGING

Relative to vitreous, osteomas are hyper-intense on T1 weighted images and hypo-intense on T2 weighted images (De Potter *et al.,* 1995). These MRI features resemble those of melanoma and are different from cortical bone.

DIFFERENTIAL DIAGNOSIS

1. **Osseous metaplasia** (Monselise *et al.,* 1985), which can occur in association with choroidal haemangiomas, melanomas, disciform lesions and disorganization of the posterior segment.
2. **Sclerochoroidal calcification**, with lesions developing under the vascular arcades, often bilaterally (Figure 9.4). Choroidal neovascularization sometimes occurs (Leys *et al.,* 1999). Sclerochoroidal calcification may be associated with hypercalcaemia. In normocalcaemic patients, the disease is usually idiopathic, but may be associated with the Bartter syndrome (metabolic alkalosis, secondary hyperaldosteronism and normocalcaemia) (Marchini *et al.,* 1998).
3. **Amelanotic choroidal naevus and melanoma** (Chapters 5 and 7).
4. **Choroidal metastases** (Chapter 19).
5. **Lymphomatous and leukaemic deposits** (Chapters 20 and 21).

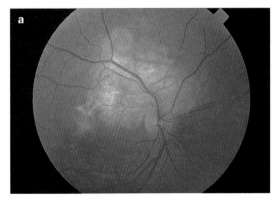 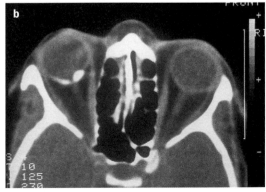

Figure 9.3 Superior choroidal osteoma in the right eye: (**a**) ophthalmoscopic appearance and (**b**) CT scan, showing opaque lesion. (Courtesy of P. Lommatzsch, Leipzig, Germany)

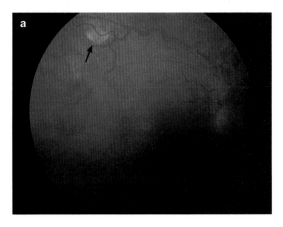

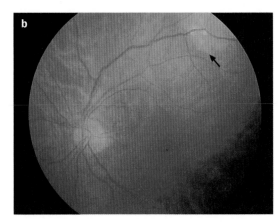

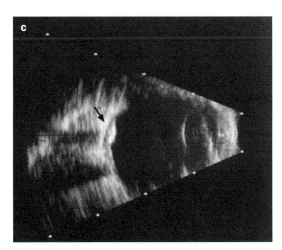

Figure 9.4 Bilateral sclerochoroidal calcification: (**a**) right eye, (**b**) left eye, (**c**) B-scan of representative lesion

MANAGEMENT

Choroidal neovascularization threatening vision may be treatable with laser photocoagulation (Morrison *et al.,* 1987).

Treatment of the osteoma itself is not usually required although regression has been reported after photocoagulation (Rose *et al.,* 1991) and after corticosteroid therapy (Katz and Gass, 1983).

PROGNOSIS

a. Disciform macular degeneration develops in about 50%.
b. Visual loss to 6/60 or worse occurs in about 60% of patients (Aylward *et al.,* 1998).

REFERENCES

Aylward, G.W., Chang, T.S., Pautler, S.E. and Gass, J.D. (1998) A long-term follow-up of choroidal osteoma. *Arch. Ophthalmol.,* **116**, 1337–41.

De Potter, P., Shields, J.A. and Shields, C.L. (1995) *MRI of the Eye and Orbit.* Philadelphia: J.B. Lippincott.

Eting, E. and Savir, H. (1992) An atypical fulminant course of choroidal osteoma in two siblings. *Am. J. Ophthalmol.,* **113**, 52–5.

Fava, G.E., Brown, G.C., Shields, J.A. and Broocker, G. (1980) Choroidal osteoma in a 6-year-old child. *J. Pediatr. Ophthalmol. Strabismus.,* **17**, 203–5.

Katz, R.S. and Gass, J.D.M. (1983) Multiple choroidal osteomas developing in association with recurrent orbital inflammatory pseudotumour. *Arch. Ophthalmol.,* **101**, 1724–7.

Leys, A., Cohen, S., Guyot-Sionnest, M., Puech, M., Stalmans, P. and Spileers, W. (1999) Personal communication; International Congress of Ocular Oncology, Philadelphia.

Magli, A., De Marco, R. and Capasso, L. (1999). Presence of bilateral limbal dermoids and choroidal osteomas in a family with inherited limbal dermoids. *Ophthalmic. Genet.,* **20**, 101–6.

Marchini, G., Tosi, R., Parolini, B., Castagna, G. and Zarbin, M. (1998) Choroidal calcification in Bartter syndrome. *Am. J. Ophthalmol.,* **126**, 727–9.

Monselise, M., Rapaport, I., Romem, M. and Barishak, Y.R. (1985) Intraocular ossification. *Ophthalmologica,* **190**, 225–9.

Morrison, D.L., Magargal, L.E., Ehrlich, D.R., Goldberg, R.E. and Robb-Doyle, E. (1987) Review of choroidal osteoma: successful krypton red laser photocoagulation of an associated subretinal neovascular membrane involving the fovea. *Ophthalmic Surg.*, **18**, 299–303.

Noble, K.G. (1990) Bilateral choroidal osteoma in three siblings. *Am. J. Ophthalmol.*, **109**, 656–60.

Rose, S.J., Burke, J.F. and Brockhurst, R.J. (1991) Argon laser photoablation of a choroidal osteoma. *Retina*, **11**, 224–8.

Traboulsi, E.I., Zin, A., Massicotte, S.J., Kosmorsky, G., Kotagal, P. and Ellis, F.D. (1999) Posterior scleral choristoma in the organoid nevus syndrome (linear nevus sebaceus of Jadassohn). *Ophthalmology*, **106**, 2126–30.

Trimble, S.N. and Schatz, H. (1983) Choroidal osteoma after intraocular inflammation. *Am. J. Ophthalmol.*, **96**, 759–64.

Trimble, S.N., Schatz, H. and Schneider, G.B. (1998) Spontaneous decalcification of a choroidal osteoma. *Ophthalmology*, **95**, 631–4.

Williams, A.T., Font, R.L., Van Dyk, H.J. and Riekhof, F.T. (1978) Osseous choristoma of the choroid simulating a choroidal melanoma. Association with a positive ^{32}P test. *Arch. Ophthalmol.*, **96**, 1874–7.

Yuzawa, M., Kawamura, A., Haruyama, M. and Matsui, M. (1994) Indocyanine green video-angiographic findings in choroidal osteoma. *Eur. J. Ophthalmol.*, **4**, 191–8.

Chapter 10

Neurofibroma, neurilemmoma and leiomyoma

Neurilemmoma, neurofibroma and leiomyoma are benign tumours. They have a predilection for the ciliary body but can arise anywhere in the uveal tract.

Most neurofibromas and some neurilemmomas occur in patients with neurofibromatosis type 1 (Huson *et al.,* 1987; Parry *et al.,* 1994). Leiomyomas do not have any systemic associations, and tend to occur in young women.

PATHOLOGY

1. **Neurilemmomas** (also known as Schwannomas) are composed of amelanotic, spindle-shaped cells, arising from Schwann cells in the ciliary nerves (Smith *et al.,* 1987; Pineda *et al.,* 1995). There may be patchy degeneration.
2. **Neurofibromas** contain Schwann cells, fibroblasts and myelinated axons. They may be circumscribed or diffuse, with the diffuse variety being more likely to be pigmented.
3. **Leiomyomas** consist of spindle-shaped smooth muscle cells with cigar-shaped nuclei

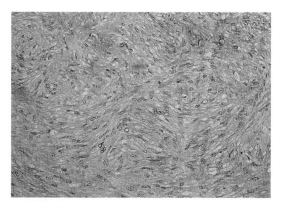

Figure 10.1 Light micrograph of leiomyoma. (Courtesy of P. Hiscott, Liverpool, UK)

(Figure 10. 1). Immunohistochemistry shows staining with anti-muscle-specific-actin antibody but not S-100. Mesectodermal leiomyomas are composed of spindle-shaped smooth muscle cells with oval nuclei and fibrillar cytoplasmic processes resembling glial tissue (Figure 10.2). There is positive staining both with muscle-specific actin and S-100 (White *et al.,* 1989).

With haematoxylin and eosin stains, the histology of some of these tumours may be very similar to an amelanotic, spindle-cell melanoma. If biopsy is performed, it is important to obtain sufficient tissue for immunohistochemistry, which often confirms the diagnosis.

Neurofibromatosis type 1

Neurofibromatosis type 1 (von Recklinghausen's disease) is caused by a mutation at 17q11. It is inherited in an autosomal dominant manner, but about half of all patients represent new mutations.

OPHTHALMIC SIGNS

- Multiple Lisch nodules of the iris.
- Prominent corneal nerves.
- Gliomas of optic nerve and chiasm.
- Hypoplasia of greater and lesser wings of the sphenoid with herniation of temporal lobe into orbit and pulsating exopthalmos.
- Retinal astrocytic hamartoma (Destro *et al.*, 1991).
- Eyelid neurofibromas, which can be pedunculated or plexiform.
- Congenital or developmental glaucoma.
- Multiple choroidal naevi (Huson *et al.*, 1987).
- RPE hyperplasia (Olsen *et al.*, 1999).

Neurofibromatosis type 2

Neurofibromatosis type 2 is caused by a mutation at locus 22q12.

OCULAR SIGNS

- Pre-senile cataract (Parry *et al.*, 1994).
- Combined hamartoma of the retina and RPE (Eliott and Schachat, 1994).
- Optic nerve sheath meningioma.

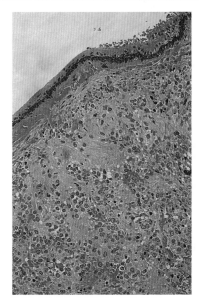

Figure 10.2 Light micrograph of mesectodermal leiomyoma. (Courtesy of P. Hiscott, Liverpool, UK)

SIGNS OF NEURILEMMOMA, NEUROFIBROMA AND LEIOMYOMA

IRIS

Neurofibromas and leiomyomas can occur anywhere in the iris, where they appear similar to melanoma. They show varying degrees of vascularity. Leiomyomas can be pigmented.

CILIARY BODY

All three types of tumour can occur in the ciliary body, forming a smooth, round tumour, usually covered by pigmented ciliary epithelium (Figure 10.3). A mesoectodermal leiomyoma can appear red (Figure 10.4). The tumour tends to indent and subluxate the lens, causing visual symptoms. Dilated episcleral vessels can be present.

CHOROID

These tumours can develop rarely in the choroid, where they mimic melanoma (Shields *et al.*, 1994), sometimes becoming large. They can also occur in the sclera or episclera (Perry, 1982; Graham *et al.*, 1989; Shields *et al.*, 1991).

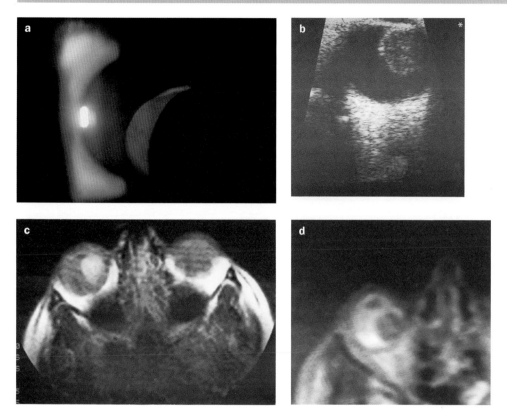

Figure 10.3 Inferonasal ciliochoroidal neurilemmoma in the right eye of a 42-year-old female: (**a**) clinical photograph, (**b**) B-scan ultrasound, (**c**) T1 weighted image and (**d**) T2 weighted image. (From Smith, P.A., Damato, B.E., Ko, M.K. and Lyness, R.W. (1989) Anterior uveal neurilemmoma-a rare neoplasm simulating melanoma. *Br. J. Ophthalmol.*, **71**, 34–40)

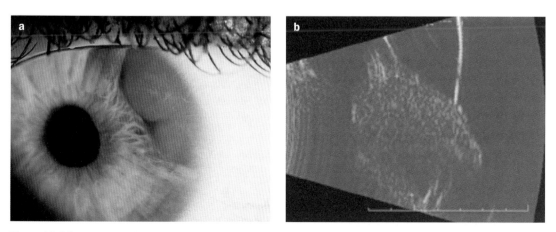

Figure 10.4 Superotemporal mesectodermal leiomyoma in the left eye of an 18-year-old female: (**a**) clinical photograph showing red colour of tumour and (**b**) B-scan ultrasonogram, showing homogenous reflectivity of medium intensity. The patient was treated by local resection with adjunctive radiotherapy and retained vision of 6/9

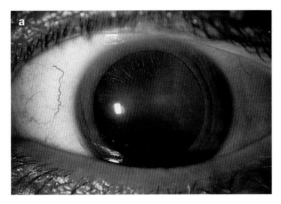
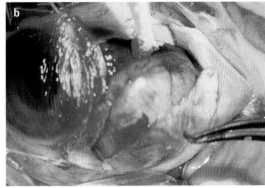

Figure 10.5 Temporal ciliochoroidal leiomyoma in the left eye of a 58-year-old female: (**a**) clinical photograph suggesting tumour pigmentation and (**b**) peroperative photograph, showing amelanotic nature of tumour

Diffuse neurofibromas cause irregular thickening of the choroid, sometimes resembling diffuse melanoma (Huson *et al.*, 1987).

INVESTIGATIONS

Imaging studies, particularly ultrasonography, are not useful diagnostically, but help to define the extent of the lesion when planning surgery. Many lesions are diagnosed only histopathologically.

TREATMENT

Circumscribed tumours can be treated by transscleral local resection (Figure 10.5). It is sometimes possible to shell out the tumour from the suprachoroidal or supraciliary space, leaving the uvea intact (Shields *et al.*, 1994).

Diffuse neurofibromas do not require treatment, unless they are large, causing retinal detachment and ocular disorganization, in which case enucleation may be appropriate.

REFERENCES

Destro, M., D'Amico, D.J., Gragoudas, E.S., Brockhurst, R.J., Pinnolis, M.K., Albert, D.M., Topping, T.M. and Puliafito, C.A. (1991) Retinal manifestations of neurofibromatosis. Diagnosis and management. *Arch. Ophthalmol.*, **109**, 662–6.

Eliott, D. and Schachat, A.P. (1994) Combined hamartoma of the retina and retinal pigment epithelium. In: S.J. Ryan (ed.), *Retina*. St Louis: Mosby, Vol. 1, Ch. 36, pp. 691–7.

Graham, C.M., McCartney, A.C. and Buckley, R.J. (1989) Intrascleral neurilemmoma. *Br. J. Ophthalmol.*, **73**, 378–81.

Huson, S., Jones, D. and Beck, L. (1987) Ophthalmic manifestations of neurofibromatosis. *Br. J. Ophthalmol.*, **71**, 235–8.

Olsen, T.W., Frayer, W.C., Myers, F.L., Davis, M.D. and Albert, D.M. (1999) Idiopathic reactive hyperplasia of the retinal pigment epithelium. *Arch. Ophthalmol.*, **17**, 50–4.

Parry, D.M., Eldridge, R., Kaiser-Kupfer, M.I., Bouzas, E.A., Pikus, A. and Patronas, N. (1994) Neurofibromatosis 2 (NF2): clinical characteristics of 63 affected individuals and clinical evidence for heterogeneity. *Am. J. Med. Genet.*, **52**, 450–61.

Perry, H.D. (1982) Isolated episcleral neurofibroma. *Ophthalmology*, **89**, 1095–8.

Pineda, R.II., Urban, R.C. Jr., Bellows, A.R. and Jakobiec, F.A. (1995) Ciliary body neurilemoma. Unusual clinical findings intimating the diagnosis. *Ophthalmology*, **102**, 918–23.

Shields, C.L., Shields, J.A. and Varenhorst, M.P. (1991) Transscleral leiomyoma. *Ophthalmology*, **98**, 84–7.

Shields, J.A., Font, R.L., Eagle, R.C. Jr., Shields, C.L. and Gass, J.D.M. (1994) Melanotic schwannoma of the choroid. Immunohistochemistry and electron microscopic observations. *Ophthalmology*, **101**, 843–9.

Shields, J.A., Shields, C.L., Eagle, R.C. Jr., and De Potter, P. (1994) Observations on seven cases of intraocular leiomyoma. The 1993 Byron Demorest Lecture. *Arch. Ophthalmol.*, **112**, 521–8.

Smith, P.A., Damato, B.E., Ko, M.K. and Lyness, R.W. (1987) Anterior uveal neurilemmoma – a rare neoplasm simulating malignant melanoma. *Br. J. Ophthalmol.*, **71**, 34–40.

White, V., Stevenson, K., Garner, A., and Hungerford, J. (1989) Mesectodermal leiomyoma of the ciliary body: case report. *Br. J. Ophthalmol.*, **73**, 12–18.

RETINAL TUMOURS

Chapter 11

Astrocytic hamartoma

Retinal astrocytic hamartomas usually occur in association with tuberous sclerosis. This is an autosomal dominant disease caused by mutations located most frequently at 9q34 (i.e., TSC1 gene, which produces hamartin) (Green *et al.,* 1994a) and 16p13 (i.e., TSC2 gene, which produces tuberin) (Green *et al.,* 1994b). About 60% of cases are caused by a new mutation.

About 50% of patients with tuberous sclerosis develop ophthalmic manifestations (Lagos and Gomez, 1967; Williams and Taylor, 1985; Robertson, 1991). In addition to retinal abnormalities, these include angiofibromas of the eyelid skin and conjunctiva, colobomas of iris and lens, megalocornea and white lashes (Figure 11.1).

Occasionally, retinal astrocytic hamartoma occurs in patients with neurofibromatosis type 1 (Destro *et al.,* 1991).

Very rarely, a solitary retinal astrocytic hamartoma develops at any age in otherwise healthy individuals and can be vascular and destructive (Arnold *et al.,* 1985; Bornfeld *et al.,* 1987).

PATHOLOGY

Astrocytic hamartomas consist of large and fibrillary astrocytes, calcospherites and blood vessels, which may be abundant (Figure 11.2).

Degeneration resulting in cyst formation and dystrophic calcification may occur.

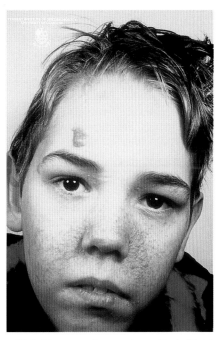

Figure 11.1 Adenoma sebaceum in a patient with tuberous sclerosis. (Courtesy of J. Dudgeon, Glasgow, UK)

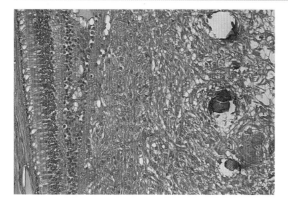

Figure 11.2 Light micrograph of retinal astrocytic hamartoma, showing fibrillary astrocytes and calcospherites. (Courtesy of P. Hiscott, Liverpool, UK)

SIGNS

- Transparent, grey, flat, indistinct sheet-like retinal astrocytomas (Nyboer *et al.,* 1976). These usually remain static but may gradually grow.
- Opaque, white/yellow, multinodular, endophytic nodules (i.e., 'mulberry tumours'), about 0.5–4 DD in diameter (Zimmer-Galler and Robertson, 1995) (Figures 11.3 and 11.4).
- Yellow calcified bodies within lesion.
- Posterior location at or near the disc, in most cases, where they are confusingly called 'giant drusen'.
- Multiple lesions in patients with tuberous sclerosis, being bilateral in about 50% of all patients with ocular lesions.

COMPLICATIONS

- Vitreous haemorrhage, which may rarely arise from small blood vessels within the astrocytic hamartoma or from associated retinal neovascularization (Kroll *et al.,* 1981).
- Neovascular glaucoma, which is rare, perhaps following necrosis of an astrocytoma or growth with retinal detachment (Bornfeld *et al.,* 1987).
- Vitreous seeding and vitritis, from optic nerve astrocytoma (De Juan *et al.,* 1984).
- Depigmented and pigmented choroidal lesions, usually in the mid-periphery (Lucchese and Goldberg, 1981).
- Optic disc swelling, perhaps resulting in atrophy.

INVESTIGATIONS

a. Binocular indirect ophthalmoscopy, for multiple retinal lesions.
b. Systemic examination for other features of tuberous sclerosis (Roach *et al.,* 1998), including dermatological examination for cutaneous lesions, using a Wood's light for depigmented lesions (Jóźwiak *et al.,* 1998).
c. MRI brain scan for intracranial lesions.
d. CT or MRI scans for visceral lesions.
e. Family studies, to identify first-degree relatives with tuberous sclerosis, since the expressivity of the disease varies greatly. Molecular genetic studies are complicated by the large size of the gene, the variety of mutations and the high rate of mosaicism (Verhoef *et al.,* 1999).

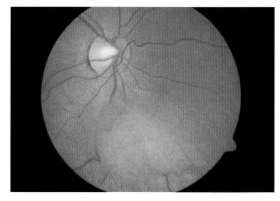

Figure 11.3 Smooth retinal astrocytic hamartoma

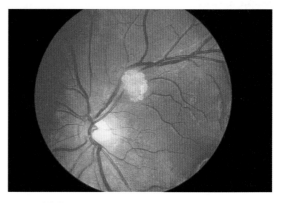

Figure 11.4 Multinodular retinal astrocytic hamartoma. (Courtesy of J. Dudgeon, Glasgow, UK)

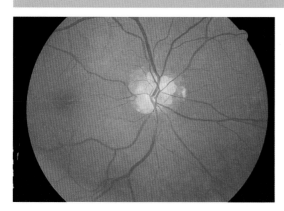

Figure 11.5 Optic disc drusen

DIFFERENTIAL DIAGNOSIS

1. **Optic disc drusen** are deeper and do not obscure disc structures (Figure 11.5).
2. **Myelinated nerve fibres** may resemble an early, flat astrocytoma.
3. **Endophytic or regressed retinoblastoma** may mimic a mulberry tumour.
4. **Retinal telangiectasia** may be difficult to differentiate from predominantly vascular retinal astrocytic hamartomas.

MANAGEMENT OF THE PRIMARY TUMOUR

Most astrocytic hamartomas are static and asymptomatic so that treatment is unnecessary.

REFERENCES

Arnold, A.C., Hepler, R.S., Yee, R.W., Maggiano, J., Eng, L.F. and Foos, R.Y. (1985) Solitary retinal astrocytoma. *Surv. Ophthalmol.*, **30**, 173–81.

Bornfeld, N., Messmer, E.P., Theodossiadis, G., Meyer Schwickerath, G. and Wessing, A. (1987) Giant cell astrocytoma of the retina. Clinicopathologic report of a case not associated with Bourneville's disease. *Retina*, **7**, 183–9.

De Juan, E. Jr, Green, W.R., Gupta, P.K. and Barañano, E.C. (1984) Vitreous seeding by astrocytic hamartoma in a patient with tuberous sclerosis. *Retina*, **4**, 100–2.

Destro, M., D'Amico, D.J., Gragoudas, E.S., Brockhurst, R.J., Pinnolis, M.K., Albert, D.M., Topping, T.M. and Puliafito, C.A. (1991) Retinal manifestations of neurofibromatosis. *Arch. Ophthalmol.*, **109**, 662–6.

Green, A.J., Johnson, P.H. and Yates, J.R. (1994a) The tuberous sclerosis gene on chromosome 9q34 acts as a growth suppressor. *Hum. Mol. Genet.*, **3**, 1833–4.

Green, A.J., Smith, M. and Yates, J.R.W. (1994b) Loss of heterozygosity on chromosome 16p13.3 in hamartomas from tuberous sclerosis patients. *Nat. Genet.*, **6**, 193–6.

Jóźwiak, S., Schwartz, R.A., Janniger, C.K., Michałowicz, R. and Chmielik, J. (1998) Skin lesions in children with tuberous sclerosis complex: their prevalence, natural course and diagnostic significance. *Int. J. Dermatol.*, **37**, 911–17.

Kroll, A.J., Ricker, D.P., Robb, R.M. and Albert, D.M. (1981) Vitreous hemorrhage complicating retinal astrocytic hamartoma. *Surv. Ophthalmol.*, **26**, 31–8.

Lagos, J.C. and Gomez, M.R. (1967) Tuberous sclerosis: reappraisal of a clinical entity. *Mayo Clin. Proc.*, **42**, 26–49.

Lucchese, N.J. and Goldberg, M.F. (1981) Iris and fundus pigmentary changes in tuberous sclerosis. *J. Pediatr. Ophthalmol. Strabismus*, **18**, 45–6.

Nyboer, J.H., Robertson, D.M. and Gomez, M.R. (1976) Retinal lesions in tuberous sclerosis. *Arch. Ophthalmol.*, **94**, 1277–80.

Roach, E.S., Gomez, M.R. and Northrup, H. (1998) Tuberous sclerosis complex consensus conference: revised clinical diagnostic criteria. *J. Child Neurol.*, **13**, 624–8.

Robertson, D.M. (1991) Ophthalmic manifestations of tuberous sclerosis. *Ann. NY Acad. Sci.*, **615**, 17–25.

Verhoef, S., Bakker, L., Tempelaars, A.M.P., Hesseling-Janssen, A.L.W., Mazurczak, T., Jozwiak, S., Fois, A., Bartalini, G., Zonnenberg, B.A., van Essen, A.J., Lindhout, D., Halley, D.J.J. and van den Ouweland, A.M.W. (1999) High rate of mosaicism in tuberous sclerosis complex. *Am. J. Hum. Genet.*, **64**, 1632–7.

Williams, R. and Taylor, D. (1985) Tuberous sclerosis. *Surv. Ophthalmol.*, **30**, 143–54.

Zimmer-Galler, I.E. and Robertson, D.M. (1995) Long-term observation of retinal lesions in tuberous sclerosis. *Am. J. Ophthalmol.*, **119**, 318–24.

Chapter 12

Retinal vascular tumours

Retinal haemangioblastoma

Retinal haemangioblastoma usually occurs in patients with von Hippel–Lindau disease (VHL). This is caused by the loss of a tumour suppressor gene on the short arm of chromosome 3 (locus 3p25-26) (Decker *et al.*, 1997). It is inherited in an autosomal dominant fashion with variable penetrance.

About two-thirds of all patients with VHL disease develop ocular manifestations (Webster *et al.*, 1999). All patients with multiple retinal capillary angiomas have von Hippel–Lindau disease. Patients with a solitary retinal haemangioblastoma (previously called 'von Hippel's disease') may or may not have the genetic mutation of VHL disease.

PATHOLOGY

Retinal capillary haemangioblastoma is a hamartoma consisting of small, thin-walled blood vessels and foamy, lipid-containing cells (Nicholson *et al.*, 1976; Ismail *et al*, 1985).

SYMPTOMS

Patients usually present with visual symptoms during the second and third decades of life. Asymptomatic retinal lesions have been detected as early as the second year of life and are present in about 80% of patients with von Hippel–Lindau syndrome by the age of 80 years.

SIGNS

- Angiomas are usually multiple, mostly superotemporal and mid-peripheral and rarely within the macula (Webster *et al.*, 1999).
- Early lesions are (1) usually tiny, red, intraretinal nodules, like microaneurysms (Figure 12.1) and (2) occasionally indistinct, mossy, red lesions, about a disc diameter in size (Schmidt and Neumann, 1995).
- Late lesions have developed into orange masses with large afferent and efferent feeder vessels extending to optic disc (Figure 12.2).
- Fibrotic angiomas are white and without feeder vessels.

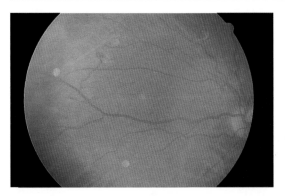

Figure 12.1 Early retinal capillary haemangioblastoma in the left eye of a 33-year-old woman

- Lesions at the optic disc (Gass and Braunstein, 1980) may be (1) endophytic, protruding into vitreous (Figure 12.3), (2) sessile, growing as a diffuse, flat lesion, or (3) exophytic, extending beneath retina (Figure12.4).

COMPLICATIONS

- Circinate or stellate exudates at the macula; even if the haemangioblastoma is located peripherally (Figure 12.2**b**).
- Exudative retinal detachment.
- Fibrovascular proliferation into vitreous, with subsequent contraction causing tractional retinal detachment, retinal tears, vitreous haemorrhage and rhegmatogenous retinal detachment (Nicholson _et al.,_ 1986) (Figure 12.5).
- Disc or retinal neovascularization.
- Cellophane maculopathy, related to a distant retinal haemangioblastoma (Laatikainen _et al.,_ 1989).
- Secondary glaucoma and phthisis, in end-stage eyes.

OCULAR INVESTIGATIONS

a. Three-mirror examination, for detecting early lesions.
b. Fluorescein angiography or fluoroscopy, which may identify early lesions and which facilitate differentiation from other lesions, such as neovascular membranes and Coats' disease.

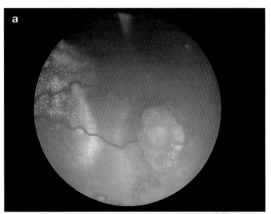

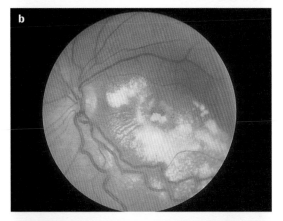

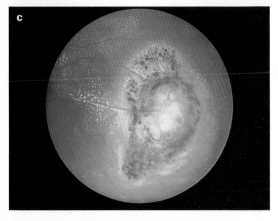

Figure 12.2 Late retinal capillary haemangioblastoma inferotemporally in the left eye: (**a**) circinate macular exudates, (**b**) tumour with feeder vessels and (**c**) scar after cryotherapy, with regression of the feeder vessels and resolution of the hard exudates. (Courtesy of W.S. Foulds, Glasgow, UK)

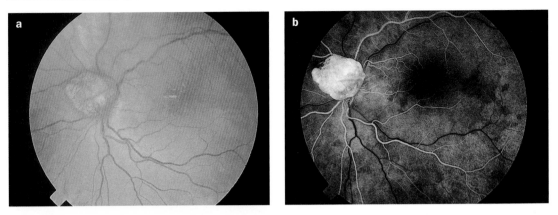

Figure 12.3 Endophytic disc angioma: (**a**) colour photograph and (**b**) fluorescein angiogram. (Courtesy of P. Lommatzsch, Leipzig, Germany)

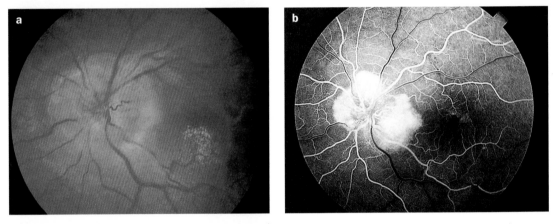

Figure 12.4 Exophytic disc haemangioblastoma in the left eye of a 21-year-old woman: (**a**) colour photograph and (**b**) fluorescein angiogram. (Courtesy of A. Halkias, Thessaloniki, Greece)

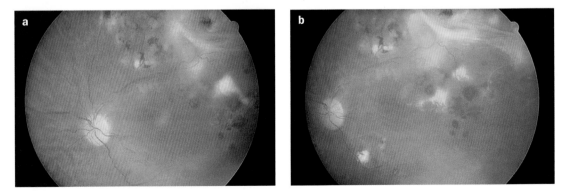

Figure 12.5 Vitreous traction from a superotemporal retinal angioma in the left eye. Note also the early lesions (**a**) before and (**b**) after photocoagulation

SYSTEMIC INVESTIGATIONS

Life-long screening for extraocular disease is indicated in all patients with retinal haemangioblastoma, including those with a solitary lesion and a negative family history (Webster *et al.,* 1999). It is also advised in all family members at risk.

SYSTEMIC FEATURES (Maher, 1994)

- Cerebellar haemangioblastomas, which affect about 25% of patients with retinal lesions, presenting in the third decade with headache, vertigo, vomiting and ataxia (Filling-Katz *et al.,* 1991).
- Spinal canal haemangioblastomas, which present with symptoms of cord compression.
- Renal cell carcinoma, the commonest cause of death, which presents with haematuria, obstruction, or an abdominal mass.
- Phaeochromocytoma.
- Islet cell carcinoma of the pancreas.
- Cysts of the testis, kidneys, ovaries and pancreas.
- Polycythaemia, which may be caused by factors released from a cerebellar tumour or renal tumour.

SCREENING PROTOCOL (Maher and Moore, 1992)

- Annual physical examination.
- Annual retinal examination from 5–60 years.
- Annual 24-hour urinary vanillyl mandelic acid (VMA) measurements for phaeochromocytoma from the age of 10 years.
- Annual abdominal ultrasonography for renal carcinoma from 16–65 years, with abdominal MRI every 3 years.
- MRI brain scans for cerebellar haemangioblastoma every 3 years from 15–60 years (Maher and Moore, 1992).

GENETIC STUDIES

A positive family history of VHL disease is present in only 20% of patients.

Intragenic VHL germline mutations can be detected by single-strand conformation poly-

morphism analysis and direct sequencing of the VHL gene. The sensitivity of these studies is approximately 80% (Maher *et al.,* 1996) but improving as newer techniques develop.

DIFFERENTIAL DIAGNOSIS

1. **Coats' disease** can resemble a peripheral retinal angioma with exudative retinal detachment.
2. **A juxtapapillary neovascular membrane** can mimic a sessile or exophytic angioma at the disc.
3. **Vasoproliferative tumour** resembles a late retinal haemangioblastoma, but is not associated with large feeder vessels (see below) .
4. **Optic disc swelling** can be falsely diagnosed in a patient with a sessile haemangioblastoma of the optic disc (Schindler *et al.,* 1975).
5. **Retinoblastoma** can have feeder vessels.
6. **Amelanotic collar-stud melanoma** can rarely be associated with a dilated retinal vein, without a feeder artery (Shields *et al.,* 1978).
7. **Retinal angiomatous lesions** can occur in patients with cat-scratch disease (Gray *et al.,* 1999).

TREATMENT

As a rule, small retinal lesions should be destroyed as early as possible, before tumour growth makes treatment more difficult.

a. Small, posterior, flat lesions can be destroyed by laser photocoagulation applied to the surface of the angioma (Lane *et al.,* 1989) (Figure 12.6). Small, anterior lesions may respond to trans-scleral cryotherapy (Watzke *et al.,* 1977) (Figure 12.2c) .
b. Lesions greater than 1–2 DD in diameter can be treated with plaque radiotherapy, delivering approximately 500 Gy to the sclera (Kreusel *et al.,* 1998) (Figure 12.7).
c. If vitreous bands are present, an alternative approach is to perform vitrectomy, destroying the angioma with endolaser photocoagulation (McDonald *et al.,* 1996).

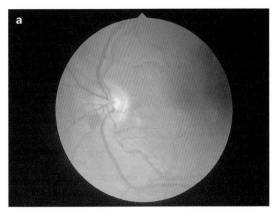
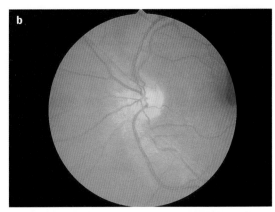

Figure 12.6 Small retinal capillary haemangioblastoma (**a**) before laser photocoagulation and (**b**) after treatment. (Courtesy of C. Lane, Cardiff, UK)

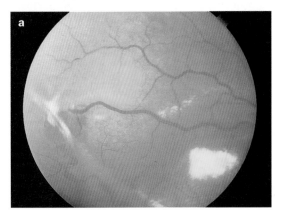
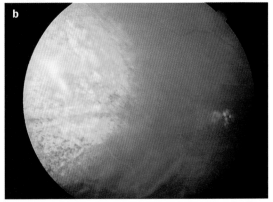

Figure 12.7 Retinal capillary haemangioblastoma with macular exudates (**a**) before ruthenium plaque radiotherapy and (**b**) after ruthenium plaque radiotherapy, showing total obliteration of the retinal and choroidal vasculature with resolution of the macular exudates. (Courtesy of N. Bornfeld, Essen, Germany)

d. Exudative retinal detachment, traction detachment and vitreous haemorrhage can follow photocoagulation, cryotherapy or brachytherapy, especially if vitreous change is present preoperatively. Tractional or rhegmatogenous retinal detachment may require vitrectomy.

The management of juxtapapillary retinal angiomas is difficult (Schindler *et al.*, 1975; Gass and Braunstein, 1980; Brown and Shields, 1985). Asymptomatic lesions should be observed, as visual loss may occur only several years later or not at all. Symptomatic lesions have been treated by photocoagulation applied either directly at the lesion or around it to create a barrier preventing maculopathy. Alternatively, external beam radiotherapy may be applied, but the results are unpredictable (Plowman and Harnett, 1988).

PROGNOSIS

About a third of all patients with retinal haemangioblastoma develop irreversible visual deficit in one or both eyes (Webster *et al.*, 1999).

Retinal cavernous angioma

This rare vascular hamartoma is characterized by the development of retinal angiomas together with extraocular abnormalities, which include (a) intracranial cavernous angiomas, involving cerebrum and pons, which may cause epilepsy and intracranial haemorrhage, and (b) cutaneous angiomas. Family studies suggest autosomal dominant inheritance with incomplete penetrance (Goldberg *et al.*, 1979), due to mutations in chromosome 7 (Marchuk *et al.*, 1995).

SIGNS

- Sessile clusters of saccular aneurysms resembling a 'bunch of grapes' without feeder vessels and without alteration of normal retinal vasculature (Sternber, 1994) (Figure 12.8**a**).
- Settling of red blood cells within the aneurysms ('pseudo-hypopyon') (Figure 12.8**b**).
- Distribution in one area, or throughout the fundus, usually in only one eye.
- Involvement of optic disc in about a third of all cases (Lewis *et al.*, 1975; Brown and Shields, 1985; Mansour *et al.*, 1988) (Figure 12.9).
- No exudation.
- No significant growth, if left untreated.

COMPLICATIONS

- Epiretinal membrane over the tumour.
- Haemorrhage, which can be into vitreous, retina or subretinal space.
- Visual loss if there is macular involvement or vitreous haemorrhage (Messmer *et al.*, 1983).

MANAGEMENT

a. Neurological examination of the patient and close relatives with MRI brain scans.
b. Avoidance of photocoagulation, which may result in haemorrhage or tumour enlargement (Klein *et al.*, 1983).

Retinal arteriovenous malformation (racemose angioma)

This may form part of the Wyburn-Mason syndrome, which is a rare, non-hereditary disease

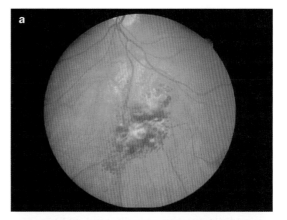
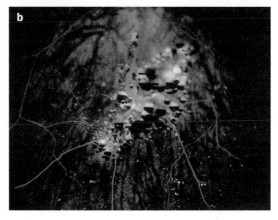

Figure 12.8 Retinal cavernous angioma: (**a**) colour photograph and (**b**) fluorescein angiogram. (Courtesy of O. Backhouse, Leeds, UK) (From Backhouse, O. and O'Neill, D. (1998) Cavernous haemangioma of the retina and skin. *Eye*, **12**, 1027–8)

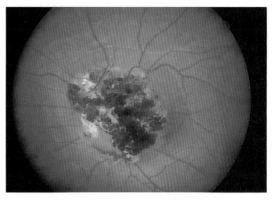

Figure 12.9 Cavernous angioma of optic disc. (Courtesy of P. Lommatzsch, Leipzig, Germany)

characterized by vascular malformations at any point in the visual pathway (Patel and Gupta, 1990). The malformations are progressive and are often detected only in adulthood.

SIGNS

- Worm-like retinal arteriovenous malformations involving one or more sectors of the fundus of one eye (Archer *et al.,* 1973), with the vessels gradually becoming more dilated, tortuous and sclerotic (Augsburger *et al.,* 1980) (Figure 12.10).
- Proptosis, which is usually mild and non-pulsatile.
- Intracranial lesions, which are present in about a third of cases, being more likely if the retinal malformation is extensive. These cause pyramidal tract lesions, subarachnoid haemorrhage, cranial nerve palsies and visual field defects, such as homonymous hemianopia (Mansour *et al.,* 1987).
- Optic atrophy, without any visible retinal abnormalities (Danis and Appen, 1984).
- Naevus flammeus and other vascular lesions in the ipsilateral trigeminal region in a minority of patients.
- Haemorrhage after dental extraction, due to vascular malformations in the jaw (Hoyt and Cameron, 1968).

COMPLICATIONS

- Vein occlusion.
- Vitreous haemorrhage.

MANAGEMENT

No treatment is required unless there are complications, which are managed in the appropriate manner.

Vasoproliferative tumour

This is a rare tumour, which can develop in either sex and at any age. It may occur in isolation or in association with other ocular conditions, such as intermediate uveitis, previous retinal detachment, ocular trauma and retinitis pigmentosa (Laqua and Wessing, 1983; Laatikainen *et al.,* 1989; Gray and Gregor, 1994; Shields *et al.,* 1995).

SIGNS

- Amelanotic, yellow, retinal or subretinal mass containing telangiectatic blood vessels (Figure 12.11).
- Location at or anterior to equator, more often inferotemporally than in other quadrants.
- Solitary, unless secondary to other disease, in which case multiple lesions can be present.

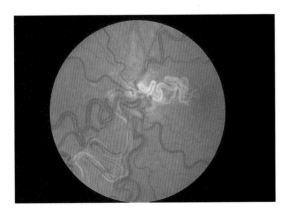

Figure 12.10 Wyburn-Mason syndrome. (Courtesy of P. Lommatzsch, Leipzig, Germany)

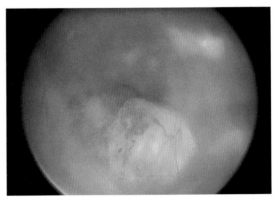

Figure 12.11 Inferotemporal vasoproliferative tumour in the right eye of a 28-year-old man

- Small retinal feeder vessels.
- A rare diffuse variety can involve large areas of retina, perhaps bilaterally, with a predilection for young females (Shields *et al.,* 1995).

COMPLICATIONS

- Exudative retinal detachment.
- Macular involvement by retinal detachment, epiretinal membrane, macular oedema or extensive hard exudates (Figure 12.12).
- Vitreous haemorrhage, which usually resolves without treatment.
- Uveitis.

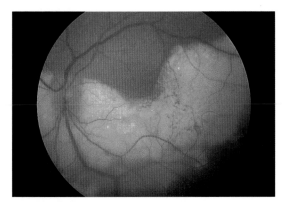

Figure 12.12 Macular exudation from an inferotemporal vasoproliferative tumour in the left eye of an 18-year-old female

MANAGEMENT

Various forms of treatment have been attempted, which include cryotherapy, diathermy and plaque radiotherapy.

PROGNOSIS

Despite treatment, visual loss often occurs as a result of macular exudation or fibrosis.

REFERENCES

Archer, D.B., Deutman, A., Ernest, J.T. and Krill, A.E. (1973) Arteriovenous communications of the retina. *Am. J. Ophthalmol.,* **75**, 224–41.

Augsburger, J.J., Goldberg, R.E., Shields, J.A., Mulberger, R.D. and Margargal, L.E. (1980) Changing appearance of retinal arteriovenous malformation. *Graefes Arch. Clin. Exp. Ophthalmol.,* **215**, 65–70.

Brown, G.C. and Shields, J.A. (1985) Tumors of the optic nerve head. *Surv. Ophthalmol.,* **29**, 239–64.

Danis, R. and Appen, R.E. (1984) Optic atrophy and the Wyburn-Mason syndrome. *J. Clin. Neuro-ophthalmol.,* **4**, 91–5.

Decker, H.J.H., Weidt, E.J. and Brieger, J. (1997) The von Hippel–Lindau tumor suppressor gene. A rare and intriguing disease opening new insight into basic mechanisms of carcinogenesis. *Cancer Genet. Cytogenet.,* **93**, 74–83.

Filling-Katz, M.R., Choyke, P.L., Oldfield, E., Charnas, L., Patronas, N.J., Glenn, G.M., Gorin, M.B., Morgan, J.K., Linehan, W.M., Seizinger, B.R. and Zbar, B. (1991) Central nervous system involvement in von Hippel–Lindau disease. *Neurology,* **41**, 41–6.

Gass, J.D. and Braunstein, R. (1980) Sessile and exophytic capillary angiomas of the juxtapapillary retina and optic nerve head. *Arch. Ophthalmol.,* **98**, 1790–7.

Goldberg, R.E., Pheasant, T.R. and Shields, J.A. (1979) Cavernous hemangioma of the retina: a four-generation pedigree with neurocutaneous manifestations and an example of bilateral retinal involvement. *Arch. Ophthalmol.,* **97**, 2321–4.

Gray, R.H. and Gregor, Z.J. (1994) Acquired peripheral retinal telangiectasia after retinal surgery. *Retina,* **14**, 10–13.

Gray, A.V., Reed, J.B., Wendel, R.T. and Morse, L.S. (1999) *Bartonella henselae* infection associated with peripapillary angioma, branch retinal artery occlusion and severe visual loss. *Am. J. Ophthalmol.,* **127**, 223–4.

Hoyt, W.F. and Cameron, R.B. (1968) Racemose angioma of the mandible, face, retina and brain: report of case. *J. Oral Surg.,* **26**, 596–601.

Ismail, S.M., Jasani, B. and Cole, G. (1985) Histogenesis of haemangioblastomas: an immunocytochemical and ultrastructural study in a case of von Hippel–Lindau syndrome. *J Clin. Pathol.,* **38**, 417–21.

Klein, M., Goldberg, M.F. and Cotlier, E. (1975) Cavernous hemangioma of the retina: report of four cases. *Ann. Ophthalmol.,* **7**, 1213–21.

Kreusel, K.M., Bornfeld, N., Lommatzsch, A., Wessing, A. and Foerster, M.H. (1998) Ruthenium-106 brachytherapy for peripheral retinal capillary hemangioma. *Ophthalmology,* **105**, 1386–92.

Laatikainen, L., Immonen, I. and Summanen, P. (1989) Peripheral retinal angioma-like lesion and macular pucker. *Am. J. Ophthalmol.,* **108**, 563–6.

Lane, C.M., Turner, G., Gregor, Z.J. and Bird, A.C. (1989) Laser treatment of retinal angiomatosis. *Eye,* **3**, 33–8.

Laqua, H. and Wessing, A. (1983) Peripheral retinal telangiectasis in adults simulating a vascular tumor or melanoma. *Ophthalmology*, **90**, 1284–91.

Lewis, R.A., Cohen, M.H. and Wise, G.N. (1975) Cavernous haemangioma of the retina and optic disc: a report of three cases and a review of the literature. *Br. J. Ophthalmol.*, **59**, 422–3.

Maher, E.R. (1994) Von Hippel–Lindau disease. *Eur. J. Cancer*, **30A**, 1987–90.

Maher, E.R. and Moore, A.T. (1992) Von Hippel–Lindau disease. *Br. J. Ophthalmol.*, **76**, 743–5.

Maher, E.R., Webster, A.R., Richards, F.M., Green, J.S., Crossey, P.A., Payne, S.J. and Moore, A.T. (1996) Phenotypic expression in von Hippel–Lindau disease: correlations with germline VHL gene mutations. *J. Med. Genet.*, **33**, 328–32.

Mansour, A.M., Jampol, L.M., Hrisomalos, N.F. and Greenwald, M. (1988) Cavernous hemangioma of the optic disc. *Arch. Ophthalmol.*, **106**, 22.

Mansour, A.M., Walsh, J.B. and Henkind, P. (1987) Arteriovenous anastomoses of the retina. *Ophthalmology*, **94**, 35–40.

Marchuk, D.A., Gallione, C.J., Morrison, L.A., Clericuzo, C.L., Hart, B.L., Kosofsky, B.E., Louis, D.N., Gusella, J.F., Davis, L.E. and Prenger, V.L. (1995) A locus for cerebral cavernous malformations maps to chromosome 7q in two families. *Genomics*, **28**, 311–14.

McDonald, H.R., Schatz, H., Johnson, R.N., Abrams, G.W., Brown, G.C., Brucker, A.J., Han, D.P., Lewis, H., Mieler, W.F. and Meyers, S. (1996) Vitrectomy in eyes with peripheral retinal angioma associated with traction macular detachment. *Ophthalmology*, **103**, 329–35.

Messmer, E., Laqua, H., Wessing, A., Spitznas, M., Weidle, E., Ruprecht, K. and Naumann, G.O.H. (1983) Nine cases of cavernous hemangioma of the retina. *Am. J. Ophthalmol.*, **95**, 383–90.

Nicholson, D.H., Anderson, L.S. and Blodi, C. (1986) Rhegmatogenous retinal detachment in angiomatosis retinae. *Am. J. Ophthalmol.*, **101**, 187–9.

Nicholson, D.H., Green, W.R. and Kenyon, K.R. (1976) Light and electron microscopic study of early lesions in angiomatosis retinae. *Am. J. Ophthalmol.*, **83**, 193–204.

Patel, U. and Gupta, S.C. (1990) Wyburn-Mason syndrome. A case report and review of the literature. *Neuroradiology.*, **31**, 544–6.

Plowman, P.N. and Harnett, A.N. (1988) Radiotherapy in benign orbital disease. I: Complicated ocular angiomas. *Br. J. Ophthalmol.*, **72**, 286–8.

Schindler, R.F., Sarin, L.K. and MacDonald, P.R. (1975) Hemangiomas of the optic disc. *Can. J. Ophthalmol.*, **10**, 305–18.

Schmidt, D. and Neumann, H.P.H. (1995) Retinal vascular hamartoma in von Hippel–Lindau disease. *Arch. Ophthalmol.*, **113**, 1163–7.

Shields, C.L., Shields, J.A., Barrett, J. and De Potter, P. (1995) Vasoproliferative tumors of the ocular fundus. Classification and clinical manifestations in 103 patients. *Arch. Ophthalmol.*, **113**, 615–23.

Shields, J.A., Joffe, L. and Guibor, P. (1978) Choroidal melanoma clinically simulating a retinal angioma. *Am. J. Ophthalmol.*, **85**, 67–71.

Sternberg, P., Jr (1994) Cavernous hemangioma. In: S.J. Ryan (ed.), *Retina*. St Louis: Mosby, Vol 1, Ch. 28, pp. 627–32.

Watzke, R.C., Weingeist, T.A. and Constantine, J.B. (1977) Diagnosis and management of von Hippel–Lindau disease. In: Peyman, G.A. *et. al.* (ed.), *Intraocular Tumors.* New York: Appleton–Century–Crofts, pp. 199–217.

Webster, A.R., Maher, E.R., Bird, A.C., Gregor, Z.J. and Moore, A.T. (1999) A clinical and molecular genetic analysis of solitary ocular angioma. *Ophthalmology,* **106**, 623–9.

Webster, A.R., Maher, E.R. and Moore, A.T. (1999) Clinical characteristics of ocular angiomatosis in von Hippel–Lindau disease and correlation with germline mutation. *Arch. Ophthalmol.*, **117**, 371–8.

Chapter 13

Retinoblastoma

Retinoblastoma is the commonest primary intra-ocular malignancy in childhood. Advances in diagnosis and treatment have greatly improved the survival rate. Chemotherapy of intraocular tumours has become increasingly popular as a means of avoiding the complications of radio-therapy.

PATHOGENESIS

The RB gene is located on the long arm of chromosome 13 at region 14 (i.e., 13q14) and is about 180 kilobases long. It codes for the RB nucleoprotein, which normally suppresses cell division (Figure 13.1).

Many different types of mutation can occur in any part of the gene (Lohmann *et al.,* 1996). If either the maternal or paternal allele of the RB gene is mutated, then the other allele produces enough functional RB protein to maintain normality. Malignancy occurs only when both the maternal and paternal alleles of the RB gene are lost (i.e., Knudson's two-hit hypothesis) so that RB protein is deficient.

The RB protein (105 kD) has a complex tertiary structure, with discrete functional domains such as N- and C-terminals and large and small pockets

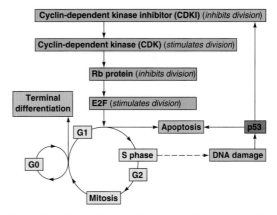

Figure 13.1 The cell cycle. After mitosis, the cell enters the G1 phase (i.e., G for Gap) and can then undergo terminal differentiation, or enter a prolonged quiescent phase (G0), or proceed to division by passing through S phase (i.e., S for synthesis) and G2 phase. The retinoblastoma protein plays a key role in determining whether or not a cell proceeds through the cell cycle towards division. p53 is activated by DNA damage and stimulates the CDKI, p21, to arrest the cell cycle until the DNA is repaired. If such repair is not possible, then p53 induces apoptosis

(Hensey *et al.,* 1994). These pockets normally bind to E2F and other cellular proteins to suppress cell division. Most gene mutations result in incomplete translation of mRNA, so that a truncated RB protein is produced, with a malfunctioning large pocket, which is unable to bind to E2F.

RB1 gene mutations can be:

a. Somatic (60%), occurring in a single retinal cell, which forms a solitary retinoblastoma.
b. Germline (40%), occurring in spermatozoa, ova, or early embryo. This type of mutation results in every cell in the body having only one normal chromosome and hence an increased probability of malignant transformation.

Germline mutations are inherited in an autosomal dominant manner and are therefore present in half of all offspring of an affected individual. The expressivity varies from one family to another, usually being about 90%. Genetic changes in families with reduced penetrance and expressivity are recognized (Schubert *et al.,* 1997).

Germinal mutations give rise to bilateral retinoblastomas in 75% of patients, unilateral retinoblastoma in 15% and no tumours (i.e., carrier state) in 10%.

In addition to retinoblastoma, germline mutations of the RB1 gene may be associated with:

a. Benign retinocytomas.
b. Midline intracranial neuroblastic tumours (e.g., trilateral retinoblastoma).
c. Osteosarcomas and other malignant soft tissue tumours.
d. The 13q deletion syndrome.

EPIDEMIOLOGY

The incidence of retinoblastoma is approximately 1/18 000 live births (Prendergrass and Davis, 1980). It is one of the commonest malignancies diagnosed in the first year of life (Gurney *et al.,* 1997). There is no sex predilection. Most patients are diagnosed in the first three years of life, usually presenting in their first year if they have bilateral disease (Augsburger *et al.,* 1995) and in the second year if they have unilateral disease.

Most new germline mutations occur in the paternal chromosome (Dryja *et al.,* 1997) and are associated with an increased parental age (Moll *et al.,* 1996). The second mutation occurs more frequently and is sensitive to environmental factors such as radiation.

PATHOLOGICAL AND CLINICAL FEATURES

RETINAL TUMOUR

HISTOLOGY

a. Retinoblastoma cells are small and basophilic with large hyperchromatic nuclei and scanty cytoplasm (Figure 13.2).
b. Flexner–Wintersteiner rosettes represent tumour differentiation and consist of columnar cells around a membrane-bound lumen, into which cytoplasmic processes project (Figure 13.2**a**).
c. Fleurettes are eosinophilic cells resembling photoreceptors attached together at their tip (Figure 13.2**b**).
d. Homer–Wright rosettes of cells form around a mass of neural fibres (Figure 13.2**c**).
e. Necrosis is manifest as an area of amorphous material or ghost cells (Figure 13.2**d**).
f. Calcification develops from necrotic tissue.
g. Pseudorosettes of viable retinoblastoma cells form around blood vessels within a necrotic area (Figure 13.2**d**).
h. Deposition of basophilic nuclear material occurs from necrotic tumour cells around blood vessels, in lakes within the tumour, in lens capsule and in Schlemm's canal.

Well-differentiated retinoblastomas tend to contain rosettes and fleurettes with little necrosis and few mitotic figures.

TUMOUR BEHAVIOUR

a. Endophytic growth into the vitreous, producing widespread seeding in the eye (Figure 13.3**a**).
b. Exophytic growth sub-retinally, with secondary retinal detachment (Figure 13.3**b**).
c. Necrosis, resulting in calcification if mild and uveitis and panophthalmitis if extensive.
d. Optic nerve invasion (Figure 13.4), possibly reaching subarachnoid space to disseminate throughout the central nervous system.
e. Choroidal invasion, which if extensive predisposes to metastatic disease and extraocular extension to orbit, bone and sinuses.

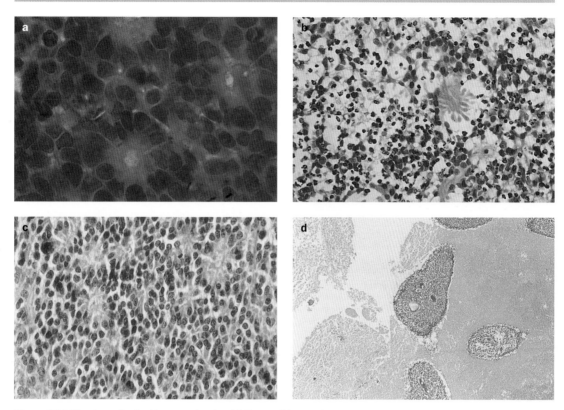

Figure 13.2 Histology of retinoblastoma showing (**a**) Flexner–Wintersteiner rosettes, (**b**) fleurettes, (**c**) Homer–Wright rosettes and (**d**) pseudorosettes. (Courtesy of W.R. Lee, Glasgow, UK)

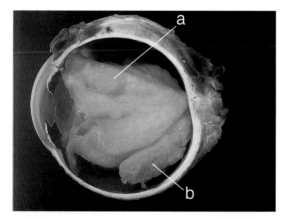

Figure 13.3 Retinoblastoma showing (**a**) endophytic and (**b**) exophytic growth. (Courtesy of W.R. Lee, Glasgow, UK)

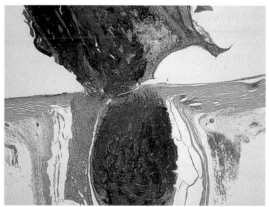

Figure 13.4 Optic nerve invasion. (Courtesy of W.R. Lee, Glasgow, UK)

f. Diffuse retinal infiltration, with widely disseminated small tumour nodules throughout the retina, without endophytic or exophytic growth (Figure 13.5).

g. Spontaneous regression, leaving a scar or an apparently benign tumour (i.e., retinocytoma). If the original tumour is large, there may be severe ocular disorganization.

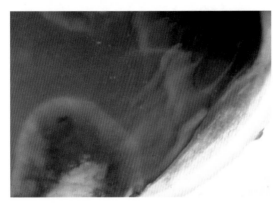

Figure 13.5 Diffuse retinoblastoma in an enucleated eye, also showing cryotherapy scars. (Courtesy of T. Kivelä, Helsinki, Finland)

PRESENTING FEATURES

1. Leukocoria, or white pupil, perhaps first noticed in family photographs (Figures 13.6 and 13.7).
2. Strabismus, due to poor vision.
3. Vitreous opacities.
4. Pseudohypopyon, without inflammation, consisting of tumour cells that have seeded into the anterior chamber (Figure 13.8).
5. Iris heterochromia, due to rubeosis iridis.
6. Spontaneous hyphaema, arising from tumour or rubeosis iridis.
7. Inflammation, due to tumour necrosis, causing uveitis and lid swelling, which may mimic orbital cellulitis (Mullaney *et al.,* 1998) (Figure 13.9).
8. Vitreous haemorrhage, which may obscure the leukocoria.
9. Glaucoma, which may be secondary to rubeosis iridis or pupil block with angle closure (Yoshizumi *et al.,* 1978).
10. Corneal oedema, caused by neovascular glaucoma.

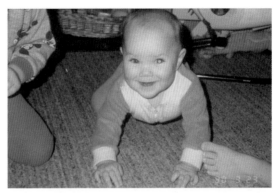

Figure 13.6 Leukocoria visible in a family photograph. (Courtesy of T. Kivelä, Helsinki, Finland)

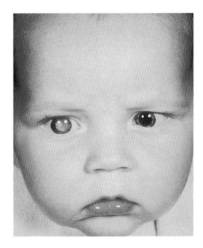

Figure 13.7 Leukocoria. (Courtesy of J. Dudgeon, Glasgow, UK)

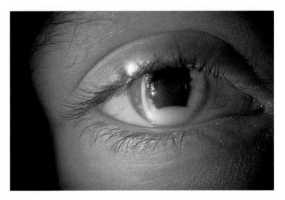

Figure 13.8 Pseudohypopyon and iris nodules in a patient with retinoblastoma. (Courtesy of J.J. Kanski, Windsor, UK)

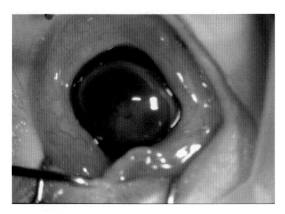

Figure 13.9 Pseudocellulitis in an eye with advanced retinoblastoma, uveitis and glaucoma. (Courtesy of T. Kivelä, Helsinki, Finland)

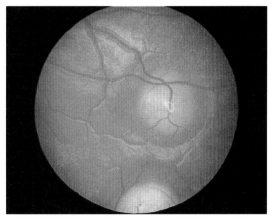

Figure 13.11 Early intraretinal retinoblastoma. (Courtesy of N. Bornfeld, Essen, Germany)

In underdeveloped countries, advanced disease may present with:

a. Buphthalmos.
b. A fungating orbital mass (Figure 13.10).
c. Metastases in regional nodes and brain.
d. Phthisis (Mullaney *et al.*, 1997).

SIGNS

1. **Early intraretinal retinoblastoma**
   - White or transparent mass, sometimes with white flecks of calcification (Figure 13.11).
   - Flat or round shape.
   - Smooth or irregular surface.

2. **Endophytic growth**
   - Friable, white pre-retinal tumours.
   - Seeding throughout the eye to form vitreous opacities (Figure 13.12).
   - Tumour nodules at the pupil margin.
   - 'Pseudohypopyon', which characteristically does not shift when the head position is altered.

3. **Exophytic growth**
   - Multilobulated, white masses beneath the retina (Figure 13.13).
   - Retinal detachment.

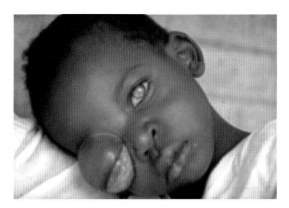

Figure 13.10 Fungating retinoblastoma in a child with bilateral disease. (Courtesy of P. Summanen, Helsinki, Finland and staff of Khartoum Eye Hospital, Sudan)

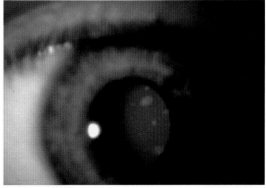

Figure 13.12 Vitreous seeds in an eye with an endophytic tumour. (Courtesy of T. Kivelä, Helsinki, Finland)

4. **Extensive retinoblastoma**
   - Rubeosis iridis, with hyphaema, secondary glaucoma and corneal oedema.
   - Vitreous haemorrhage.

5. **Tumour necrosis**
   - Uveitis.
   - Severe periocular inflammation.
   - Redness and swelling of the eyelids.

6. **Orbital invasion**
   - Massive proptosis.
   - Invasion of bone and sinuses.

7. **Diffuse retinoblastoma** (Bhatnagar and Vine, 1991)
   - Unilateral.
   - Presentation between the age of 5 and 12 years.
   - Snowball opacities in the anterior chamber and vitreous.
   - Pseudohypopyon and hyphaema.
   - Red eye, which may be the presenting sign.
   - Minimal calcification, undetectable with CT (Foster and Mukai, 1996).

8. **Spontaneous regression**
   - Usually produces severe inflammation resulting in phthisis.
   - Sometimes asymptomatic, resulting in an inactive scar which clinically resembles an irradiated retinoblastoma (Figure 13.14). This can undergo malignant trans-

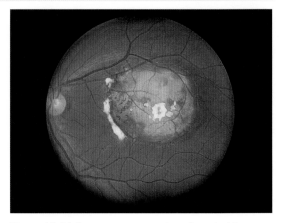

Figure 13.14 Spontaneous regression of a retinoblastoma, showing calcification. (Courtesy of J.A. Shields and C.L. Shields, Philadelphia, USA)

formation at any age (Eagle *et al.,* 1989; Balmer *et al.,* 1991).

9. **Adult retinoblastoma** (Mietz *et al.,* 1997)
   - Very rare.
   - Unilateral or bilateral.
   - Usually peripheral.
   - Often associated with clinical features resembling uveitis, which may be the presenting feature.
   - May arise from a retinocytoma.

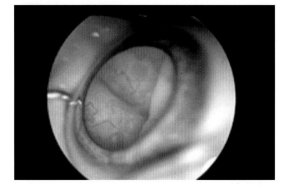

Figure 13.13 Exophytic retinoblastoma, with subretinal tumour. (Courtesy of T. Kivelä, Helsinki, Finland)

PRIMITIVE NEURAL ECTODERMAL TUMOUR (TRILATERAL RETINOBLASTOMA)

A primitive neural ectodermal tumour (PNET) develops in about 3% of patients with germline RB1 mutations (Kingston *et al.,* 1985; Amoaku *et al.,* 1996). It is usually located in the pineal gland but may arise in the parasellar region.

This tumour usually has similar histological features to retinoblastoma.

CLINICAL FEATURES

- Headache.
- Vomiting.

- Epileptic fits.
- Meningism.
- Hydrocephalus.
- Fever.

About 50% of PNETs are detected at the time of diagnosis of the intraocular tumour. Parasellar tumours tend to present earlier than pineal tumours.

METASTATIC RETINOBLASTOMA

Metastatic death usually occurs within two years of diagnosis and treatment of the primary tumour, with survival being shorter in patients with unilateral retinoblastoma, who tend to present late.

MAIN SITES OF METASTASIS

a. Regional nodes.
b. Lung.
c. Brain.
d. Bone.

PREDICTIVE FACTORS OF METASTATIC DISEASE

a. Orbital invasion (Messmer et al., 1991).
b. Optic nerve invasion, with the risk being proportional to the length of nerve involved (Magramm et al., 1989).
c. Massive choroidal invasion (Olver et al., 1991).
d. Tumour volume greater than 1 cm^3.

SECOND MALIGNANT NEOPLASM

If no external beam radiotherapy has been administered, then by the age of 40 years just over 5% of patients with germline mutations develop a second malignant neoplasm (SMN) (Eng et al., 1993). The commonest types of SMN are osteosarcoma of the skull and long bones (Figure 13.15), cutaneous melanoma and a variety soft tissue sarcomas (Moll et al., 1997). There is also an increased

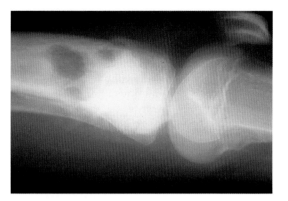

Figure 13.15 Osteosarcoma developing in the femur of a patient with bilateral retinoblastoma. (Courtesy of T. Kivelä, Helsinki, Finland)

incidence of breast cancer and Hodgkin's disease (Wong et al., 1997).

External beam radiotherapy is associated with an increased incidence of a second malignancy developing in the irradiated field, in a dose-related fashion (Wong et al., 1997) so that about 35% of patients die within 40 years of radiotherapy (Eng et al., 1993) (Figure 13.16). The incidence of second malignancy is greater if the radiotherapy is administered before the age of 12 months (Abramson and Frank, 1998), but it is not known whether this increase is related to early radiotherapy or early development of retinoblastoma (Kony et al., 1997).

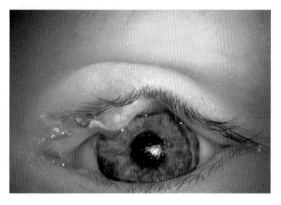

Figure 13.16 Sebaceous gland carcinoma developing 5 years after radiotherapy and enucleation for germinal retinoblastoma. (Courtesy of T. Kivelä, Helsinki, Finland)

HISTORY

It is important to ask about:

a. Birth weight, oxygen treatment and other risk factors for retinopathy of prematurity.
b. Exposure to puppies, which indicates a possibility of toxocariasis.
c. Family history of retinoblastoma, which if positive would suggest a germline mutation.
d. Family history of ocular malformations.

CLINICAL EXAMINATION

OCULAR

Both eyes are examined with binocular indirect ophthalmoscopy with indentation, documenting all findings with colour drawings and, if possible, colour photography using a hand-held, wide angle camera (Retcam 120, Massie Research Laboratories Inc., Pleasanton, California, USA). Slitlamp examination of the anterior segment, and measurement of the intraocular pressure and corneal diameter are performed at the same time.

SYSTEMIC

Full clinical examination and special investigations are performed to establish a diagnosis and detect any RB1 mutation or other disease needing treatment.

SCREENING FOR OTHER DISEASE

a. Stigmata of the rubella syndrome and tuberous sclerosis, which may cause pseudoretinoblastoma.
b. Features of chromosomal abnormalities, such as 13q deletion syndrome, which include microcephaly with psychomotor and mental deficits, hypertelorism, microphthalmos, large low-set ears, short neck, anogenital defects and abnormal digits.
c. Other primary systemic tumours, which may very rarely metastasize to the eye.

SYSTEMIC INVESTIGATIONS

SCREENING FOR PRIMITIVE NEURAL ECTODERMAL TUMOUR

A PNET needs to be excluded in patients with a germline mutation. Initial CT with follow-up MRI has been recommended (Bagley *et al.*, 1996) (Figure 13.17).

SCREENING FOR METASTATIC DISEASE

1. **Lumbar puncture**, if there is optic nerve or orbital involvement; placing the CSF in

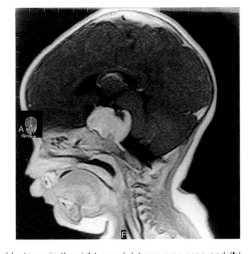

Figure 13.17 MRI scan showing a PNET in addition to a large retinoblastoma in the right eye: (**a**) transverse scan and (**b**) sagittal scan. (Courtesy of J. Pe'er, Jerusalem, Israel)

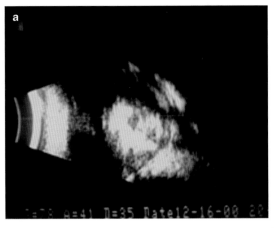 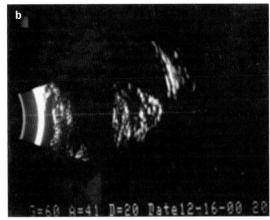

Figure 13.18 B-scan ultrasonography of a retinoblastoma: (**a**) high gain, showing multiple high and low intensity echoes, with orbital shadowing and (**b**) low gain, showing persistence of echoes from calcification. (Courtesy of H. Atta, Aberdeen, UK)

tubes containing fixative (Mackay *et al.,* 1984).

2. **Bone marrow aspiration** from iliac crest, if there is massive choroidal or orbital involvement.

3. **Whole body scans**, if there is a significant risk of metastatic disease.

OCULAR INVESTIGATIONS

ULTRASONOGRAPHY

A-scans and B-scans demonstrate calcification as multiple, small, highly reflective echoes, which persist after the gain is reduced and which cause orbital shadowing (Figure 13.18). Measurement of tumour dimensions is important for treatment planning and monitoring.

RADIOGRAPHY

A plain X-ray often demonstrates calcification in eyes with retinoblastoma but has been superseded by ultrasonography and CT.

COMPUTERIZED TOMOGRAPHY

Computerized tomography demonstrates calcification in about 90% of retinoblastomas (Figure 13.19) and may detect extraocular extension

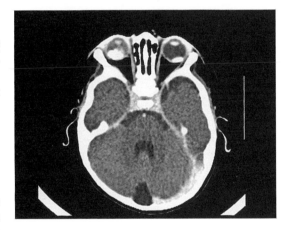

Figure 13.19 CT scan showing bilateral retinoblastomas with calcification. (Courtesy of H.E. Willshaw, Birmingham, UK)

(Haik *et al.,* 1985). CT may also reveal a trilateral retinoblastoma. In patients having retinoblastoma with orbital cellulitis, inflammatory swelling can mimic tumour invasion into nerve or orbit, which regresses with systemic steroids (Shields *et al.,* 1991; Mullaney *et al.,* 1998).

MAGNETIC RESONANCE IMAGING

Retinoblastoma is hyper-intense on T1 weighted images, especially if the tumour is well differen-

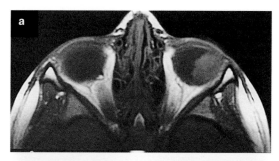

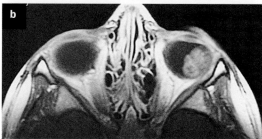

Figure 13.20 T1 weighted MRI images of a sporadic retinoblastoma (**a**) pre- and (**b**) post-contrast injection. (Courtesy of P. De Potter, Brussels, Belgium)

tiated and hypo-intense on T2 weighted images (Barkhof *et al.,* 1997) (Figure 13.20). Gadolinium enhancement is irregular if there are large areas of tumour necrosis. Calcification is demonstrated less reliably than with CT and appears as hypo-intense spots on T1 weighted images, more easily visible after enhancement.

MRI is about as effective as ultrasonography or CT in detecting optic nerve invasion.

FINE NEEDLE ASPIRATION BIOPSY

FNAB of retinoblastoma is controversial because it is generally believed to carry a significant risk of tumour seeding into the orbit. It is therefore contraindicated, as a rule. Some authorities perform FNAB in very rare cases and then only as a last resort (Shields *et al.,* 1993). To reduce the risk of seeding, some workers have devised special precautions, such as passing the needle through the cornea and peripheral iris (Augsburger *et al.,* 1985) and sealing the wound with tissue glue. (Char and Miller, 1984).

INCISIONAL BIOPSY

Incisional biopsy of an intraocular tumour is absolutely contraindicated. The procedure is useful in confirming the diagnosis when there is a large fungating orbital tumour.

AQUEOUS AND SERUM STUDIES

Measurement of aqueous-to-serum ratios of lactate dehydrogenase is not usually performed, but may be helpful in difficult cases. Determination of esterase D activity has been superseded by direct genetic tests.

GENETIC STUDIES

Genetic studies require a sample of fresh tumour tissue, taken from the enucleated eye, and a blood sample, for analysis of DNA extracted from leukocytes. It may also be useful to examine blood samples from relatives and a sperm sample from the patient's father (Sippel *et al.,* 1998).

There are many techniques for detecting RB mutations (Harbour, 1998), a few of which include:

a. Genetic linkage analysis, which is possible if blood samples from several affected relatives are available.
b. Cytogenetic analysis, which only demonstrates large chromosomal deletions, present in a small proportion of patients.
c. The protein truncation test, which may prove to be useful in detecting the large majority of mutations.

OBSTACLES TO THE DETECTION OF RB MUTATIONS

a. Large RB gene.
b. Mutation in any part of the gene.
c. Cost and laborious nature of genetic tests.
d. Mosaicism, which can give rise to false negative results (Lohmann *et al.,* 1997; Sippel *et al.,* 1998). In this condition, non-tumoral cells (e.g., leukocytes, germ cells) are composed of two populations of cells: those bearing the mutated RB gene and those containing a normal RB gene within the same parental chromosome.

DIFFERENTIAL DIAGNOSIS

Almost half of all referrals to an oncology centre with suspected retinoblastoma have other conditions, the commonest being Coats' disease, persistent hyperplasia primary vitreous and presumed ocular toxocariasis (Shields *et al.,* 1991).

INHERITED DISEASE

1. **Dominant exudative vitreoretinopathy** is an autosomal dominant disease, which is bilateral but asymmetrical. It tends to cause retinal traction and detachment as well as subretinal exudation, which, unlike retinoblastoma, is yellow.
2. **Norrie's disease** is a rare, X-linked recessive condition, causing bilateral total retinal detachments and presenting as white, retrolental masses. These boys are usually deaf and mentally retarded.
3. **Incontinentia pigmenti** (of the Bloch–Sulzberger type) is an X-linked dominant condition causing a wide variety of ocular and systemic abnormalities, which are usually lethal in males (Figure 13.21). Females can present with leukocoria due to total retinal detachment and cataract.

DEVELOPMENTAL DISEASE

1. **Persistent hyperplastic primary vitreous** (PHPV) is a unilateral disease, caused by abnormal persistence of mesenchymal tissue. This is usually in the retrolental space (Figure 13.22**b**) but may be at the optic nerve head (Figure 13.22**a**). PHPV presents within a few weeks of birth with unilateral leukocoria, usually in a microphthalmic eye. In the mild form, there is a small white opacity at the back of a clear lens, with a visible hyaloid artery. In the severe form, there is a mass of fibrovascular tissue, pulling the ciliary processes, which are elongated and visible (Figure 13.23). The lens is cataractous and the anterior chamber is shallow. Retinal detachment and retinal dysplasia are often present.
2. **Retinopathy of prematurity** can present as unilateral or bilateral leukocoria, caused by

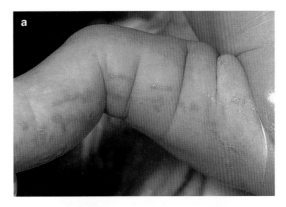

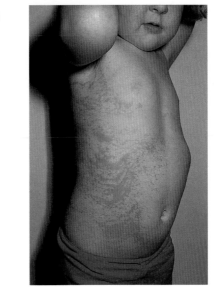

Figure 13.21 Cutaneous manifestations of incontinentia pigmenti: (**a**) early changes and (**b**) late appearances. (Courtesy of J.J. Kanski, Windsor, UK)

a retrolental mass of fibrovascular tissue. There is usually a history of prematurity, small birth weight and oxygen therapy.
3. **Cataracts** can be mistaken for leukocoria. They are usually present at birth, in one or both eyes, and can be due to conditions such as maternal rubella, inflammation, or trauma.
4. **White fundus lesions**, such as coloboma of the choroid, medullated nerve fibres (Figure 13.24) and the morning glory syndrome are easily recognized by indirect ophthalmoscopy.

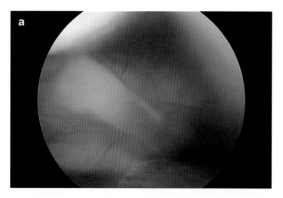
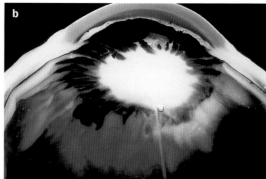

Figure 13.22 PHPV (**a**) posteriorly, obscuring optic disc (courtesy of L. Desjardins, Paris, France) and (**b**) anteriorly in an enucleated eye, showing elongation of ciliary processes (courtesy of W.R. Lee, Glasgow, UK)

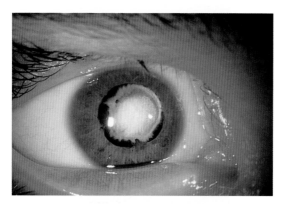

Figure 13.23 Clinical photograph showing elongation of ciliary processes in anterior PHPV. (Courtesy of J.J. Augsburger, Cincinnati, USA)

INFLAMMATION

1. **Toxocariasis** can cause a large, white retinal inflammatory mass, with a hazy vitreous containing traction bands, which contract to cause retinal detachment and cataract. Alternatively, a subretinal granuloma may develop with a clear vitreous (Figure 13.25). This disease is never present at birth. About 90% of patients have a positive serum ELISA for *Toxocara canis* at 1:16 dilution as compared to almost none of the retinoblastoma patients.

2. **Posterior uveitis** due to cytomegalovirus, herpes simplex, or *Toxocara* infection may mimic diffuse infiltrating retinoblastoma,

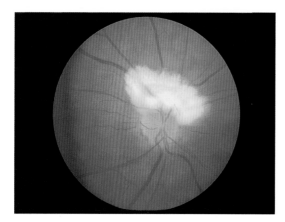

Figure 13.24 Opaque nerve fibres

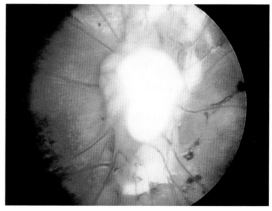

Figure 13.25 Toxocara. (Courtesy of J. Dudgeon, Glasgow, UK)

pseudohypopyon, iris nodules and true uveitis occurring as a result of tumour necrosis.

3. **Infectious orbital cellulitis** is usually caused by ethmoid sinusitis or septicaemia and can be mistaken for orbital cellulitis caused by tumour necrosis.

4. **Congenital toxoplasmosis** produces a characteristic choroidal scar.

NEOPLASIA

1. **Retinal astrocytic hamartoma** does not calcify until the age of 8–9 years (Drewe *et al.*, 1985) (Chapter 11).

2. **Medulloepithelioma** tends to be more anterior than retinoblastoma (Chapter 18).

3. **Leukaemia** (McManaway and Neely, 1994) also causes pseudohypopyon. (Chapter 21).

4. **Rhabdomyosarcoma** may very rarely occur within the eye in childhood. The tumour may be localized or diffuse, developing in the iris or ciliary body (Font and Zimmerman, 1972; Wilson *et al.*, 1990).

TRAUMA

1. **Traumatic retinal detachment** needs to be differentiated from diffuse retinoblastoma so as to avoid the need for systemic chemotherapy after inappropriate vitrectomy.

2. **Massive reactive gliosis of the retina** can form a tumour in an eye that has become disorganized in childhood as a result of infection or injury. Calcification and bone can develop in the gliotic tissue (Figure 13.26).

IDIOPATHIC DISEASE

1. **Coats' disease** is the most common cause of enucleation with a misdiagnosis of retinoblastoma. It tends to present at an older age than retinoblastoma, to be unilateral and to be more common in males, but these features are not reliable at differentiating between the two conditions. Dilated and telangiectatic retinal blood vessels, which are characteristic of Coats' disease, can also be

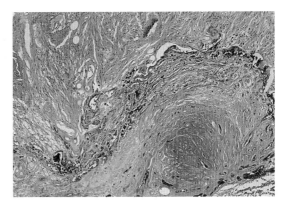

Figure 13.26 Retinal gliosis (H&E)

present with retinoblastoma. With Coats' disease, however, the blood vessels are entirely visible, from arteriole to venule (Figure 13.27), whereas with retinoblastoma they disappear into the tumour. Typically, the retina in Coats' disease shows a yellow colour (13.28), but this can also occur with retinoblastoma. For these reasons, ancillary tests are usually required. In Coats' disease: (a) ultrasonography is convenient and

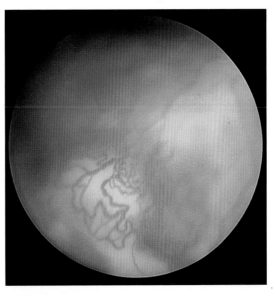

Figure 13.27 Coats' disease showing dilated telangiectatic retinal vessels, which are entirely visible joining arterioles to venules in an uninterrupted fashion. Note also the yellow subretinal exudation. (Courtesy of W.S. Foulds, Glasgow, UK)

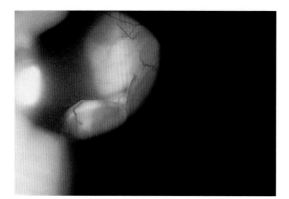

Figure 13.28 Coats' disease with extensive, yellow exudative retinal detachment. (Courtesy of J.J. Kanski, Windsor, UK)

demonstrates the absence of a subretinal mass or calcification; (b) CT shows homogenous subretinal densities without contrast media enhancement and without calcification and (c) MRI shows the subretinal fluid to be uniformly hyper-intense on T2 weighted images (in contrast to retinoblastoma). MRI is especially useful if there is subretinal haemorrhage, because it allows sequential examination without exposing the patient to ionizing radiation (Haik, 1991).

2. **Juvenile xanthogranuloma** is an infiltration of foamy histiocytes and multinucleated Touton giant cells, containing lipid droplets. It usually presents as a nodular or diffuse, white mass on the surface of the iris, often

with neovascularization, hyphaema, uveitis and secondary glaucoma (Zimmerman, 1965). The condition usually responds to topical steroids, although low-dose radiotherapy may be necessary in some cases (Parmley *et al.*, 1998). Lesions can also occur at the limbus (Yanoff and Perry, 1995), eyelid, retina, choroid and optic nerve (Wertz *et al.*, 1982; DeBarge *et al.*, 1994) (Figure 13.29).

TREATMENT

TREATMENT OF PRIMARY TUMOUR

The treatment of retinoblastoma is ideally performed at a specialist centre, where a wide range of therapeutic modalities can be applied, individually or in combination, and with the involvement of a multidisciplinary team of workers.

SMALL TUMOURS

a. **Photocoagulation** is indicated for small tumours, with a width of up to 3–4 mm, a thickness of not more than 1.5 mm and not showing any vitreous seeding or optic nerve involvement (Shields *et al.*, 1990) (Figure 13.30). Trans-scleral diode laser photocoagulation may be preferable for some anterior tumours (Abramson *et al.*, 1998) (Chapter 25).

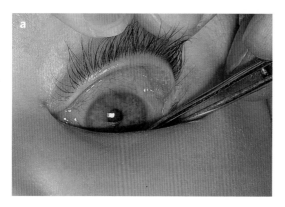
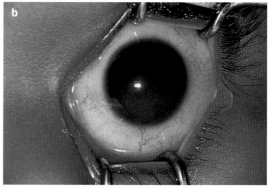

Figure 13.29 Juvenile xanthogranuloma: (**a**) yellow mass in the superior iris (courtesy of J. Dudgeon, Glasgow, UK) and (**b**) with diffuse hyphaema (courtesy of J.A. Shields and C.L. Shields, Philadelphia, USA)

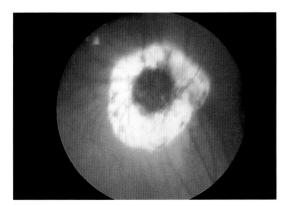

Figure 13.30 Laser treatment of an early retinoblastoma. (Courtesy of J. Dudgeon, Glasgow, UK)

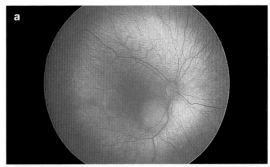

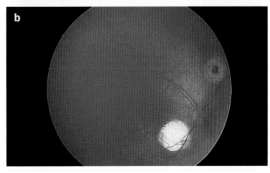

Figure 13.31 Two early retinoblastoma nodules (**a**) before and (**b**) after transpupillary thermotherapy. (Courtesy of P. De Potter, Brussels, Belgium)

b. **Transpupillary thermotherapy**, with or without chemotherapy, causes less visual loss than photocoagulation and is preferable for small, posterior tumours (Shields *et al.*, 1999; Lueder and Goyal, 1996; Bornfeld *et al.*, 1997) (Figure 13.31) (Chapter 25).

c. **Cryotherapy**, if repeated, can be effective with tumours up to 3.5 mm and 2.0 mm thick but is reserved for pre-equatorial tumours because of the risk of causing optic nerve and macular damage (Shields and Shields, 1990). A retinal break sometimes develops within the cryotherapy scar, causing rhegmatogenous retinal detachment.

d. **Chemotherapy** alone can be attempted for a macular tumour, in the hope of conserving central vision (Hungerford, 1999).

MEDIUM SIZED TUMOURS

a. **Brachytherapy** is indicated for tumours too large to treat by photo- or cryotherapy but not more than about 12 mm wide or 6 mm thick. This treatment is contraindicated if there is anything more than minimal vitreous seeding well within the radiational field (Shields *et al.*, 1993) (Figure 13.32) (Chapter 23).

b. **Systemic chemotherapy** followed by local therapy has become more popular as a means of avoiding radiotherapy (Figure 13.33) (Chapter 25).

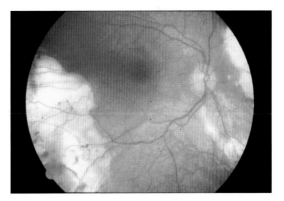

Figure 13.32 Plaque radiotherapy of two retinoblastoma nodules, showing good tumour regression with preservation of the macula. (Courtesy of T. Kivelä, Helsinki, Finland)

c. **External beam radiotherapy** is now applied only when it offers the last hope of conserving some useful vision, that is, when a tumour is unsuitable for brachytherapy, because of large size, close proximity to disc, or vitreous seeding. This is because it may induce second malignant neoplasms in patients with germinal mutations. It also causes orbital bone growth arrest, especially in younger patients (Imhof *et al.*, 1996) (Chapter 23).

Regression after radiotherapy is categorized as follows:

Type 0: No visible change.
Type 1: Cottage cheese mass of calcification (Figure 13.34).
Type 2: Fish-flesh lesion (Figure 13.33).
Type 3: Mixed pattern.
Type 4: Flat scar, which tends to occur after brachytherapy.

LARGE TUMOURS

a. **Chemotherapy** can shrink tumours so that they are treatable by conservative methods (i.e., 'chemoreduction') (Murphree *et al.*, 1996; Gallie *et al.*, 1996; Shields *et al.*, 1997). The technique is indicated if there is hope for useful vision and if the tumour is too large for conservative therapy alone. Contraindications include rubeosis iridis, neovascular glaucoma and tumour extension to optic nerve, anterior chamber or orbit. Total retinal detachment can resolve completely and is not a contraindication (Shields *et al.*, 1997). Chemotherapy administered for a large tumour in one eye may facilitate treatment of small tumours in the fellow eye (Figure 13.35).

b. **Enucleation** is indicated in the presence of rubeosis, vitreous haemorrhage, or optic nerve invasion. Diffuse retinoblastoma is generally treated by enucleation because of diagnostic uncertainty, poor visual prognosis and increased risk of recurrence (Girard *et al.*, 1989). Enucleation is also performed if chemoreduction fails or if a good status in the fellow eye makes such aggressive therapy undesirable. The surgical technique is described in Chapter 24.

Although with advanced tumours retention of the eye is now achieved more frequently, conservation of vision is disappointing (Kingston *et al.*, 1996).

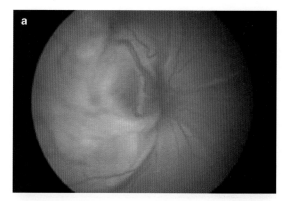

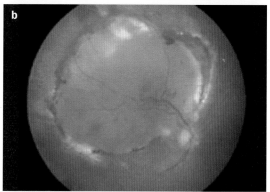

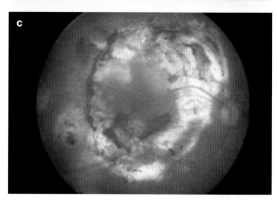

Figure 13.33 (**a**) Retinoblastoma with total retinal detachment at the right macula of a 1-year-old girl. The other eye had even more advanced disease. (**b**) Partial tumour regression with complete resolution of the retinal detachment after three cycles of systemic vincristine, etoposide and carboplatin. High-dose cyclosporine was used to block multidrug resistance and cryotherapy was administered before each cycle to disrupt the blood ocular barrier. (**c**) Two years after diagnosis, the tumour was mostly reduced to a flat scar with a small residual tumour, which was being treated with frequency doubled YAG and infra-red phototherapy every 8 weeks. (Courtesy of B. Gallie, Toronto, Canada)

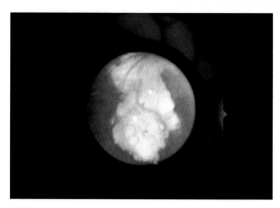

Figure 13.34 Type 1 regression after external beam radiotherapy. (Courtesy of T. Kivelä, Helsinki, Finland)

Table 13.1 Reese–Ellsworth classification of retinoblastoma

Group 1	A	Solitary tumour less than 4 DD wide, at or behind equator
	B	Multiple tumours, none over 4 DD wide, all at or behind equator
Group 2	A	Solitary tumour, 4–10 DD wide, at or behind equator
	B	Multiple tumours, 4–10 DD wide, at or behind equator
Group 3	A	Any tumour anterior to equator
	B	Solitary tumour, larger than 10 DD, behind equator
Group 4	A	Multiple tumours, some larger than 10 DD wide
	B	Any lesion extending to ora serrata
Group 5	A	Massive tumours involving over half the retina
	B	Vitreous seeding

EXTRAOCULAR EXTENSION

a. **External beam radiotherapy** is indicated if tumour extends extraocularly or to the cut end of the optic nerve. This is the case even in patients with hereditary retinoblastoma, because the risk of death from intracranial spread is greater than that of a future second malignant neoplasm (Chapter 23).

b. **Initial chemoreduction followed by enucleation** is indicated if there is a large, fungating orbital tumour, as it may allow less mutilating surgery to be performed (Murphree and Munier, 1994; Kiratli *et al.*, 1998).

The Reese–Ellsworth classification was developed to predict ocular outcome after external beam radiotherapy (Table 13.1). It underestimates the results that can be now achieved with anterior tumours or vitreous seeding so that newer classifications are being developed. Nevertheless, most groups have used this classification to report the results of treatment, particularly radiotherapy (Toma *et al.*, 1995; Blach *et al.*, 1996; Hernandez *et al.*, 1996).

TREATMENT OF PNET

PNET is treated with systemic and intrathecal chemotherapy sometimes combined with craniospinal irradiation (Nelson *et al.*, 1992).

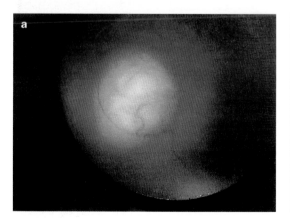
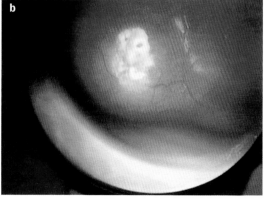

Figure 13.35 Regression of a retinoblastoma after one cycle of systemic chemotherapy for a large retinoblastoma in the fellow eye. (Courtesy of H.E. Willshaw, Birmingham, UK)

TREATMENT OF METASTATIC DISEASE

Metastatic retinoblastoma is treated with high-dose chemotherapy, total body irradiation, intrathecal chemotherapy and bone marrow rescue (i.e., extracorporeal preservation of bone marrow during chemotherapy) (Kingston *et al.,* 1987; White, 1991; Saarinen *et al.,* 1991).

The 'JOE' chemotherapy regime is widely used and consists of:

a. JM8 (carboplatin).
b. Oncovin (vincristine).
c. Etoposide (VP-16).

Some workers also add cyclosporine (Gallie *et al.,* 1996), which inhibits the multidrug resistance protein, p170, but failure can still occur if a second multidrug resistance protein is present (Chan *et al.,* 1997).

COMPLICATIONS OF CHEMOTHERAPY

a. Bone marrow suppression, with immunodeficiency and haemorrhage.
b. Nephropathy.
c. Deafness.
d. 11q23-translocated leukaemia (Winick *et al.,* 1993). This has been reported after treatment of other tumours by etoposide but with higher doses than are administered for retinoblastoma (Winick *et al.,* 1993).

Some authorities argue that if the vision in the fellow eye is good it is difficult to justify the risks associated with systemic chemotherapy. A number of methods are being developed for local administration of chemotherapy. These include peribulbar injection (Abramson *et al.,* 1999), episcleral balloon administration (in experimental animals) (Mendelsohn *et al.,* 1998) and selective ophthalmic artery injection (Kaneko and Moori, 1999) (Figure 13.36).

FOLLOW-UP

OBJECTIVES

a. To ensure that the tumour has responded adequately to conservative treatment.

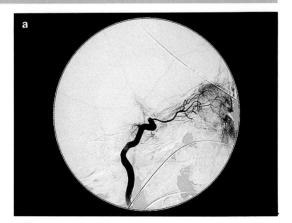

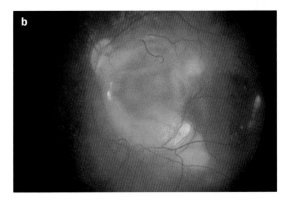

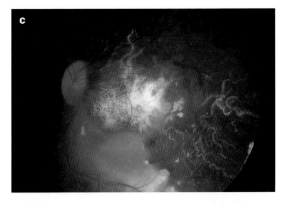

Figure 13.36 Selective ophthalmic artery perfusion: (**a**) preliminary angiogram, (**b**) pre-treatment fundus photograph, showing a large retinoblastoma at the left macula and (**c**) post-treatment appearance showing tumour regression. (Courtesy of A. Kaneko, Tokyo, Japan)

b. To detect local tumour recurrence after conservative treatment (Abramson *et al.*, 1994).

c. To detect any new tumours, which are especially common after treatment during the first year of life (Abramson *et al.*, 1994). Such new tumours tend to occur peripherally and are rare after the age of 6 years (Abramson *et al.*, 1992).

PROTOCOL AFTER CONSERVATIVE THERAPY

- Examination 3–6 weeks after treatment;
- then every 1–3 months for the first year;
- then every 3–4 months during the second year;
- then every 4–6 months until the age of 4–6 years;
- then annually, perhaps until the age of 8–12 years, although there is no consensus about the age at which follow-up should be stopped.

Examination protocols vary from centre to centre and also depend on the type of treatment used and hence the chances of further tumour activity. Recurrence of an intraocular tumour has rarely been reported more than 30 months after treatment (Abramson *et al.*, 1986).

PROTOCOL AFTER ENUCLEATION

Any orbital recurrence after enucleation is most likely to occur during the first 18 months (Rubin *et al.*, 1985). Scanning is generally performed once a year in high-risk cases, perhaps more frequently in selected patients.

PROTOCOL FOR PATIENTS WITH GERMINAL MUTATION

To screen for PNET in patients with hereditary retinoblastoma, some workers recommend regular MRI brain scans until the age of 4 years.

With regards to second malignant neoplasms in patients with germinal mutations, some practitioners advise early presentation if any symptoms persist for more than a week (Murphree and Munier, 1994), whereas others recommend observation by an oncologist (Abramson and Frank, 1998).

Retinocytoma requires life-long monitoring, since it can progress to retinoblastoma at any age.

FAMILY CARE

ESTIMATED RISKS

The risk of transmitting the disease depends on the family history and whether or not the retinoblastoma is solitary (Draper *et al.*, 1992).

If a patient has multiple retinoblastomas, the chances of having the mutation are:

- 50% in each sibling, if the family history is positive.
- 2% in each sibling, if the family history is negative.
- 50% in each offspring.
- 50% in each child of any offspring with clinical retinoblastoma.
- 5% in each child of any apparently healthy offspring (because 10% are carriers).

If a patient has a solitary retinoblastoma, the chances of having the mutation are:

- 1% in each sibling if the family history is negative. This diminishes with the number of unaffected siblings.
- 50% in each sibling if the family history is positive.
- 1% in each offspring if the family history is negative.
- 50% in each offspring if the family history is positive.

SCREENING PROTOCOLS

a. Screening of relatives at risk for the first five years of life, starting as soon as possible after birth.

b. Ophthalmoscopic examination of both parents if the family history is negative, as evidence of regressed retinoblastoma improves estimation of the probability of clinical disease in siblings and offspring.

c. Consideration of pre-natal detection of RB1 mutation in relatives at risk by chorionic villous sampling by amniocentesis.

d. Pre-natal detection of retinoblastoma in relatives at risk by ultrasonography can be attempted.

e. Collection of blood specimens from several affected and unaffected family members, to facilitate genetic studies, thereby avoiding unnecessary clinical examinations in relatives not having the mutation (Gallie, 1997).

f. DNA analysis of tumour tissue and peripheral blood cells, to identify germline mutations in patients with solitary retinoblastoma and no family history (Lohmann *et al.*, 1997).

When terminal illness develops in a child, it is important to address all the psychological difficulties that are likely to develop in the patient and the rest of the family (Black, 1998).

REFERENCES

Abramson, D.H. (1997) Unilateral retinoblastoma in adults. *Ophthalmology*, **104**, 1207.

Abramson, D.H., Franck, C.M. and Dunkel, I.J. (1999) A phase I/II study of subconjunctival carboplatin for intraocular retinoblastoma. *Ophthalmology*, **106**, 1947–50.

Abramson, D.H., Ellsworth, R.M., Grumbach, N., Sturgis-Buckhout, L. and Haik, B.G. (1986) Retinoblastoma: correlation between age at diagnosis and survival. *J. Pediatr. Ophthalmol. Strabismus*, **23**, 174–7.

Abramson, D.H. and Franck, C.M. (1998) Second nonocular tumors in survivors of bilateral retinoblastoma: a possible age effect on radiation-related risk. *Ophthalmology*, **105**, 573–80.

Abramson, D.H., Gamell, L.S., Ellsworth, R.M., Kruger, E.F., Servodidio, C.A., Turner, L. and Sussman, D. (1994) Unilateral retinoblastoma: new intraocular tumours after treatment. *Br. J. Ophthalmol.*, **78**, 698–701.

Abramson, D.H., Greenfield, D.S. and Ellsworth, R.M. (1992) Bilateral retinoblastoma. Correlations between age at diagnosis and time course for new intraocular tumors. *Ophthalmic Paediatr. Genet.*, **13**, 1–7.

Abramson, D.H., Servodidio, C.A., De Lillo, A.R., Gamell, L.S., Kruger, E.F. and McCormick, B. (1994) Recurrence of unilateral retinoblastoma following radiation therapy. *Ophthalmic Genet.*, **15**, 107–13.

Abramson, D.H., Servodidio, C.A. and Nissen, M. (1998) Treatment of retinoblastoma with the transscleral diode laser. *Am. J. Ophthalmol.*, **126**, 733–5.

Amoaku, W.M., Willshaw, H.E., Parkes, S.E., Shah, K.J. and Mann, J.R. (1996) Trilateral retinoblastoma. A report of five patients. *Cancer*, **78**, 858–63.

Augsburger, J.J., Oehlschläger, U. and Manzitti, J.E. (1995) Multinational clinical and pathologic registry of retinoblastoma. Retinoblastoma International Collaborative Study report 2. *Graefes Arch. Clin. Exp. Ophthalmol.*, **233**, 469–75.

Augsburger, J.J., Shields, J.A., Folberg, R., Lang, W., O'Hara, B.J. and Claricci, J.D. (1985) Fine needle aspiration biopsy in the diagnosis of intraocular cancer. Cytologic-histologic correlations. *Ophthalmology*, **92**, 39–49.

Bagley, L.J., Hurst, R.W., Zimmerman, R.A., Shields, J.A., Shields, C.L. and De Potter, P. (1996) Imaging in the trilateral retinoblastoma syndrome. *Neuroradiology*, **38**, 166–70.

Balmer, A., Munier, F. and Gailloud, C. (1991) Retinoma. Case studies. *Ophthal. Paediatr. Genet.*, **12**, 131–7.

Barkhof, F., Smeets, M. van der Valk, Tan, K.E.W.P., Hoogenraad, F., Peeters, J. and Valk, J. (1997) MR imaging in retinoblastoma. *Eur. Radiol.*, **7**, 726–31.

Bhatnagar, R. and Vine, A.K. (1991) Diffuse infiltrating retinoblastoma. *Ophthalmology*, **98**, 1657–61.

Blach, L.E., McCormick, B. and Abramson, D.H. (1996) External beam radiation therapy and retinoblastoma: long-term results in the comparison of two techniques. *Int. J. Radiat. Oncol. Biol. Phys.*, **35**, 45–51.

Black, D. (1998) Coping with loss. The dying child. *Br. Med. J.*, **316**, 1376–8.

Bornfeld, N., Schüler, A., Bechrakis, N., Henze, G. and Havers, W. (1997) Preliminary results of primary chemotherapy in retinoblastoma. *Klin. Padiatr.*, **209**, 216–21.

Bremner, R., Du, D.C., Connolly-Wilson, M.J., Bridge, P., Ahmad, K.F., Mostachfi, H., Rushlow, D., Dunn, J.M. and Gallie, B.L. (1997) Deletion of *RB* exons 24 and 25 causes low-penetrance retinoblastoma. *Am. J. Hum. Genet.*, **61**, 556–70.

Chan, H.S.L., Lu, Y., Grogan, T.M., Haddad, G., Hipfner, D.R., Cole, S.P.C., Deeley, R.G., Ling, V. and Gallie, B.L. (1997) Multidrug resistance protein (MRP) expression in retinoblastoma correlates with the rare failure of chemotherapy despite cyclosporine for reversal of P-glycoprotein. *Cancer Res.*, **57**, 2325–30.

Char, D.H. and Miller, T.R. (1984) Fine needle biopsy in retinoblastoma. *Am. J. Ophthalmol.*, **97**, 686–90.

DeBarge, L.R., Chan, C-C., Greenberg, S.C., McLean, I.W., Yannuzzi, L.A. and Nussenblatt, R.B. (1994) Chorioretinal, iris and ciliary body infiltration by juvenile xanthogranuloma masquerading as uveitis. *Surv. Ophthalmol.*, **39**, 65–71.

Draper, G.J., Sanders, B.M., Brownbill, P.A. and Hawkins, M.M. (1992) Patterns of risk of hereditary retinoblastoma and applications to genetic counselling. *Br. J. Cancer*, **66**, 211–19.

Drewe, R.H., Hiscott, P. and Lee, W.R. (1985) Solitary astrocytic hamartoma simulating retinoblastoma. *Ophthalmologica*, **190**, 158–67.

Dryja, T.P., Morrow, J.F. and Rapaport, J.M. (1997) Quantification of the paternal allele bias for new germline mutations in the retinoblastoma gene. *Hum. Genet.*, **100**, 446–9.

Eagle, R.C.Jr., Shields, J.A., Donoso, L. and Milner, R.S. (1989) Malignant transformation of spontaneously regressed retinoblastoma, retinoma/retinocytoma variant. *Ophthalmology*, **96**, 1389–95.

Eng, C., Li, F.P., Abramson, D.H., Ellsworth, R.M., Wong, F.L., Goldman, M.B., Seddon, J., Tarbell, N. and Boice, J.D. Jr. (1993) Mortality from second tumors among long-term survivors of retinoblastoma. *J. Natl Cancer Inst.*, **85**, 1121–8.

Font, R.L. and Zimmerman, L.E. (1972) Electron microscopic verification of primary rhabdomyosarcoma of the iris. *Am. J. Ophthalmol.*, **74**, 110–17.

Foster, B.S. and Mukai, S. (1996) Intraocular retinoblastoma presenting as ocular and orbital inflammation. *Int. Ophthalmol. Clin.*, **36**, 153–60.

Gallie, B.L. (1997) Predictive testing for retinoblastoma comes of age. *Am. J. Hum. Genet.*, **61**, 279–81.

Gallie, B.L., Budning, A., DeBoer, G., Thiessen, J.J., Koren, G., Verjee, Z., Ling, V. and Chan, H.S.L. (1996) Chemotherapy with focal therapy can cure intraocular retinoblastoma without radiotherapy. *Arch. Ophthalmol.*, **114**, 1321–8.

Girard, B., Le Hoang, P., D'Hermies, F., Quere, M.A. and Rousselie, F. (1989). Le rétinoblastome infiltrant diffus. *J. Fr. Ophtalmol.*, **12**, 369–81.

Gurney, J.G., Ross, J.A., Wall, D.A., Bleyer, W.A., Severson, R.K. and Robison, L.L. (1997) Infant cancer in the U.S.: Histology-specific incidence and trends, 1973 to 1992. *J. Pediatr. Hematol. Oncol.*, **19**, 428–32.

Haik, B.G. (1991) Advanced Coats' disease. *Trans. Am. Ophthalmol. Soc.,* **89**, 371–476.

Haik, B.G., Saint Louis, L., Smith, M.E., Abramson, D.H. and Ellsworth, R.M. (1985) Computed tomography of the nonrhegmatogenous retinal detachment in the pediatric patient. *Ophthalmology*, **92**, 1133–42.

Harbour, J.W. (1998) Overview of RB gene mutations in patients with retinoblastoma. Implications for clinical genetic screening. *Ophthalmology*, **105**, 1442–7.

Hensey, C.E., Hong, F., Durfee, T., Qian, Y-W., Lee, E.Y. and Lee, W-H. (1994) Identification of discrete structural domains in the retinoblastoma protein. Amino-terminal domain is required for its oligomerization. *J. Biol. Chem.*, **269**, 1380–7.

Hernandez, J.C., Brady, L.W., Shields, J.A., Shields, C.L., DePotter, P., Karlsson, U.L., Markoe, A.M., Amendola, B.E. and Singh, A. (1996) External beam radiation for retinoblastoma: results, patterns of failure and a proposal for treatment guidelines. *Int. J. Radiat. Oncol., Biol. Phys.*, **35**, 125–32.

Hungerford, J.L. (1999) Personal communication; International Congress of Ocular Oncology, Philadelphia.

Imhof, S.M., Mourits, M.P., Hofman, P., Zonneveld, F.W., Schipper, J., Moll, A.C. and Tan, K.E.W.P. (1996) Quantification of orbital and mid-facial growth retardation after megavoltage external beam irradiation in children with retinoblastoma. *Ophthalmology*, **103**, 263–8.

Kaneko, A. and Moori, M. (1999) Personal communication; International Congress of Ocular Oncology, Philadelphia.

Kingston, J.E., Hungerford, J.L., Madreperla, S.A. and Plowman, P.N. (1996) Results of combined chemotherapy and radiotherapy for advanced intraocular retinoblastoma. *Arch. Ophthalmol.*, **114**, 1339–43.

Kingston, J.E., Plowman, P.N. and Hungerford, J.L. (1985) Ectopic intracranial retinoblastoma in childhood. *Br. J. Ophthalmol.*, **69**, 742–8.

Kingston, J.E., Hungerford, J.L. and Plowman, P.N. (1987) Chemotherapy in metastatic retinoblastoma. *Ophthal. Paediatr. Genet.*, **8**, 69–72.

Kiratli, H., Bilgiç, S. and Özerdem, U. (1998) Management of massive orbital involvement of intraocular retinoblastoma. *Ophthalmology*, **105**, 322–6.

Kony, S.J., de Vathaire, F., Chompret, A., Shamsaldim, A., Grimaud, E., Raquin, M-A., Oberlin, O., Brugières, L., Feunteun, J., Eschwège, F., Chavaudra, J., Lemerle, J. and Bonaïti-Pellié, C. (1997) Radiation and genetic factors in the risk of second malignant neoplasms after a first cancer in childhood. *Lancet*, **350**, 91–5.

Lohmann, D.R., Brandt, B., Höpping, W., Passarge, E. and Horsthemke, B. (1996) The spectrum of RB1 germ-line mutations in hereditary retinoblastoma. *Am. J. Hum. Genet.*, **58**, 940–9.

Lohmann, D.R., Brandt, B., Passarge, E. and Horsthemke, B. (1997) Molekulare genetik und Diagnostik des Retinoblastoms. Bedeutung für die Ophthalmologische Praxis. *Ophthalmologe*, **94**, 263–7.

Lohmann, D.R., Gerick, M., Brandt, B., Oelschläger, U., Lorenz, B., Passarge, E. and Horsthemke, B. (1997) Constitutional RB1-gene mutations in patients with isolated unilateral retinoblastoma. *Am. J. Hum. Genet.*, **61**, 282–94.

Lueder, G.T. and Goyal, R. (1996) Visual function after laser hyperthermia and chemotherapy for macular retinoblastoma. *Am. J. Ophthalmol.*, **121**, 582–4.

MacKay, C.J., Abramson, D.H. and Ellsworth, R.M. (1984) Metastatic patterns of retinoblastoma. *Arch. Ophthalmol.*, **102**, 391–6.

Magramm, I., Abramson, D.H. and Ellsworth, R.M.

(1989) Optic nerve involvement in retinoblastoma. *Ophthalmology*, **96**, 217–22.

McManaway, J.W. and Neely, J.E. (1994) Choroidal and orbital leukemic infiltrate mimicking advanced retinoblastoma. *J. Pediatr. Ophthalmol. Strabismus*, **31**, 394–6.

Mendelsohn, M.E., Abramson, D.H., Madden, T., Tong, W., Tran, H.T. and Dunkel, I.J. (1998) Intraocular concentrations of chemotherapeutic agents after systemic or local administration. *Arch. Ophthalmol.*, **116**, 1209–12.

Messmer, E.P., Heinrich, T., Höpping, W., de Sutter, E., Havers, W. and Sauerwein, W. (1991) Risk factors for metastases in patients with retinoblastoma. *Ophthalmology*, **98**, 136–41.

Mietz, H., Hutton, W.L. and Font, R.L. (1997) Unilateral retinoblastoma in an adult: report of a case and review of the literature. *Ophthalmology*, **104**, 43–7.

Moll, A.C., Imhof, S.M., Bouter, L.M. and Tan, K.E.W.P. (1997) Second primary tumors in patients with retinoblastoma. A review of the literature. *Ophthal. Genet.*, **18**, 27–34.

Moll, A.C., Imhof, S.M., Kuik, D.J., Bouter, L.M., Den Otter, W., Bezemer, P.D., Koten, J.W. and Tan, K.E.W.P. (1996) High parental age is associated with sporadic hereditary retinoblastoma: the Dutch retinoblastoma register 1862–1994. *Hum. Genet.*, **98**, 109–12.

Mullaney, P.B., Karcioglu, Z.A., Al-Mesfer, S. and Abboud, E.B. (1997) Presentation of retinoblastoma as phthisis bulbi. *Eye*, **11**, 403–8.

Mullaney, P.B., Karcioglu, Z.A., Huaman, A.M. and Al-Mesfer, S. (1998) Retinoblastoma associated orbital cellulitis. *Br. J. Ophthalmol.*, **82**, 517–21.

Murphree, A.L. and Munier, F.L. (1994) Retinoblastoma. In: S.J. Ryan (ed.), *Retina*. St Louis: Mosby, Vol. 1, Ch. 27, pp. 571–626.

Murphree, A.L., Villablanca, J.G., Deegan, W.F. IIIrd, Sato, J.K., Malogolowkin, M., Fisher, A., Parker, R., Reed, E. and Gomer, C.J. (1996) Chemotherapy plus local treatment in the management of intraocular retinoblastoma. *Arch. Ophthalmol.*, **114**, 1348–56.

Nelson, S.C., Friedman, H.S., Oakes, W.J., Halperin, E.C., Tien, R., Fuller, G.N., Hockenberger, B., Scroggs, M.W., Moncino, M., Kurzberg, J. *et al.* (1992) Successful therapy for trilateral retinoblastoma. *Am. J. Ophthalmol.*, **114**, 23–9.

Olver, J.M., McCartney, A.C.E., Kingston, J. and Hungerford, J. (1991) Histological indicators of the prognosis for survival following enucleation for retinoblastoma. In: N. Bornfeld, E.S. Gragoudas, W. Höpping, P.K. Lommatzsch, A. Wessing and L. Zografos (eds), *Tumors of the Eye*. Amsterdam: Kugler, pp. 59–67.

Parmley, V.C., George, D.P. and Fannin, L.A. (1998) Juvenile xanthogranuloma of the iris in an adult. *Arch. Ophthalmol.*, **116**, 377–9.

Prendergrass, T.W. and Davis, S. (1980) Incidence of retinoblastoma in the United States. *Arch. Ophthalmol.*, **98**, 1204–10.

Rubin, C.M., Robison, L.L., Cameron, J.D., Woods, W.G., Nestbit, M.E. Jr., Krivit, W., Kim, T.H., Letson, R.D. and Ramsay, N.K.C. (1985) Intraocular retinoblastoma group V: an analysis of prognostic factors. *J. Clin. Oncol.*, **3**, 680–5.

Saarinen, U.M., Sariola, H. and Hovi, L. (1991) Recurrent disseminated retinoblastoma treated by high-dose chemotherapy, total body irradiation and autologous bone marrow rescue. *Am. J. Pediatr. Hematol. Oncol.*, **13**, 315–19.

Schubert, E.L., Strong, L.C. and Hansen, M.F. (1997) A splicing mutation in RB1 in low penetrance retinoblastoma. *Hum. Genet.*, **100**, 557–63.

Shields, J.A. and Shields, C.L. (1990) Treatment of retinoblastoma with cryotherapy. *Trans. Am. Acad. Ophthalmol. Otolaryngol.*, **42**, 977–80.

Shields, J.A., Shields, C.L. Parsons, H., and Giblin, M.E. (1990) The role of photocoagulation in the management of retinoblastoma. *Arch. Ophthalmol.*, **108**, 205–8.

Shields, J.A., Parsons, H.M., Shields, C.L. and Shah, P. (1991) Lesions simulating retinoblastoma. *J. Pediatr. Ophthalmol. Strabismus*, **28**, 338–40.

Shields, C.L., Santos, M.C.M., Diniz, W., Gündüz, K., Mercado, G., Cater, J.R. and Shields, J.A. (1999) Thermotherapy for retinoblastoma. *Arch. Ophthalmol.*, **117**, 885–93.

Shields, C.L., Shields, J.A., De Potter, P., Himelstein, B.P. and Meadows, A.T. (1997) The effect of chemoreduction on retinoblastoma-induced retinal detachment. *J. Pediatr. Ophthalmol. Strabismus*, **34**, 165–9.

Shields, C.L., Shields, J.A., De Potter, P., Minelli, S., Hernandez, C., Brady, L.W. and Cater, J.R. (1993) Plaque radiotherapy in the management of retinoblastoma. *Ophthalmology*, **100**, 216–24.

Shields, J.A., Shields, C.L., Ehya, H., Eagle, R.C. Jr. and De Potter, P. (1993) Fine-needle aspiration biopsy of suspected intraocular tumors. The 1992 Urwick Lecture. *Ophthalmology*, **100**, 1677–84.

Shields, C.L., Shields, J.A., Needle, M., De Potter, P., Kheterpal, S., Hamada, A. and Meadows, A.T. (1997) Combined chemoreduction and adjuvant treatment for intraocular retinoblastoma. *Ophthalmology*, **104**, 2101–11.

Shields, J.A., Shields, C.L., Suvarnamani, C., Schroeder, R.P. and De Potter, P. (1991) Retinoblastoma manifesting as orbital cellulitis. *Am. J. Ophthalmol.*, **112**, 442–9.

Sippel, K.C., Fraioli, R.E., Smith, G.D., Schalkoff, M.E., Sutherland, J., Gallie, B.L. and Dryja, T.P. (1998) Frequency of somatic and germ-line mosaicism in retinoblastoma: implications for genetic counseling. *Am. J. Hum. Genet.*, **62**, 610–19.

Toma, N.M., Hungerford, J.L., Plowman, P.N., Kingston, J.E. and Doughty, D. (1995) External beam radiotherapy for retinoblastoma: II. Lens sparing technique. *Br. J. Ophthalmol.*, **79**, 112–17.

Wertz, F.D., Zimmerman, L.E., McKeown, C.A., Croxatto, J.O., Whitmore, P.V. and LaPiana, F.G. (1982) Juvenile xanthogranuloma of the optic nerve, disc, retina and choroid. *Ophthalmology*, **89**, 1331–5.

White, L. (1991) Chemotherapy in retinoblastoma: current status and future directions. *Am. J. Pediatr. Hematol. Oncol.*, **13**, 189–201.

Wilson, M.E., McClatchey, S.K. and Zimmerman, L.E. (1990) Rhabdomyosarcoma of the ciliary body. *Ophthalmology*, **97**, 1484–8.

Winick, N.J., McKenna, R.W., Shuster, J.J., Schneider, N.R., Borowitz, M.J., Bowman, W.P., Jacaruso, D., Kamen, B.A. and Buchanan, G.R. (1993) Secondary acute myeloid leukemia in children with acute lymphoblastic leukemia treated with etoposide. *J. Clin. Oncol.*, **11**, 209–17.

Wong, F.L., Boice, J.D. Jr., Abramson, D.H., Tarone, R.E., Kleinerman, R.A., Stovall, M., Goldman, M.B., Seddon, J.M., Tarbell, N., Fraumeni, J.F. Jr. and Li, F.P. (1997) Cancer incidence after retinoblastoma. Radiation dose and sarcoma risk. *JAMA*, **278**, 1262–7.

Yanoff, M. and Perry, H.D. (1995) Juvenile xanthogranuloma of the corneoscleral limbus. *Arch. Ophthalmol.*, **113**, 915–17.

Yoshizumi, M.O., Thomas, J.V. and Smith, T.R. (1978) Glaucoma-inducing mechanisms in eyes with retinoblastoma. *Arch. Ophthalmol.*, **96**, 105–10.

Zimmerman, L.E. (1965) Ocular lesions of juvenile xanthogranuloma. Nevoxanthoedothelioma. *Am. J. Ophthalmol.*, **60**, 1011–35.

EPITHELIAL TUMOURS

Chapter 14

Congenital hypertrophy of the retinal pigment epithelium

Congenital hypertrophy of the retinal pigment epithelium can be solitary or multiple.

Solitary typical congenital hypertrophy of the RPE (CHRPE) is rare and does not have any systemic associations (Shields *et al.,* 1992; Buettner, 1994).

Multiple atypical CHRPE lesions occur in association with familial adenomatous polyposis (FAP). This disease is caused by a mutation in the long arm of chromosome 5, which is inherited in an autosomal dominant manner. In FAP, large numbers of adenomatous polyps develop in the colon, stomach and duodenum, usually after the age of 20 years (Figure 14.1). Malignant transformation of the polyps into adenocarcinomas usually occurs between the ages of 20 and 40 years. If FAP is associated with desmoid tumours, osteomas, and sebaceous cysts it is referred to as Gardner's syndrome.

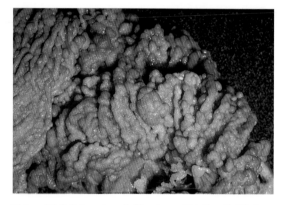

Figure 14.1 Polyposis coli. (Courtesy of J.J. Kanski, Windsor, UK)

PATHOLOGY

The retinal pigment epithelial cells are large and completely filled with large melanosomes. The abnormal cells usually form a single layer, but there can be benign, abnormal proliferation (i.e., hyperplasia) with multi-layering (Wirz *et al.,* 1982). The underlying Bruch's membrane is thickened and the overlying retina shows atrophy of the receptor cell layer. Areas with atrophy of RPE cells (i.e., 'lacunae') appear later. At the margin of the

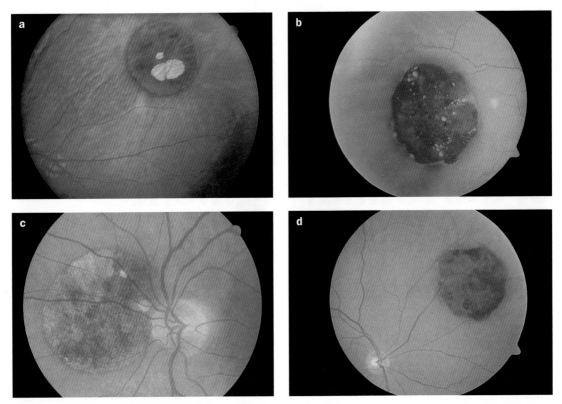

Figure 14.2 Clinical photographs of CHRPE lesions showing variation in pigmentation, atrophy and halo: (**a**) large central lacunae and marginal halo, (**b**) multiple, small lacunae, (**c**) irregular atrophy and absence of halo, (**d**) absence of both lacunae and halo

lesion, depigmented RPE cells may give the appearance of a halo.

SYMPTOMS

CHRPE is asymptomatic and detected on routine examination.

SIGNS

TYPICAL CHRPE

- Black, grey or dark brown colour (Figure 14.2).
- Diameter of several millimetres, although there is much variation.
- Flat shape.
- Oval or wavy contour.
- Discrete margins, often with a narrow, depigmented line (i.e., 'halo').

- White 'lacunae' within the lesion, revealing sclera and choroidal vessels. The atrophy may predominate, and may be complete (i.e., 'polar bear spot') (Figure 14.3).
- Diffuse darkening of the surrounding choroid, mimicking a shadow cast by an elevated lesion on indirect ophthalmoscopy (Figure 14.2**a**).
- Gradual enlargement in some cases (Boldrey and Schwartz, 1982).
- Development of a nodular tumour (Shields and Shields, 1999).
- Retinal vascular occlusion, which is very rare (Cleary *et al.,* 1976).

ATYPICAL CHRPE

- Four or more lesions in any or all quadrants of one or both eyes (Romania *et al.,* 1989).
- Oval, fusiform or linear shape (Figure 14.4).

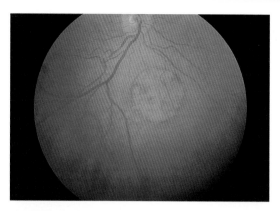

Figure 14.3 Atrophic CHRPE lesion (i.e., 'polar bear spot')

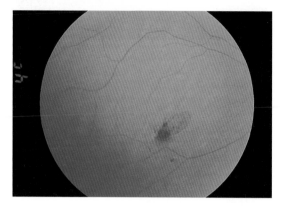

Figure 14.4 Small, oval lesions in a patient with FAP. (Courtesy of C. Dodd, Manchester, UK)

- Usually small.
- Lightly pigmented or non-pigmented.
- Depigmented halo or 'comet's tail' radiating posteriorly.

The RPE lesions associated with FAP may be difficult to see, so that three-mirror examination is advised.

INVESTIGATIONS

VISUAL FIELD EXAMINATION

There is usually a relative scotoma, which may enlarge and eventually become absolute.

FLUORESCEIN ANGIOGRAPHY

The pigmented areas are hypofluorescent, with hyperfluorescence corresponding to the halo and any lacunae (Figure 14.5).

ULTRASONOGRAPHY

Ultrasonography confirms the absence of any thickened lesion.

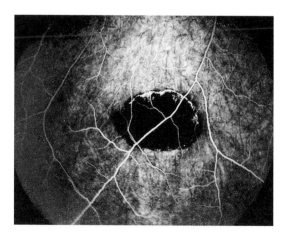

Figure 14.5 Fluorescein angiogram of a CHRPE lesion showing hypofluorescence with a hyperfluorescent halo

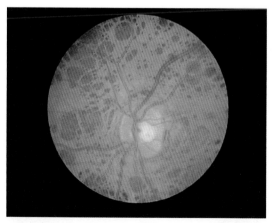

Figure 14.6 Bear tracks

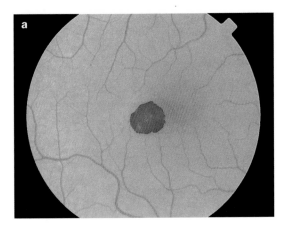

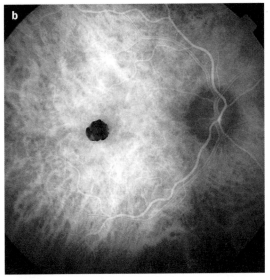

Figure 14.7 Presumed RPE hamartoma: (**a**) colour photograph and (**b**) ICG angiogram. (Courtesy of G. Modorati, Milan, Italy)

DIFFERENTIAL DIAGNOSIS

1. **Grouped pigmentation** or 'bear tracks' of the RPE are multiple, usually clustered in one part of the eye, and without halos or lacunae (Figure 14.6). This abnormality is generally believed not to have any systemic associations (Shields *et al.*, 1992). One study reports autosomal dominant inheritance of bilateral grouped pigmentation in families with a high risk of colonic cancer (Berthemy *et al.*, 1998).
2. **RPE hamartoma** consists of a small, flat deeply pigmented lesion with sharp margins (Figure 14.7). This is a presumed diagnosis (also referred to as congenital RPE hyperplasia).
3. **Choroidal naevi** (Chapter 5).
4. **Inflammatory scars** have irregular margins (Figure 14.8).

SYSTEMIC EVALUATION

The presence of multiple CHRPE lesions in a patient with a family history of FAP or colonic cancer merits referral to a gastroenterologist for screening. If polyposis coli is found to be present, further management will include total colectomy and regular screening for gastroduodenal tumours. The absence of CHRPE lesions does not guarantee that the patient has not inherited the gene.

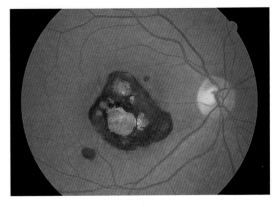

Figure 14.8 Inflammatory scarring at right macula

REFERENCES

Berthemy, S., Romanet, J.P. and Mouillon, M. (1998) Bilateral bear tracks hypertrophy of the retinal pigment and familial adenomatous polyposis. *Ophthal. Res.*, **30** (Suppl 1), 57.

Boldrey, E.E. and Schwartz, A. (1982) Enlargement of congenital hypertrophy of the retinal pigment epithelium. *Am. J. Ophthalmol.*, **94**, 64–6.

Buettner, H. (1994) Congenital hypertrophy of the retinal pigment epithelium. In: S.J. Ryan (ed.), *Retina*. St Louis: Mosby, Vol. 1, Ch. 35, pp. 685–90.

Cleary, P.E., Gregor, Z.J. and Bird, A.C. (1976) Retinal vascular changes in congenital hypertrophy of the retinal pigment epithelium. *Br. J. Ophthalmol.*, **60**, 499–503.

Romania, A., Zakov, Z.N., McGannon, E., Schroeder, T., Heyen, F. and Jagelman, D.G. (1989) Congenital hypertrophy of the retinal pigment epithelium in familial adenomatous polyposis. *Ophthalmology*, **96**, 879–84.

Shields, J.A. and Shields, C.L. (1999) *Tumors and Related Lesions of the Retinal Pigment Epithelium*. Philadelphia: Lippincott, Williams & Wilkins, p. 294.

Shields, J.A., Shields, C.L., Shah, P.G., Pastore, D.J. and Imperiale, S.M. Jr. (1992) Lack of association among typical congenital hypertrophy of the retinal pigment epithelium, adenomatous polyposis, and Gardner syndrome. *Ophthalmology*, **99**, 1709–13.

Wirz, K., Lee, W.R. and Coaker, T. (1982) Progressive changes in congenital hypertrophy of the retinal pigment epithelium. *Graefes Arch. Clin. Exp. Ophthalmol.*, **219**, 214–21.

Chapter 15

Combined hamartoma of the retina and retinal pigment epithelium

Combined hamartoma of the retina and retinal pigment epithelium (RPE) is uncommon. It usually occurs in the juxtapapillary region but may be located in the peripheral fundus. Presentation is usually in early adult life but can be at any age, including infancy.

PATHOLOGY

The lesion consists of glial cells, blood vessels and RPE cells, which tend to invade the retina (Font *et al.,* 1989). Contracture causes wrinkling of the retina, macular oedema and, rarely, retinoschisis, retinal tears and detachment.

This tumour is believed to be a hamartoma, although it could be a malformation or a reactive process (Olsen *et al.,* 1999). There seems to be an association with neurofibromatosis type 2 (Eliott and Schachat, 1994).

SYMPTOMS

a. Visual loss, due to involvement of the optic nerve or fovea by the lesion, retinal contraction, or neovascular membrane formation.
b. Floaters, due to vitreous haemorrhage.

SIGNS

Juxtapapillary lesion (Schachat *et al.,* 1984; Font *et al.,* 1989; Eliott and Schachat, 1994)

- Grey/brown hyperpigmentation (Figure 15.1).
- Slight elevation.
- Wrinkling of the retina, with tortuosity of the retinal blood vessels (Figure 15.1).
- Superficial, white, glial tissue (Figure 15.2).
- Intraretinal hard exudates and oedema.
- Optic disc malformation (Figure 15.2).
- Progressive enlargement (Font *et al.,* 1989).

Peripheral lesion (Schachat *et al.,* 1984; Font *et al.,* 1989; Eliott and Schachat, 1994)

- Linear ridge.
- Stretching of blood vessels peripheral to ridge.

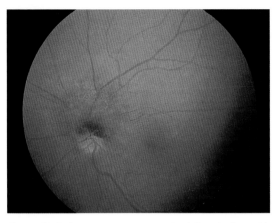

Figure 15.1 Hamartoma superior to the left optic disc, with hyperpigmentation, vascular tortuosity and retinal folds extending to fovea

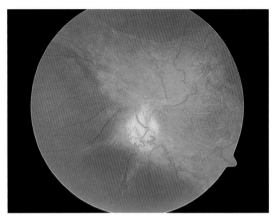

Figure 15.2 Hamartoma superior to the left optic disc, showing retinal gliosis and malformation of the optic disc

COMPLICATIONS

- Choroidal neovascularization at the margin of the lesion, perhaps with vitreous haemorrhage.
- Strabismus, due to poor vision and amblyopia in children.
- An afferent pupillary defect, if the optic nerve is abnormal.

INVESTIGATIONS

FLUORESCEIN ANGIOGRAPHY

Distorted blood vessels are clearly visible against the hypofluorescent pigmentation (Figure 15.3). There is delayed fluid leakage from these abnormal vessels and from any neovascular membrane, if this is present.

DIFFERENTIAL DIAGNOSIS

1. **Choroidal naevus** may be associated with a neovascular membrane, but does not usually cause retinal contraction.
2. **Melanoma** may be mimicked by apparent growth (Font *et al.,* 1989).
3. **Epiretinal membrane** may closely resemble combined hamartoma, especially if pigmented (Robertson and Buettner, 1977), but is preretinal and therefore removable surgically.
4. **Retinopathy of prematurity** may resemble a peripheral lesion.

MANAGEMENT

Children with amblyopia may benefit from occlusion of the fellow eye. Cryotherapy to a peripheral lesion may prevent recurrence of troublesome vitreous haemorrhage. Epiretinal membrane sur-

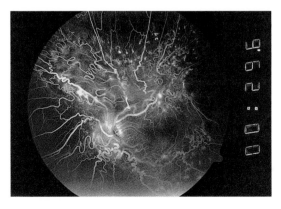

Figure 15.3 Fluorescein angiogram of the same eye as Figure 15.2, showing vascular tortuosity

gery may occasionally improve vision (Schachat *et al.,* 1984).

REFERENCES

Eliott, D. and Schachat, A.P. (1994) Combined hamartoma of the retina and retinal pigment epithelium. In: S.J. Ryan (ed.), *Retina*. St Louis: Mosby, Vol. 1, Ch. 36, pp. 691–7.

Font, R.L., Moura, R.A., Shetlar, D.J., Martinez, J.A. and McPherson, A.R. (1989) Combined hamartoma of sensory retina and retinal pigment epithelium. *Retina*, **9**, 302–11.

Olsen, T.W., Frayer, W.C., Myers, F.L., Davis, M.D. and Albert, D.M. (1999) Idiopathic reactive hyperplasia of the retinal pigment epithelium. *Arch. Ophthalmol.*, **117**, 50–4.

Robertson, D.M. and Buettner, H. (1977) Pigmented pre-retinal membranes. *Am. J. Ophthalmol.*, **83**, 824–9.

Schachat, A.P., Shields, J.A., Fine, S.L., Sanborn, G.E., Weingeist, T.A., Valenzuela, R.A., Brucker, A.J. and The Macular Society Research Committee (1984) Combined hamartomas of the retina and retinal pigment epithelium. *Ophthalmology*, **91**, 1609–15.

Chapter 16

Intraocular cysts

Primary intraocular cysts are usually asymptomatic, being detected on routine examination.

PATHOLOGY

1. **Primary cysts** (Lois *et al.,* 1998b) may occur in the following locations:
   a. Iris pigment epithelium, at the pupil margin (i.e., 'iris flocculi'), mid-zonal iris region, or iridociliary angle.
   b. Non-pigmented ciliary epithelium, particularly the pars plana.
   c. Iris stroma, where they are lined with stratified epithelium with goblet cells (Capo *et al.,* 1993; Lois *et al.,* 1998c).
2. **Secondary (implantation) cysts** form as a result of epithelial downgrowth, either following trauma or surgery, such as amniocentesis (Rummelt *et al.,* 1993).

Many normal eyes have sub-clinical iridociliary cysts, mostly inferiorly and temporally (Kunimatsu *et al.,* 1999). Asymptomatic pars plana cysts are common. They can also occur in association with multiple myeloma (Baker and Spencer, 1974).

Free floating vitreous cysts are rare and can arise in a variety of ways (e.g., ciliary epithelium, adenoma, medulloepithelioma, or embryonic remnants) (Nork and Millecchia, 1998).

SYMPTOMS

Cysts are usually asymptomatic, being detected on routine examination, although some patients complain of pain or blurred vision. Complications occur in a minority of patients and include cataract, lens subluxation, uveitis and secondary glaucoma from angle closure or pigment dispersion.

SIGNS

PUPILLARY MARGIN CYSTS

- Solitary or multiple.
- Small.
- Inflated or collapsed (i.e., 'iris flocculi').
- Pigmented.
- Unilateral or bilateral (Figure 16.1).

A family has been reported in which autosomal dominant iris flocculi have been associated with fatal, dissecting aortic aneurysm (Lewis and Merin, 1995).

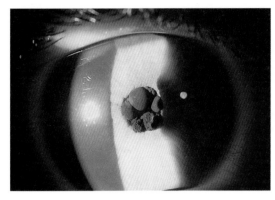

Figure 16.1 Pupil margin cysts. (Courtesy of N. Lois, J.A. Shields and C.L. Shields, Philadelphia, USA)

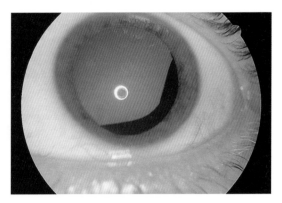

Figure 16.2 Mid-zonal cyst, which wobbled on eye movement

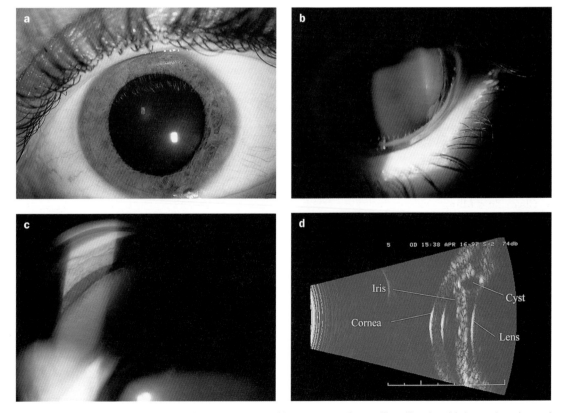

Figure 16.3 Iridociliary cyst: (**a**) bulging of the peripheral iris, (**b**) appearance after pupillary dilatation, (**c**) three-mirror view and (**d**) high-frequency ultrasonography

MID-ZONAL CYSTS

- Location between the iris and lens (Figure 16.2).
- Smooth.
- Brown.
- Fusiform shape, which alters with mydriasis.
- Wobbling of the cyst with eye movements.
- Mostly inferotemporal.
- Multiple, small cysts in other meridians of the same eye, usually.
- Sometimes bilateral, but asymmetrical.

IRIDOCILIARY CYSTS

- Bulge in the peripheral iris (Figure 16.3**a**).
- Inferotemporal location.
- Strong female preponderance.
- Usually visible if the pupil is maximally dilated (Figure 16.3**b**) especially with three-mirror examination (Figure 16.3**c**).
- Pigmented or transparent.
- Dislodged in some cases, either floating freely in the anterior chamber or vitreous or settling in the anterior chamber angle (Figure 16.4).

STROMAL IRIS CYSTS

- Detection mostly in children, usually in infancy (Figure 16.5).
- Atrophy of the overlying iris tissue.
- Inferotemporal location.
- Clear fluid-filling cyst, occasionally with a fluid-debris level.
- Slow growth in adults but more rapid enlargement in children.
- Complications, such as poor vision, amblyopia, corneal touch, band keratopathy, subluxated lens, cataract (Lois *et al.*, 1998c), and secondary 'mucogenic' glaucoma (Albert *et al.*, 1992).

SECONDARY (IMPLANTATION) CYSTS

- Transparent if filled with clear fluid, or pearly white if filled with keratin debris (Figure 16.6).
- Visible superficial scar in some cases.

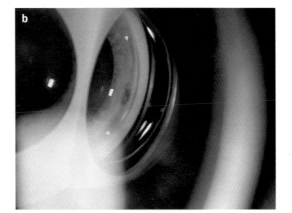

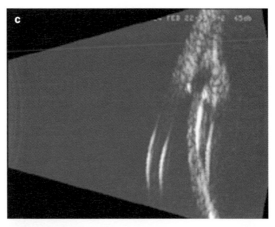

Figure 16.4 Migratory cyst wedged in angle: (**a**) slitlamp view, (**b**) three-mirror view and (**c**) high-frequency ultrasonography

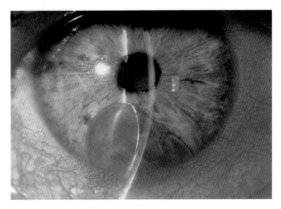

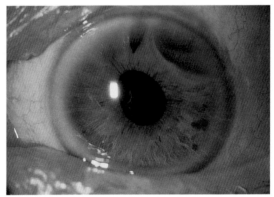

Figure 16.5 Stromal cyst. (Courtesy of N. Lois, C.L. Shields and J.A. Shields, Philadelphia, USA)

Figure 16.6 Implantation cyst after lens extraction

INVESTIGATIONS

TRANSILLUMINATION

Retroillumination with the slitlamp will often show pigmented cysts to transilluminate.

HIGH-FREQUENCY ULTRASONOGRAPHY

Cysts have a dark, echo-free lumen, with bright, echogenic, thin walls (Figure 16.3**d**) (Marigo *et al.*, 1999).

DIFFERENTIAL DIAGNOSIS

1. **Ciliary body melanoma** may be cystic or pseudocystic (Lois *et al.*, 1998a) (Figure 16.7) (Chapter 7).
2. **Cavitary ciliary body melanocytoma** containing cystoid spaces (Chapter 6).
3. **Iris melanoma** can be associated with an adjacent cyst (Figures 1.9 and 16.8) (Chapter 7).
4. **Medulloepithelioma** (Chapter 18).
5. **Lacrimal gland choristoma** of the ciliary body may contain large cysts (Rowley and Karwatowski, 1997).

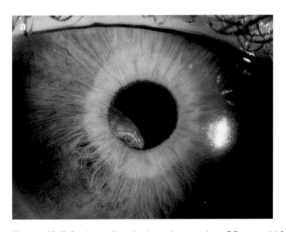

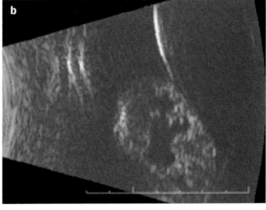

Figure 16.7 Cavitary ciliary body melanoma in a 36-year-old female: (**a**) colour photograph and (**b**) high-frequency ultrasonography. The patient underwent iridocyclectomy and adjunctive plaque radiotherapy with retention of vision of 6/9

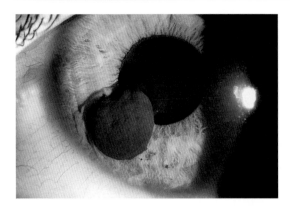

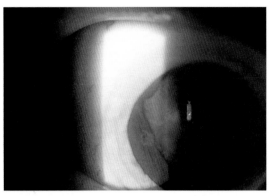

Figure 16.8 Iris melanoma with adjacent cyst in a 26-year-old female (see Figure 1.9 for ultrasonography). The cyst regressed after proton beam radiotherapy and the patient retained vision of 6/6 2 years after treatment

Figure 16.9 Rupture of mid-zonal cyst by argon laser photocoagulation. This was performed in an (unsuccessful) attempt to prevent the progression of pre-existing cataract. Subsequent lens extraction was uncomplicated

6. **Adenoma of the iris pigment epithelium** (Shields *et al.,* 1985).
7. **Lens coloboma** can be mimicked by lens indentation by a transparent cyst.
8. **Miotic-induced iris cysts**, which occur in children after prolonged use of strong miotics without concurrent phenylephrine (Chin *et al.,* 1964).

MANAGEMENT

a. Primary epithelial cysts are observed unless symptomatic, in which case they can be ruptured with argon or Nd-YAG laser photocoagulation (Figure 16.9).

b. Stromal iris cysts can be collapsed by needle aspiration and destroyed with cryotherapy (Lois *et al.,* 1998c). Recurrence can occur, making repeated treatment necessary. Local excision is another approach (Paridaens *et al.,* 1992; Rummelt and Naumann, 1992).

c. Implantation cysts are treated by local resection, taking special care not to rupture the cyst, possibly aspirating some of the contents with a fine needle passed through an area where the cyst is attached to the eye wall. The resection is performed either with full-thickness scleral excision and a tectonic graft, or using a lamellar flap (Figure 16.10) (Chapter 24).

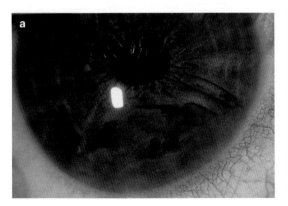

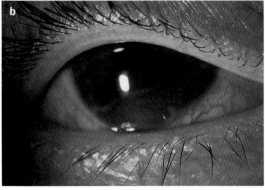

Figure 16.10 Inferior iris cyst in the right eye of a 47-year-old male: (**a**) preoperatively and (**b**) after local resection, when the vision was 6/9

REFERENCES

Albert, D.L., Brownstein, S. and Kattleman, B.S. (1992) Mucogenic glaucoma caused by an epithelial cyst of the iris stroma. *Am. J. Ophthalmol.*, **114**, 222–4.

Baker, T.R. and Spencer, W.H. (1974) Ocular findings in multiple myeloma. A report on two cases. *Arch. Ophthalmol.*, **91**, 110–13.

Capo, H., Palmer, E. and Nicholson, D.H. (1993) Congenital cysts of the iris stroma. *Am. J. Ophthalmol.*, **116**, 228–32.

Chin, N.B., Gold, A. and Breinin, G.M. (1964) Iris cysts and miotics. *Arch. Ophthalmol.*, **71**, 611–16.

Kunimatsu, S., Araie, M., Ohara, K. and Hamada, C. (1999) Ultrasound biomicroscopy of ciliary body cysts. *Am. J. Ophthalmol.*, **127**, 48–55.

Lewis, R.A. and Merin, L.M. (1995) Iris flocculi and familial aortic dissection. *Arch. Ophthalmol.*, **113**, 1330–1.

Lois, N., Shields, C.L., Shields, J.A., Eagle, R.C. Jr. and De Potter, P. (1998a) Cavitary melanoma of the ciliary body. A study of eight cases. *Ophthalmology*, **105**, 1091–8.

Lois, N., Shields, C.L., Shields, J.A. and Mercado, G. (1998b) Primary cysts of the iris pigment epithelium. Clinical features and natural course in 234 patients. *Ophthalmology*, **105**, 1879–85.

Lois, N., Shields, C.L., Shields, J.A., Mercado, G. and De Potter, P. (1998c) Primary iris stromal cysts. A report of 17 cases. *Ophthalmology*, **105**, 1317–22.

Marigo, F.A., Esaki, K., Finger, P.T., Ishikawa, H., Greenfield, D.S., Liebman, J.M. and Ritch, R. (1999) Differential diagnosis of anterior segment cysts by ultrasound biomicroscopy. *Ophthalmology*, **106**, 2131–5.

Nork, T.M. and Millecchia, L.L. (1998) Treatment and histopathology of a congenital vitreous cyst. *Ophthalmology*, **105**, 825–30.

Paridaens, A.D.A., Deuble, K. and McCartney, A.C.E. (1992) Spontaneous congenital non-pigmented epithelial cysts of the iris stroma. *Br. J. Ophthalmol.*, **76**, 39–42.

Rowley, S.A. and Karwatowski, W.S.S. (1997) Lacrimal gland choristoma of the ciliary body. *Arch. Ophthalmol.*, **115**, 1482–3.

Rummelt, V. and Naumann, G.O.H. (1992) Block excision of congenital and infantile nonpigmented epithelial iris cysts. Report on eight infants. *Ger. J. Ophthalmol.*, **1**, 361–6.

Rummelt, V., Rummelt, C. and Naumann, G.O.H. (1993) Congential nonpigmented epithelial iris cyst after amniocentesis. Clinicopathological report on two children. *Ophthalmology*, **100**, 776–81.

Shields, C.L., Shields, J.A., Cook, G.R., Von Fricken, M.A. and Augsburger, J.J. (1985) Differentiation of adenoma of the iris pigment epithelium from iris cyst and melanoma. *Am. J. Ophthalmol.*, **100**, 678–81.

Chapter 17

Adenoma and adenocarcinoma

Adenomas and adenocarcinomas can occur in the pigment epithelium of the iris, ciliary body or retina and in the non-pigmented ciliary epithelium (Ts'o and Albert, 1972; Folberg, 1994; Shields *et al.*, 1996).

Although asymptomatic adenomas are common, adenocarcinomas are very rare. They are often clinically misdiagnosed as melanoma. The histological diagnosis of these tumours can also be difficult.

PATHOLOGY

   a. Variable cellular patterns (Figure 17.1).
   b. Mucopolysaccharide in cytoplasmic vacuoles and extracellular matrix in ciliary body tumours.
   c. Hyaline stroma.
   d. Tumour necrosis.
   e. Osseous metaplasia.

The usual histological signs of malignancy (i.e., mitotic rate, cellular pleomorphism, and invasion) do not always allow differentiation between adenoma and adenocarcinoma.

The prognosis for survival is good if the tumour is localized within the eye (Edelstein *et al.*, 1998).

If there is extraocular extension, the patient can die as a result of intracranial invasion or metastatic disease (Laver *et al.*, 1999).

SYMPTOMS

Patients may have an asymptomatic tumour detected on routine examination, or may present with deterioration of vision caused by lens changes or retinal abnormality.

SIGNS

IRIS PIGMENT EPITHELIUM

- Small, pigmented lesion having a smooth or multinodular surface, developing on the posterior iris surface or in the angle (Shields *et al.*, 1999).
- Pigment scatter causing secondary glaucoma (Shields and Shields, 1999).

PIGMENTED CILIARY EPITHELIUM

- Dark grey or black tumour in the ciliary body (Shields *et al.*, 1996), perhaps with invasion of

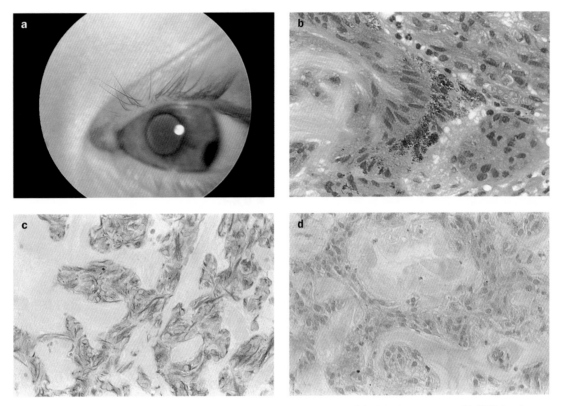

Figure 17.1 Pigmented adenocarcinoma of the left iris in an 11-year-old boy: (**a**) clinical appearance, (**b**) H&E showing a mixed cellular pattern, (**c**) positive staining CAM 5.2 for epithelial peptides and (**d**) negative staining with HMB-45 for melanoma

the anterior chamber and, unusually, the corneal endothelium (Figure 17.2).

- Multinodular appearance in some cases.
- Cyst formation in the adjacent ciliary body.
- Complications such as pigment scatter, indentation and subluxation of the lens, cataract, vitreous seeding and vitreous haemorrhage.

NON-PIGMENTED CILIARY EPITHELIUM
(Shields *et al.*, 1996)

- White or light brown colour.
- Irregular shape.
- Complications including (a) subluxation and indentation of the lens, (b) cataract, (c) cells and flare in the anterior chamber and vitreous, (d) extraocular extension (Rodrigues *et al.*, 1988) resulting in proptosis and/or epibulbar

tumour (Laver *et al.*, 1999) and (e) tumour necrosis resulting in endophthalmitis and orbital cellulitis.

Many ciliary epithelial adenocarcinomas develop in blind, traumatized eyes (Laver *et al.*, 1999).

Consider adenocarcinoma if a blind, disorganized eye develops proptosis or an epibulbar mass.

RETINAL PIGMENT EPITHELIUM

- Black colour, although some are dark brown or amelanotic (Shields *et al.*, 1999b).
- Steep and distinct margins (Figure 17.3).
- Slow growth of adenomas (Loose *et al.*, 1999).

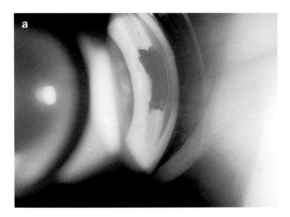

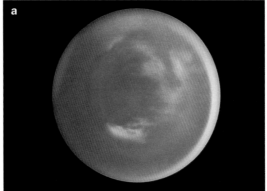

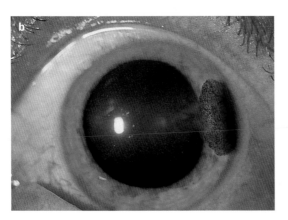

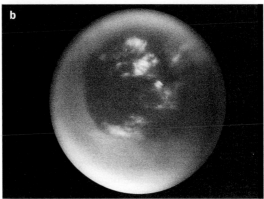

Figure 17.3 Adenocarcinoma of the retinal pigment epithelium of the right eye of a 50-year-old man treated by trans-scleral local resection. (Courtesy of W.S. Foulds, Glasgow, UK)

- Invasion of sensory retina.
- Dilated retinal feeder vessels (Shields *et al.*, 1999b).
- Complications such as haemorrhage, exudative retinal detachment, phthisis, and extraocular extension.
- Vitreous seeding.

INVESTIGATIONS

Adenomas and adenocarcinomas tend to be diagnosed histologically, after local resection or enucleation for suspected melanoma. Fine needle aspiration biopsy can be useful in selected cases if there are doubts about performing local resection.

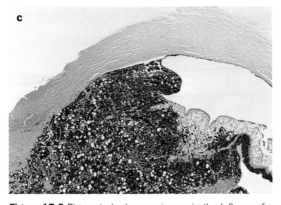

Figure 17.2 Pigmented adenocarcinoma in the left eye of a 72-year-old female: (**a**) three-mirror examination showing the tumour arising in the ciliary body and invading the anterior chamber, (**b**) slitlamp view, showing Pagetoid spread of the tumour across the corneal endothelium and (**c**) light micrograph showing the pigmented nature of the tumour, the presence of microcysts and the spread along the corneal endothelium (H&E)

DIFFERENTIAL DIAGNOSIS

1. **An exaggerated reactive RPE hyperplasia** can occur in RPE scars (e.g. after the presumed ocular histoplasmosis syndrome). There may not be a positive history of ocular disease (Jampel *et al.,* 1986).
2. **Amelanotic melanoma and benign tumours of the ciliary body** are usually covered by pigment epithelium and have a smooth surface.
3. **Medulloepithelioma** (Chapter 18).
4. **Epibulbar squamous cell carcinoma** may resemble a non-pigmented ciliary epithelial adenocarcinoma with extraocular extension.
5. **Choroidal melanoma** has more indistinct margins (Chapter 7).
6. **Melanocytoma** may resemble a juxtapapillary or ciliary body tumour of the pigmented epithelium.
7. **Fuchs' adenoma** is a benign hyperplasia of the non-pigmented ciliary epithelium (Iliff and Green, 1972). This white tumour is common, but usually sub-clinical, having a diameter of less than 5 mm and a thickness of about 1 mm (Figure 17.4). Rarely, it is large enough to mimic melanoma.

MANAGEMENT

Observation has been recommended by some authorities, but others prefer to perform an excisional biopsy, which usually consists of iridocyclectomy (Chapter 24).

REFERENCES

Edelstein, C., Shields, C.L., Shields, J.A. and Eagle, R.C. Jr (1998) Presumed adenocarcinoma of the retinal pigment epithelium in a blind eye with a staphyloma. *Arch. Ophthalmol.,* **116**, 525–8.

Folberg, R. (1994) Other tumors of the retinal pigment epithelium. In: S.J. Ryan (ed.), *Retina.* St Louis: Mosby, Vol. 1, Ch. 37, pp. 698–700.

Iliff, W.J. and Green, W.R. (1972) The incidence and histology of Fuchs' adenoma. *Arch. Ophthalmol.,* **88**, 249–54.

Jampel, H.D., Schachat, A.P., Conway, B., Shaver, R.P., Coston, T.O., Isernhagen, R. and Green, W.R. (1986) Retinal pigment epithelial hyperplasia assuming

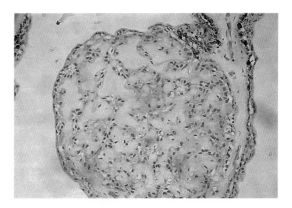

Figure 17.4 Light micrograph of a Fuchs' adenoma. (Courtesy of P. Hiscott, Liverpool, UK)

tumor-like proportions. Report of two cases. *Retina,* **6**, 105–12.

Laver, N.M., Hidayat, A.A. and Croxatto, J.O. (1999) Pleomorphic adenocarcinomas of the ciliary epithelium. Immunohistochemical and ultrastructural features of 12 cases. *Ophthalmology,* **106**, 103–10.

Loose, I.A., Jampol, L.M. and O'Grady, R. (1999) Pigmented adenoma mimicking a juxtapapillary melanoma. *Arch. Ophthalmol.,* **117**, 120–2.

Rodrigues, M., Hidayat, A. and Karesh, J. (1988) Pleomorphic adenocarcinoma of ciliary epithelium simulating an epibulbar tumor. *Am. J. Ophthalmol.,* **106**, 595–600.

Shields, J.A., Eagle, R.C. Jr, Shields, C.L. and De Potter, P. (1996) Acquired neoplasms of the nonpigmented ciliary epithelium (adenoma and adenocarcinoma). *Ophthalmology,* **103**, 2007–16.

Shields, J.A. and Shields, C.L. (1999) *Atlas of Intraocular Tumors.* Philadelphia: Lippincott, Williams & Wilkins, pp. 300–7 and 316–21.

Shields, J.A., Shields, C.L., Gündüz, K. and Eagle, R.C. Jr. (1999a) Adenoma of the ciliary body epithelium. The 1998 Albert Ruedemann Sr, Memorial Lecture, Part 1. *Arch. Ophthalmol.,* **117**, 592–7.

Shields, J.A., Shields, C.L., Gündüz, K. and Eagle, R.C. Jr. (1999b) Neoplasms of the retinal pigment epithelium. The 1998 Albert Ruedemann Sr, Memorial Lecture, Part 2. *Arch. Ophthalmol.,* **117**, 601–8.

Shields, J.A., Shields, C.L., Mercado, G., Gündüz, K. and Eagle, R.C. Jr. (1999) Adenoma of the iris pigment epithelium: a report of 20 cases. The 1998 Pan-American lecture. *Arch. Ophthalmol.,* **117**, 736–41.

Ts'o, M.O.M. and Albert, D.M. (1972) Pathological condition of the retinal pigment epithelium: neoplasms and nodular non-neoplastic lesions. *Arch. Ophthalmol.,* **88**, 27–38.

Chapter 18

Medulloepithelioma

Medulloepithelioma, previously called 'diktyoma', is a rare, congenital tumour arising from the inner layer of the optic cup (i.e., medullary epithelium). It usually presents in childhood but can become manifest in adulthood (Broughton and Zimmerman, 1978; Canning *et al.,* 1988; Shields *et al.,* 1996; Husain *et al.,* 1998).

PATHOLOGY

a. Cords and sheets of nonpigmented and pigmented epithelial cells (Figure 18.1a)

(Wakakura and Lee, 1990). Malignant medulloepitheliomas may be histologically indistinguishable from retinoblastoma.

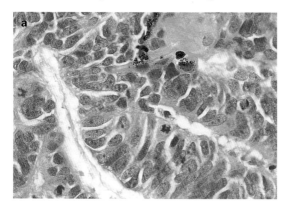

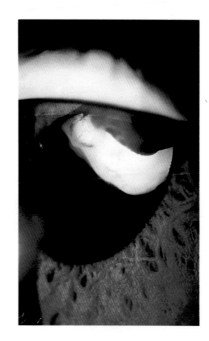

Figure 18.1 Superotemporal medulloepithelioma in the left eye of a seven-year-old boy: (**a**) light micrograph showing sheets of epithelial cells (H&E) (courtesy of W.R. Lee, Glasgow, UK) and (**b**) clinical photograph showing a white ciliary body tumour

b. Cystic spaces filled with hyaluronic acid and undifferentiated neuroblastic cells.
c. Heterologous tissues such as cartilage, brain tissue and striated muscle in some cases (i.e., 'teratoid medulloepithelioma') (Zimmerman *et al.*, 1972).

Most medulloepitheliomas are malignant. They can eventually fill the eye and extend extraocularly. Death can occur as a result of intracranial invasion or, rarely, metastatic disease (Broughton and Zimmerman, 1978).

PRESENTATION

a. Visual loss.
b. Pain or photophobia.
c. Ciliary body or anterior chamber mass.
d. Leukocoria.
e. Proptosis in advanced cases.

SIGNS

- White, pink, yellow or brown colour (Figure 18.2).
- Lens coloboma, due to the absence of zonules in the affected quadrant.
- Rubeosis.
- Solid or polycystic mass.
- Free floating cysts, which may settle in the anterior chamber or vitreous.
- Sheet-like tumour growth behind the lens, resembling a cyclitic membrane.

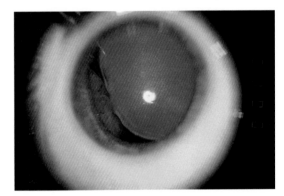

Figure 18.2 Lightly pigmented polycystic medullo-epithelioma. (Courtesy of J.A. Shields and C.L. Shields, Philadelphia, USA)

- Grey-white opacities, like chalk particles, consisting of cartilage (Shields *et al.*, 1996).

COMPLICATIONS

- Glaucoma, perhaps with buphthalmos, as a result of anterior displacement of the lens-iris diaphragm, rubeosis, or neoplastic invasion of the trabecular meshwork.
- Cataract.
- Retinal detachment.

DIFFERENTIAL DIAGNOSIS

1. **Retinoblastoma** may have similar features both clinically and histologically, but is rarely located so far anteriorly (Chapter 13).
2. **Glioneuroma** is a very rare choristoma consisting of disorganized retinal and neural tissue and arising at the anterior margin of the optic nerve cup, usually in association with a coloboma. The tumour presents at birth or infancy in most cases (Addison and Font, 1984). Clinically, there is a white, anterior chamber mass, usually inferotemporally, which can extend extraocularly.
3. **Lacrimal gland choristoma** (Klüppel *et al.*, 1999) usually presents in infancy as a pink mass. Cysts may be visible and may enlarge, mimicking growth. Intrascleral involvement is often present and the overlying episclera may appear pigmented.
4. **Metastasis** to eye.
5. **Ciliary body melanoma** might be the erroneous diagnosis if the medulloepithelioma presents in adulthood as a pigmented tumour (Husain *et al.*, 1998). The MRI features of the two types of tumour are similar.

MANAGEMENT

Small tumours can be observed, unless there is documented growth. Localized lesions may be treated by local resection, although there is a high risk of recurrence. Diffuse, large or recurrent tumours may require enucleation. Exenteration may be indicated if there is orbital extension.

PROGNOSIS

Most eyes are enucleated, often because the correct diagnosis was not made clinically. A small number of patients die of their disease, usually because of intracranial spread (Broughton and Zimmerman, 1978).

REFERENCES

Addison, D.J. and Font, R.L. (1984) Glioneuroma of iris and ciliary body. *Arch. Ophthalmol.*, **102**, 419–21.

Broughton, W.L. and Zimmerman, L.E. (1978) A clinico-pathologic study of 56 cases of intraocular medulloepitheliomas. *Am. J. Ophthalmol.*, **85**, 407–18.

Canning, C.R., McCartney, A.C.E. and Hungerford, J. (1988) Medulloepithelioma (diktyoma) *Br. J. Ophthalmol.*, **72**, 764–7.

Husain, S.E., Husain, N., Boniuk, M. and Font, R.L. (1998) Malignant nonteratoid medulloepithelioma of the ciliary body in an adult. *Ophthalmology*, **105**, 596–9.

Klüppel, M., Müller, W. and Sundmacher, R. (1999) Lacrimal gland choristoma of the iris. *Arch. Ophthalmol.*, **117**, 110–11.

Shields, J.A., Eagle, R.C. Jr, Shields, C.L. and De Potter, P. (1996) Congenital neoplasms of the nonpigmented ciliary epithelium (medulloepithelioma) *Ophthalmology*, **103**, 1998–2006.

Wakakura, M. and Lee, W.R. (1990) Ultrastructural pleomorphism in medulloepithelioma of the ciliary body: a comparative study of tumour cells and fetal ciliary epithelium. *Jpn J. Ophthalmol.*, **34**, 364–80.

Zimmerman, L.E., Font, R.L. and Andersen, S.R. (1972) Rhabdomyosarcomatous differentiation in malignant intraocular medulloepitheliomas. *Cancer*, **30**, 817–35.

SYSTEMIC TUMOURS

Chapter 19

Ocular metastasis

Metastasis is the commonest type of intraocular malignancy but is usually microscopic or unrecognized clinically, either because of the patient's poor general health (Bloch and Gartner, 1971; Eliassi-Rad *et al.,* 1996) or because it is asymptomatic (Wiegel *et al.,* 1999).

EPIDEMIOLOGY

The primary sites and their approximate frequencies (Ferry and Font, 1974; Wharam *et al.,* 1994; Shields *et al.,* 1997) depend on the patient's sex:

a. In females, metastases arise in breast (70–80%), lung (10%), at an unknown site (10%) and at other sites (<1% each) .
b. In males, the primary site is lung (40–60%), unknown (25%) and other (10%).

Rare sources include gastrointestinal tract, prostate (Keizur *et al.,* 1995), pancreas (Castillo *et al.,* 1995), kidney (Kindermann *et al.,* 1981), testis, cutaneous melanoma (Bell *et al.,* 1995), thyroid (Ainsworth *et al.,* 1992) and carcinoid (Harbour *et al.,* 1994; Fan *et al.,* 1995).

Presentation with ocular metastasis before the diagnosis and treatment of the primary tumour occurs in about 10% of patients with breast carcinoma and in more than 50% of patients with lung and renal cancers.

PATHOLOGY

Metastases usually occur in the post-equatorial choroid, but can develop in the ciliary body, iris, optic disc, retina, vitreous and conjunctiva. They tend to grow rapidly, with uveal tumours not allowing the overlying retinal pigment epithelium to proliferate, so that their amelanotic nature can be recognized ophthalmoscopically.

SYMPTOMS

a. Visual loss, due to macular involvement, exudative retinal detachment or subluxation of the lens.
b. Photopsia.
c. Pain, which is most common in patients with metastases from lung cancer.
d. Floaters.

SIGNS

CHOROID AND CILIARY BODY

- Placoid or slightly domed shape (Figure 19.1).
- Oval or irregular margins.
- Indistinct edges.
- Yellow or white colour, except for carcinoid, renal and thyroid secondaries, which can be light brown or orange (Figure 19.2), and cutaneous melanomas, which can be brown or black.
- Severely atrophic RPE, perhaps with black clumps of residual pigment and 'orange pigment'.
- Absence of large tumour vessels.

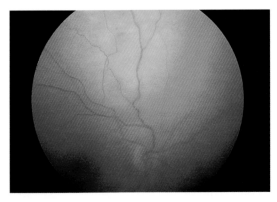

Figure 19.1 Superior choroidal metastasis from breast carcinoma in the right eye of a 49-year-old female

- Post-equatorial location.
- Multifocality, in a *minority* of patients (i.e., about 30%).
- Bilaterality in about 30% of patients with breast carcinoma, 20% of patients with lung cancer and 10% of patients with other primaries.

COMPLICATIONS

- Retinal detachment, which tends to be more extensive than expected for a melanoma of a similar size.
- Dilated episcleral vessels, if there is ciliary body involvement.
- Neovascular glaucoma, with advanced disease.
- Cataract.

IRIS

- White colour (Figure 19.3).
- Irregular surface.
- Hyphaema, which occurs frequently.
- Anterior uveitis.
- Pseudohypopyon, in some cases (Shields *et al.*, 1995).

RETINA AND VITREOUS

Retinal metastases are very rare. They form peri-vascular infiltrates, which break through the inner limiting membrane to form vitreous deposits

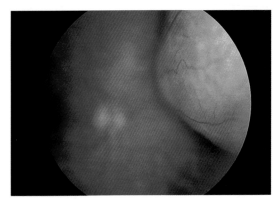

Figure 19.2 Neuroendocrine metastasis in the right eye of a 56-year-old male. The tumour was successfully treated by trans-scleral local resection

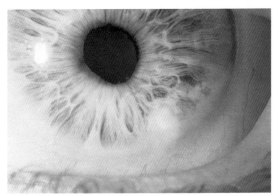

Figure 19.3 Iris metastasis from adenocarcinoma of the lung in the right eye of a 67-year-old male

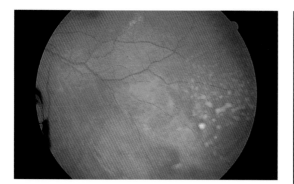

Figure 19.4 Fundus photograph of an early retinal metastasis in a 42-year-old woman with breast carcinoma. Note the perivascular sheathing and vitreous deposits. (Courtesy of A.M. Leys, Leuven, Belgium)(Case report published in *Arch. Ophthalmol.*, 1990, **108**, 1448–52)

(Figure 19.4) or which coalesce to form a confluent intraretinal white mass (Figure 19.5) (Leys *et al.,* 1990).

Cutaneous melanoma can metastasize to the retina and vitreous, to form multiple, round, brown clumps of tumour cells (Robertson *et al.,* 1981) (Figure 19.6). There may also be neovascular glaucoma (Gündüz *et al.,* 1998)

OPTIC DISC

Metastases to the optic disc are rare and tend to be amelanotic with an irregular surface, perhaps

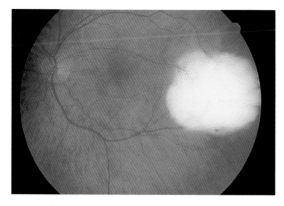

Figure 19.5 Confluent retinal metastasis in a 49-year-old man with small cell carcinoma of the lung. (Courtesy of A.M. Leys, Leuven, Belgium)(Case report published in *Arch. Ophthalmol.*, 1990, **108**, 1448–52)

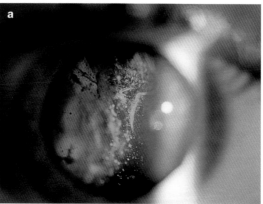

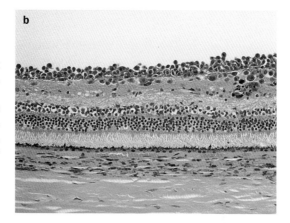

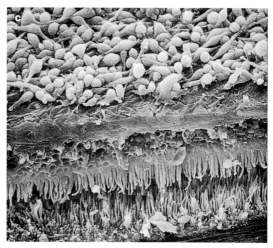

Figure 19.6 Vitreous metastasis from cutaneous melanoma in the right eye of a 38-year-old female: (**a**) slitlamp view, (**b**) light micrograph showing metastatic cells on the inner surface of the retina and (**c**) scanning electron micrograph. (Courtesy of W.R. Lee, Glasgow, UK)

mimicking central retinal vein occlusion, acute ischaemic optic neuropathy, or swelling due to meningioma (Backhouse *et al.,* 1998) (Figure 19.7).

CONJUNCTIVA

Conjunctival metastases are very rare. They can arise from cutaneous melanoma (Kwapiszeski and Savitt, 1997) and other tumours. They tend to occur in the presence of widespread disease (Kiratli *et al.,* 1996).

INVESTIGATIONS

FLUORESCEIN ANGIOGRAPHY

Choroidal metastases show early hypofluorescence with diffuse late staining. A 'dual circulation' does not occur (Figure 19.8).

ICG ANGIOGRAPHY

With choroidal metastases there is early hypofluorescence with late isofluorescence (Shields *et al.,* 1995) and less evidence of RPE change than with fluorescein angiography (Harino *et al.,* 1995) (Figure 19.9).

ULTRASONOGRAPHY

Ultrasonography shows moderately high acoustic reflectivity throughout the tumour, which is suggestive but not pathognomonic of metastasis (Figure 19.10). Sequential ultrasonography is useful for documenting response to treatment, but it is important to take account of any overlying retinal detachment.

COMPUTERIZED TOMOGRAPHY

This is not diagnostic but demonstrates the distribution of metastases in the eye and orbit.

MAGNETIC RESONANCE IMAGING

Compared to vitreous, metastases tend to be hyperintense on T1 weighted images and hypo- or isointense on T2 weighted images (De Potter *et al.,*

1995) (Figure 19.11). These features are not diagnostic. Gadolinium enhancement is less marked than with melanoma.

BIOPSY

A biopsy is essential for diagnosis, so a tissue specimen should be obtained either from the primary tumour or from an extraocular metastasis or, if this is not present, from the intraocular tumour.

Fine needle aspiration biopsy (Augsburger, 1988) or incisional biopsy (Isaacs and McAllister, 1995) can be appropriate when the site of the primary tumour is unknown. It is important to obtain enough tissue for immunohistochemistry (Figure 19.12). The following stains can be useful:

a. HMB-45 for melanoma.
b. Cytokeratin for carcinoma.
c. Chromogranin and synaptophysin for carcinoid and other neuroendocrine tumours.
d. Prostate specific antigen for prostatic carcinoma.
e. Human chorionic gonadotrophin (HCG) for germ cell tumour.

DIFFERENTIAL DIAGNOSIS

1. **Choroidal melanoma** (Chapter 7).
2. **Choroidal haemangioma** (Chapter 8).
3. **Choroidal osteoma** (Chapter 9).
4. **Iridocyclitis**, which can be mimicked by metastatic deposits.

Note: Do not assume that an intraocular lesion is a metastasis just because there is a previous history of malignancy; dual pathology is not uncommon.

SYSTEMIC ASSESSMENT

If the site of the extraocular primary tumour is known, investigations are guided by the need for staging.

If the site of the primary tumour is not known, assessment may include the following:

a. Full history and physical examination.
b. Mammography in females.
c. Chest radiography and sputum cytology.

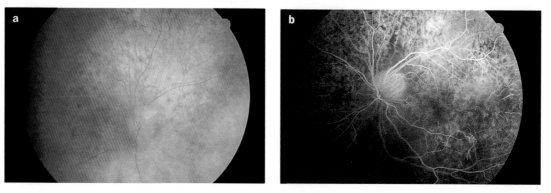

Figure 19.7 Optic disc metastasis in a 48-year-old female with breast carcinoma: (**a**) fundus photograph showing disc swelling and characteristic white 'antlers', (**b**) fluorescein angiogram showing diffuse hyperfluorescence. (Courtesy of A.M. Leys, Leuven, Belgium)

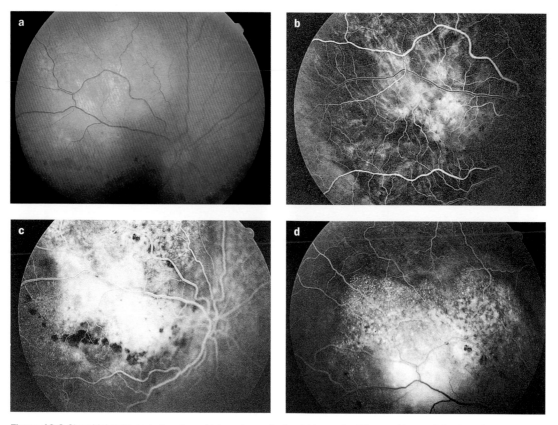

Figure 19.8 Choroidal metastasis from bronchial carcinoma in the right eye of a 57-year-old man: (**a**) colour photograph and fluorescein angiographs, (**b**) at 21 seconds showing generalized hypofluorescence with early hyperfluorescence centrally, (**c**) at 44 seconds showing diffuse hyperfluorescence with masking by residual pigment epithelium and (**d**) at 272 seconds showing persistent hyperfluorescence with drusen near the margins of the tumour

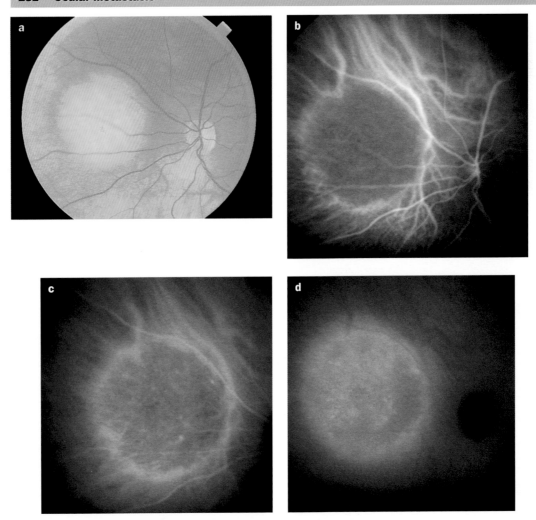

Figure 19.9 Nasal choroidal metastasis in the left eye: (**a**) colour photograph, (**b**) early phase, showing hypofluorescence, (**c**) venous phase, showing persistent hypofluorescence with marginal hyperfluorescence and (**d**) late phase showing diffuse fluorescence. (Courtesy of B.A. Lafaut, Ghent, Brussels)

d. Serum biochemistry, including alkaline phosphatase.
e. Abdominal CT scan.
f. Faecal occult blood (not only for primary gastrointestinal tumours but also for metastases).
g. Urinalysis, for red blood cells.

In all patients, it is important to determine whether other metastases are present in the brain, so that appropriate radiotherapy can be given at the same time. Screening for metastases in weight-bearing bones is also indicated, so that pathological fractures and loss of mobility may be prevented.

TREATMENT OF THE OCULAR TUMOUR

NON-TREATMENT

Some metastases are inactive and if peripheral and asymptomatic may be kept under observation without treatment.

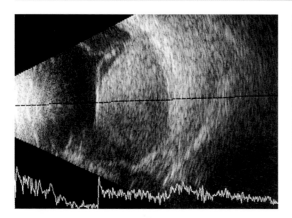

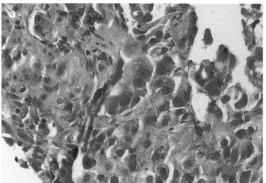

Figure 19.10 A- and B-scan ultrasonography of a choroidal metastasis showing moderately high internal acoustic reflectivity throughout the tumour

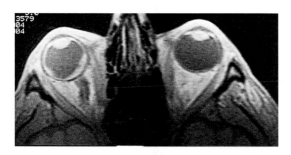

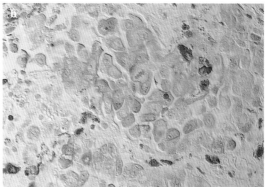

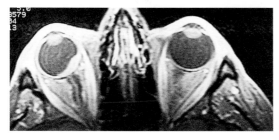

Figure 19.11 MRI scan of a choroidal metastasis from adenocarcinoma of the lung showing axial T1 weighted images with fat suppression technique (**top**) pre-contrast and (**bottom**) post-contrast. (Courtesy of P. De Potter, Brussels, Belgium)

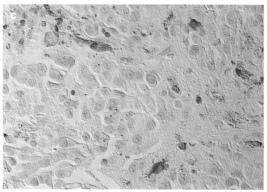

Figure 19.12 Light micrographs of a trans-scleral incisional biopsy of a choroidal metastasis in the right eye of a 59-year-old man: (**a**) H&E, showing amelanotic cells with large nuclei and prominent nucleoli, (**b**) positive staining with CAM 5.2, indicating carcinoma, (**c**) negative staining with HMB-45, virtually excluding melanoma. (Courtesy of P. Hiscott, Liverpool, UK)

SYSTEMIC CHEMOTHERAPY

Some types of tumour, such as breast carcinoma and choriocarcinoma, are likely to be chemosensitive whereas thyroid carcinoma may respond to radioiodine treatment. With these tumours, if the patient is about to receive systemic treatment, it is reasonable to withhold radiotherapy as the intraocular tumour might regress.

EXTERNAL BEAM RADIOTHERAPY

This is indicated for chemoresistant tumours, such as squamous cell ·or large cell carcinoma of the lung, and breast carcinoma after chemotherapy. Treatment is advised if vision is threatened.

Most patients receive a total of 30 Gy, delivered in daily fractions of 3 Gy, four or five days a week (Chapter 23). If the prognosis for survival is good, as in breast carcinoma, then a higher dose is given, such as 45–50 Gy, delivered in 2–2.25 Gy fractions. For unilateral tumours, the external beam radiotherapy is administered using a 4 × 4 cm anterior direct field (Chapter 23). Treatment of both eyes using a lateral beam is indicated for bilateral metastases. Some workers also suggest bilateral treatment for patients with unilateral metastases, to treat any occult metastases in the fellow eye (Tkocz *et al.*, 1997), but this is controversial.

PLAQUE RADIOTHERAPY

If a choroidal metastasis is small and solitary, plaque radiotherapy delivering about 50–70 Gy to the tumour apex may be more convenient for the patient, being completed in about a week (Shields *et al.*, 1997). This treatment can also be useful if there is residual or recurrent tumour after external beam radiotherapy or chemotherapy (Chapter 23).

ENUCLEATION

Enucleation will not improve the prognosis for survival and is indicated only if there is extensive intraocular disease causing a blind, painful eye.

PROGNOSIS

SYSTEMIC

The prognosis for survival averages 3–5 months with lung tumours, 8–12 months with breast carcinoma and several years with carcinoid. Some patients may therefore live long enough to develop radiational complications arising from the treatment of their metastatic tumour.

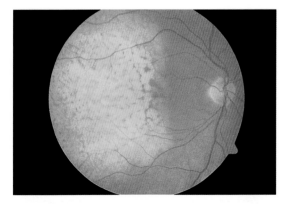

Figure 19.13 Regressed choroidal metastasis after external beam radiotherapy in a 64-year-old woman with breast carcinoma

OCULAR

After radiotherapy, ocular metastases regress completely in most patients, leaving areas of choroidal atrophy with many pigment clumps (Figure 19.13). A good response to radiotherapy is more likely if the history is short (i.e., less than 2 months) and if the tumour is small with minimal retinal detachment. Any visual improvement usually occurs within a few weeks.

Early side-effects include mild lid erythema and temporary visual loss due to retinal oedema. Cataract and radiation retinopathy can develop from the second year onwards. Radiational complications are more likely if the patient is diabetic (Viebahn *et al.*, 1991) or receiving concurrent chemotherapy (Parsons *et al.*, 1994).

Rapid regrowth of the intraocular tumour can occur, especially after chemotherapy, so that patients should be monitored closely.

REFERENCES

Ainsworth, J.R., Damato, B.E., Lee, W.R. and Alexander, W.D. (1992) Follicular thyroid carcinoma metastatic to the iris. *Arch. Ophthalmol.*, **110**, 19–20.

Augsburger, J.J. (1988) Fine needle aspiration biopsy of suspected metastatic cancers to the posterior uvea. *Trans. Am. Ophthalmol. Soc.*, **86**, 499–560.

Backhouse, O., Simmons, I., Frank, A. and Cassels-Brown, A. (1998) Optic nerve breast metastasis mimicking meningioma. *Aust. NZ J. Ophthalmol.*, **26**, 247–9.

Bell, R.W.D., Ironside, J.W., Fleck, B.W. and Singh, J. (1995) Cutaneous malignant melanoma metastatic to the choroid: a clinicopathological case report. *Eye*, **9**, 650–3.

Bloch, R.S. and Gartner, S. (1971) The incidence of ocular metastatic carcinoma. *Arch. Ophthalmol.*, **85**, 673–5.

Castillo, J., Ascaso, F.J., Aguelo, J.M., Minguez, E., Cristóbal, J.A. and Palomar, A. (1995) Métastases choroïdiennes bilatérales d'un carcinome du pancréas. *J. Fr. Ophtalmol.*, **18**, 795–8.

De Potter, P., Shields, J.A. and Shields, C.L. (1995) *MRI of the Eye and Orbit*. Philadelphia: J.B. Lippincott, Ch. 6, pp. 59, 78–82.

Eliassi-Rad, B., Albert, D.M. and Green, W.R. (1996) Frequency of ocular metastases in patients dying of cancer in eye bank populations. *Br. J. Ophthalmol.*, **80**, 125–8.

Fan, J.T., Buettner, H., Bartley, G.B. and Bolling, J.P. (1995) Clinical features and treatment of seven patients with carcinoid tumor metastatic to the eye and orbit. *Am. J. Ophthalmol.*, **119**, 211–18.

Ferry, A.P. and Font, R.L. (1974) Carcinoma metastatic to the eye and orbit. I. A clinicopathological study of 227 cases. *Arch. Ophthalmol.*, **92**, 276–86.

Gündüz, K., Shields, J.A., Shields, C.L. and Eagle, R.C. Jr (1998) Cutaneous melanoma metastatic to the vitreous cavity. *Ophthalmology*, **105**, 600–5.

Harbour, J.W., De Potter, P., Shields, C.L. and Shields, J.A. (1994) Uveal metastasis from carcinoid tumor. Clinical observations in nine cases. *Ophthalmology*, **101**, 1084–90.

Harino, S., Miyamoto, K., Okada, M., Ogawa, K., Saito, Y., Tada, R., Okamoto, N. and Fukuda, M. (1995) Indocyanine green videoangiographic findings in choroidal metastatic tumor. *Graefes Arch. Clin. Exp. Ophthalmol.*, **233**, 339–46.

Isaacs, T.W. and McAllister, I.L. (1995) Adenocarcinoma metastatic to the choroid: diagnosis by trans-scleral biopsy. *Eye*, **9**, 643–7.

Keizur, J.J., Kane, C.J., North, R. and Leidich, R.B. (1995) Adenocarcinoma of the prostate metastatic to the choroid of the eye. *Prostate*, **27**, 336–9.

Kindermann, W.R., Shields, J.A., Eiferman, R.A., Stephens, R.F. and Hirsch, S.E. (1981) Metastatic renal cell carcinoma to the eye and adnexae: a report of three cases and review of the literature. *Ophthalmology*, **88**, 1347–50.

Kiratli, H., Shields, C.L., Shields, J.A. and De Potter, P. (1996) Metastatic tumours to the conjunctiva: report of 10 cases. *Br. J. Ophthalmol.*, **80**, 5–8.

Kwapiszeski, B.R. and Savitt, M.L. (1997) Conjunctival metastasis from a cutaneous melanoma as the initial sign of dissemination. *Am. J. Ophthalmol.*, **123**, 266–8.

Leys, A.M., Van Eyck, L.M., Nuttin, B.J., Pauwels, P.A., Delabie, J.M. and Libert, J.A. (1990) Metastatic carcinoma to the retina. Clinicopathologic findings in two cases. *Arch. Ophthalmol.*, **108**, 1448–52.

Parsons, J.T., Bova, F.J., Fitzgerald, C.R., Mendenhall, W.M. and Million, R.R. (1994) Radiation retinopathy after external-beam irradiation: analysis of time-dose factors. *Int. J. Radiat. Oncol. Biol. Phys.*, **30**, 765–73.

Robertson, D.M., Wilkinson, C.P., Murray, J.L. and Gordy, D.D. (1981) Metastatic tumor to the retina and vitreous cavity from primary melanoma of the skin: treatment with systemic and subconjunctival chemotherapy. *Ophthalmology*, **88**, 1296–301.

Shields, C.L., Shields, J.A. and De Potter, P. (1995) Patterns of indocyanine green videoangiography of choroidal tumours. *Br. J. Ophthalmol.*, **79**, 237–45.

Shields, C.L., Shields, J.A., De Potter, P., Quaranta, M., Freire, J., Brady, L.W. and Barrett, J. (1997) Plaque radiotherapy for the management of uveal metastasis. *Arch. Ophthalmol.*, **115**, 203–9.

Shields, C.L., Shields, J.A., Gross, N.E., Schwartz, G.P. and Lally, S.E. (1997) Survey of 520 eyes with uveal metastases. *Ophthalmology*, **104**, 1265–76.

Shields, J.A., Shields, C.L., Kiratli, H. and De Potter, P. (1995) Metastatic tumors to the iris in 40 patients. *Am. J. Ophthalmol.*, **119**, 422–30.

Tkocz, H.-J., Hoffmann, S., Schnabel, K., Niewald, M., Ruprecht, K.-W., Schmidt, W. and Mink, D. (1997) Bilateral radiotherapy in cases of one-sided choroidal metastases. In: T. Wiegel, N. Bornfeld, M.H. Foerster and W. Hinkelbein (eds), *Radiotherapy of Ocular Disease*. Basle: Karger, pp. 160–4.

Viebahn, M., Barricks, M.E. and Osterloh, M.D. (1991) Synergism between diabetic and radiation retinopathy: case report and review. *Br. J. Ophthalmol.*, **75**, 629–32.

Wharam, M.D. Jr. and Schachat, A.P. (1994) Choroidal metastasis. In: S.J. Ryan (ed.), *Retina*. St Louis: Mosby, Vol. 1, Ch. 52, pp. 835–45.

Wiegel, T., Kreusel, K.M., Bornfeld, N., Bottke, D., Stange, M., Foerster, M.H. and Hinkelbein, W. (1998) Frequency of asymptomatic choroidal metastasis in patients with disseminated breast cancer: results of a prospective screening programme. *Br. J. Ophthalmol.*, **82**, 1159–61.

Chapter 20

Lymphoid tumours

Lymphoid tumours can arise in conjunctiva or uvea and can be benign, malignant or indeterminate.

Conjunctival reactive lymphoid hyperplasia

Reactive lymphoid hyperplasia (or benign conjunctival lymphoid proliferation) is a benign condition, which is characterized histologically by:

a. Well-differentiated T- and B-lymphocytes, the latter showing polyclonality for heavy chains (i.e., IgG, IgA and IgM) and κ and λ light chains.
b. Lymphoid follicles with germinal centres containing proliferating cells.
c. Systemic vasculitis in some patients.

The clinical manifestations are similar to lymphoma (Figure 20.1).

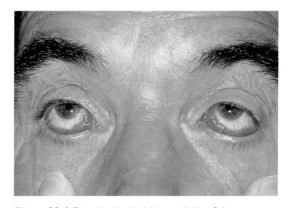

Figure 20.1 Reactive lymphoid hyperplasia of the conjunctiva showing pink lesions in fornices

Uveal reactive lymphoid hyperplasia

Uveal reactive lymphoid hyperplasia (Ryan *et al.*, 1972; Grossniklaus *et al.*, 1998; Cockerham *et al.*, 2000) is increasingly referred to as 'uveal lymphoid infiltration' and 'lymphoid tumour'. Patients are usually more than 40 years old.

PATHOLOGY

The tumour diffusely involves the uvea and tends to spread subconjunctivally.

SYMPTOMS

a. Visual loss.
b. Diplopia.
c. Epibulbar nodules.
d. Pain.

SIGNS

- Unilateral disease in most patients (Ryan *et al.*, 1972).
- Cells in anterior chamber and vitreous.
- Solitary or multifocal creamy-yellow choroidal infiltrates, with depigmentation of the RPE (Jakobiec *et al.*, 1987).
- Uveal thickening, which may be diffuse or nodular (Figure 20.2**a**).
- Proptosis.
- Salmon-pink conjunctival nodules (Jakobiec *et al.*, 1987) (Figure 20.2**b**).

COMPLICATIONS

- Exudative retinal detachment (Escoffery *et al.*, 1985).
- Glaucoma (Gass, 1967; Cockerham, *et al.*, 2000).
- Iris heterochromia.

- Scleritis, in some patients (Desroches *et al.*, 1983).

OCULAR INVESTIGATIONS

Ultrasonography demonstrates uveal thickening with low internal reflectivity, and extraocular nodules, both anteriorly and around the optic nerve.

Fluorescein angiography often shows choroidal folds (Johnson *et al.*, 1999).

SCREENING FOR SYSTEMIC LYMPHOMA

a. History and full clinical examination.
b. Chest radiography.
c. Full blood count.
d. Abdominal CT scan.
e. Bone marrow biopsy.

DIFFERENTIAL DIAGNOSIS

1. **Uveitis** may mimic uveal lymphoid hyperplasia because of the presence of anterior chamber cells.
2. **Multifocal choroidal lesions** can occur, as in conditions such as multifocal choroiditis, punctate inner choroiditis, acute multifocal posterior placoid pigment epitheliopathy and birdshot choroiditis (Figure 20.3).

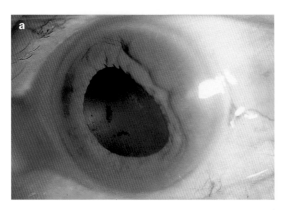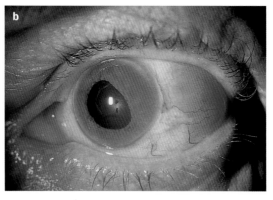

Figure 20.2 Reactive lymphoid hyperplasia of the uvea, with (**a**) iris and (**b**) conjunctival nodules. Ophthalmoscopy showed choroidal involvement

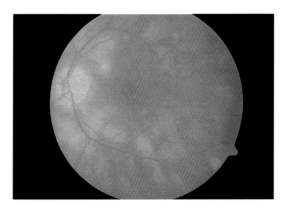

Figure 20.3 Birdshot choroiditis showing multiple pale choroidal lesions

3. **Diffuse uveal melanoma** shows similar diffuse choroidal thickening on ultrasonography.
4. **Uveal metastasis** may have a similar creamy appearance.
5. **Scleritis** can occur as part of uveal lymphoid infiltration.
6. **Post-transplant lymphoproliferative disorder** (Boubenider *et al.*, 1997) can give rise to solitary or multiple white iris nodules (Croley *et al.*, 1999). The condition occurs as a result of Epstein–Barr virus (EBV) transfection and may resolve if the immunosuppression is reduced.

MANAGEMENT

The ocular tumours typically respond to systemic steroids (Desroches *et al.*, 1983; Jakobiec *et al.*, 1987) or low dose radiotherapy (i.e., 20 Gy) (Char, 1997).

About 50% of patients retain vision of 6/60 (Grossniklaus *et al.*, 1998). Systemic lymphoma develops in a minority of patients (Grossniklaus *et al.*, 1998).

Conjunctival lymphoma

Methods for examining conjunctival lymphoid proliferations have improved greatly in recent years (Coupland *et al.*, 1998).

PATHOLOGY

The most common types of conjunctival lymphoma (Coupland *et al.*, 1998) can be categorized according to the REAL classification (Harris *et al.*, 1994).

a. Extranodal marginal-zone B-cell lymphoma (otherwise known as MALT lymphoma (Medeiros and Harris, 1990; Wotherspoon *et al.*, 1993; White *et al.*, 1995), which accounts for about two-thirds of all conjunctival lymphomas (Figure 20.4). It is associated with a good prognosis.
b. Follicle centre lymphoma, with monoclonal proliferations of small and large cells forming follicles.
c. Diffuse large cell lymphoma, showing high mitotic rates and invasion of surrounding tissues, including bone.

METHODS FOR CONFIRMING MALIGNANCY

a. Demonstration of monoclonal immunoglobulin light and heavy chains by immunohistochemistry.
b. Demonstration of monoclonal immunoglobulin gene rearrangements in tumour cell DNA, using the polymerase chain reaction (PCR) technique.

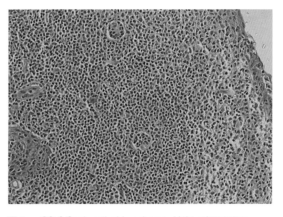

Figure 20.4 Conjunctival lymphoma. Light microscopy showing infiltration of epithelium by lymphoma cells

SYMPTOMS

a. Painless conjunctival swelling or redness.
b. Photophobia.
c. Irritation.
d. Epiphora.

SIGNS

- Orange–pink masses in the upper or lower fornix (i.e., salmon patches) (Figure 20.5).
- Bilateral disease in most patients, perhaps with involvement of the second eye demonstrated only by laboratory examination.
- Occasionally, diffuse conjunctival infiltration mimicking chronic inflammation (Akpek *et al.,* 1999b).
- Rarely, scleritis and 'choroidal white-dot syndrome' (Hoang-Xuan *et al.,* 1996).

DIFFERENTIAL DIAGNOSIS

1. **Chronic conjunctivitis.**
2. **Scleritis.**
3. **Uveitis.**

TREATMENT

Conjunctival lymphoma is treated by external beam radiotherapy, delivering 30–35 Gy using an anterior electron field with lens sparing (Dunbar *et al.,* 1990) (Chapter 23). If the lymphoma shows aggressive histology, then this may be combined with systemic chemotherapy (Shipp *et al.,* 1997).

Periodic review is required because of the risk of local and systemic recurrences.

PROGNOSIS

CLINICAL INDICATORS OF A POOR PROGNOSIS (Jenkins, 1999)

- Bilateral disease.
- Lacrimal gland or eyelid involvement.
- Age greater than 65 years.
- Short history (i.e., < 12 months).
- Pain.
- Optic neuropathy.
- Involvement of paranasal sinuses.

PATHOLOGICAL INDICATORS OF A POOR PROGNOSIS (Coupland *et al.,* 1998)

- High grade lymphoma (i.e., diffuse large cell lymphoma and T-cell lymphoma).
- Advanced stage at presentation.
- Proliferation rate greater than 20% (independent of type of lymphoma).
- Over-expression of p53.
- Presence of CD5+ cells.
- Association with the acquired immune deficiency syndrome (AIDS).

Primary intraocular lymphoma

PATHOLOGY

Primary intraocular lymphoma forms part of 'primary central nervous system lymphoma (PCNSL)' (Freeman *et al.,* 1993; Verbraeken *et al.,* 1997), which is increasing in incidence (Lutz and Coleman, 1994). This can present with any of the following:

a. One or more discrete, intracranial nodules.
b. Diffuse meningeal or periventricular lesions.
c. Localized intradural spinal masses.
d. Subretinal infiltrates and vitreous cells.

The lymphoma cells are large, pleomorphic B-lymphocytes having a large, multilobular nucleus, a prominent nucleolus, and scanty cytoplasm (Figure 20.6). In the eye, reactive T cells are also present in the adjacent choroid and retina as well as in the vitreous.

Patients with intraocular lymphoma usually present after the age of 35 years, unless they are immunocompromised, in which case they can present earlier (Rivero *et al.,* 1999).

SYMPTOMS

a. Blurred vision.
b. Floaters.
c. Photophobia.

SIGNS

- Bilateral ocular involvement, often asymmetrically (Peterson *et al.*, 1993).
- Mild anterior chamber inflammation, with flare and keratic precipitates.
- Vitreous cells, typically occurring in sheets.
- Multifocal, round or oval, white/yellow infiltrates between RPE and Bruch's membrane (Figure 20.7). These can rarely form a ring encircling the equator of each eye, with the appearance being pathognomonic of intraocular lymphoma (Figure 20.8) (Gass *et al.*, 1984). Resolution of these infiltrates is followed by RPE atrophy (Figure 20.8**d**) with a subsequent risk of disciform lesions (Dean *et al.*, 1996).
- Diffuse retinal or subretinal infiltrates (Figure 20.9).
- Retinal perivasculitis (Brown *et al.*, 1994), which may be haemorrhagic.

COMPLICATIONS

- Retinal arteriolar occlusion.
- Macular oedema.
- Exudative retinal detachment.
- Secondary glaucoma.
- Optic neuropathy leading to atrophy (Dunker *et al.*, 1996) (Figure 20.7**a**).
- Pseudohypopyon, which is rare.

Most patients presenting with ocular lymphoma eventually develop CNS lymphoma within 2 or 3 years. CNS disease can also precede or coincide with the intraocular lymphoma.

CLINICAL FEATURES OF CNS DISEASE

- Headache, personality change, or focal deficit, caused by an intracranial mass.
- Vague neuropathies, from leptomeningeal disease.
- Bilateral motor and sensory deficits affecting the arms or legs, secondary to spinal cord disease.

Fewer than 10% of patients are diagnosed with visceral metastases, which are usually sub-clinical.

INVESTIGATIONS

FLUORESCEIN ANGIOGRAPHY

a. Hyperfluorescent window defects corresponding to areas of RPE atrophy associated with underlying tumour infiltrates, many of which are invisible ophthalmoscopically (Figure 20.9**b**).
b. Hypofluorescent lesions.
c. Retinal vasculitis.
d. Macular oedema.

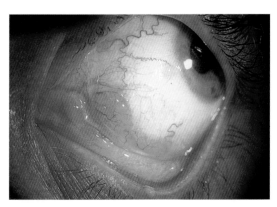

Figure 20.5 Conjunctival lymphoma showing salmon-pink nodules

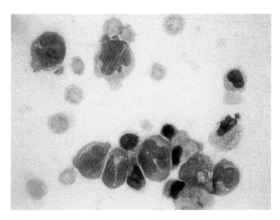

Figure 20.6 Vitreous biopsy showing lymphoma cells having a large, irregular nucleus. (Courtesy of P. Smith, Liverpool, UK)

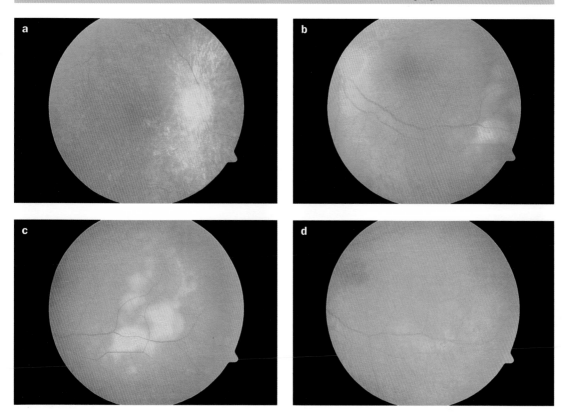

Figure 20.7 Clinical photographs of a 67-year-old female showing (**a**) optic atrophy in the right eye, caused by lymphoma, (**b**) subretinal deposits inferotemporal to the left macula, (**c**) lymphomatous deposits at higher magnification and (**d**) minimal RPE scarring after regression of the deposits following treatment with intravitreal methotrexate

ULTRASONOGRAPHY (Ursea *et al.*, 1997)

a. Vitreous debris.
b. Elevated choroidal lesions.
c. Widening of the optic nerves.

BIOPSY

Before starting treatment, it is essential to confirm the diagnosis of intraocular lymphoma by pars plana vitrectomy (Akpek *et al.*, 1999a), vitreous biopsy using a 20-gauge needle, or fine needle aspiration biopsy of subretinal nodules (Pavan *et al.*, 1995). False negative results occur frequently, because lymphoma cells are delicate and may be scanty, outnumbered by reactive cells and histiocytes. Reliability is improved by adding tissue culture medium to the collection chamber and by examination of the sample by an experienced cytopathologist within 30 minutes. Vitreous samples can be examined for a raised interleukin-10 level (Buggage *et al.*, 1999), and for altered B- and T-gene rearrangements (White *et al.*, 1999). Despite all precautions, FNAB of subretinal nodules may yield only necrotic cells because viable lymphoma cells are present only near the choriocapillaris (Figure 20.10)

Note: Steroids are cytotoxic to lymphoma cells and increase the chances of a false negative vitreous biopsy. They should therefore be stopped a few days before biopsy.

SCREENING FOR CNS AND SYSTEMIC DISEASE

a. Clinical neurological examination.
b. Contrast-enhanced MRI brain scans, which if negative need to be repeated regularly.

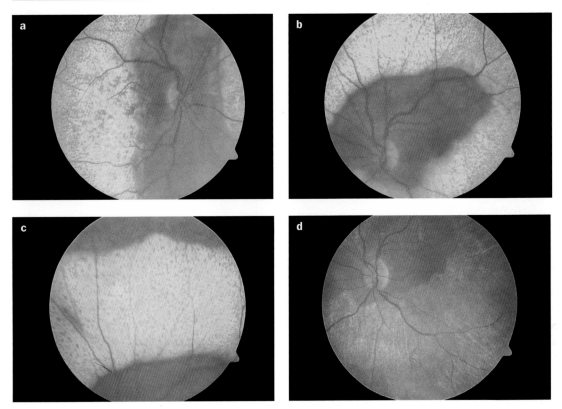

Figure 20.8 Clinical photographs of a 62-year-old female: (**a**) annular subretinal lymphomatous tumour in the right eye, with clear vitreous, (**b**) similar deposits in the left eye, (**c**) peripheral view showing normal peripheral choroid, (**d**) tumour regression after external beam radiotherapy leaving RPE scars. The vision 18 months after treatment was Counting Fingers in the right eye and 6/12 in the left eye

c. Lumbar puncture, which may need to be repeated.
d. Chest X-ray.
e. Abdominal CT scan.
f. Bone marrow biopsy.

DIFFERENTIAL DIAGNOSIS

1. **Uveitis** in elderly individuals is usually idiopathic or caused by herpes zoster or simplex (Chatzistefanou *et al.*, 1998). Many patients with intraocular lymphoma have been treated for 'vitritis' for long periods before the proper diagnosis is made.
2. **Sarcoidosis** is excluded by chest X-ray, serum angiotensin converting enzyme (ACE) and lysozyme levels, and pulmonary function tests.
3. **Intraocular foreign body** is another cause of refractory uveitis.
4. **Reactive lymphoid hyperplasia** (see above).
5. **Leukaemic infiltration** (Chapter 21).
6. **Multifocal creamy lesions**, caused by conditions such as birdshot chorioretinopathy and acute posterior multifocal placoid pigment epitheliopathy.
7. **Viral retinitis** can present as haemorrhagic retinal vasculitis.

TREATMENT OF OCULAR DISEASE

a. External beam radiotherapy is the usual treatment, delivering 40–50 Gy to both eyes (Chapter 23).
b. Intravitreal methotrexate injection is useful for recurrent disease (Figure 20.7). Some

authorities suggest that it may be preferable to radiotherapy as a first line treatment. The methotrexate is injected at a dose of 400 μg twice weekly for one month, then once a week for a month, then monthly for one year (Fishburne *et al.*, 1997).

TREATMENT OPTIONS FOR CNS DISEASE

a. Radiotherapy (i.e., 45–50 Gy) to the brain and spinal cord. Some authorities reserve this for recurrence so as to avoid late radiational complications (Freilich *et al.,* 1996; Sandor *et al.*, 1998).
b. High dose systemic chemotherapy with autologous bone marrow transplantation (Valluri *et al.*, 1995).
c. High dose systemic and intrathecal chemotherapy, using intra-arterial mannitol to disrupt the blood–brain barrier (de Smet *et al.*, 1996).

If there is no evidence of CNS disease, opinion is divided as to whether patients should be treated prophylactically or monitored closely.

PROGNOSIS

There is usually a good response to treatment, but recurrence commonly occurs. Less than a third of patients survive five years (Peterson *et al.*, 1993).

Secondary intraocular lymphoma

Most patients have overt systemic disease by the time they develop ocular manifestations, which primarily involve the choroid (Oh *et al.*, 1998).

OCULAR SIGNS

* Uveal deposits (Jensen *et al.*, 1994) (Figure 20.11).
* Widespread retinal flecks resembling fundus flavimaculatus (Gass *et al.*, 1987).

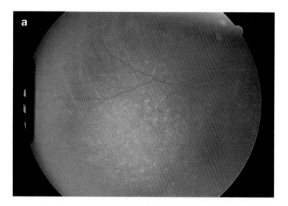
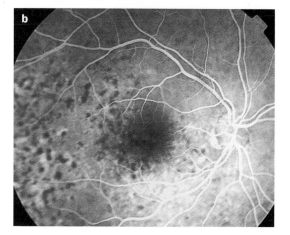
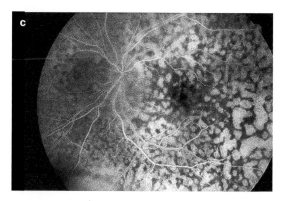

Figure 20.9 Diffuse lymphomatous infiltration: (**a**) colour photograph, (**b**) fluorescein angiogram of the right eye of a 70-year-old female with ocular and CNS lymphoma and (**c**) fluorescein angiogram of the left eye of a 60-year-old female with ocular lymphoma and no cerebral or systemic disease. (Courtesy of the Department of Ophthalmology, Pitié-Salpêtrière Hospital, Paris, France)

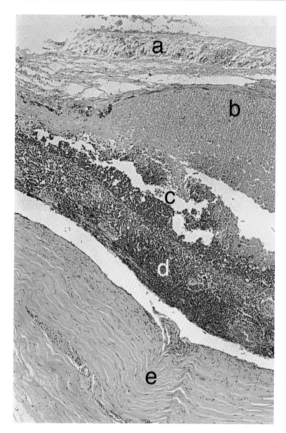

Figure 20.10 Light micrograph of primary intraocular lymphoma nodules similar to those shown in Figure 20.8: (**a**) retina, (**b**) necrotic cells, (**c**) lymphoma cells near choriocapillaris, (**d**) reactive lymphocytic infiltration in choroid and (**e**) sclera. (Courtesy of P. Hiscott, Liverpool, UK)

Hodgkin's lymphoma

Hodgkin's lymphoma originates in lymph nodes, eventually spreading to spleen, liver, bone marrow and other sites. Most patients are less than 40 years old at the time of diagnosis. Histologically, this disease is characterized by the presence of pathognomonic multinucleated giant cells (Reed–Sternberg cells).

OCULAR SIGNS (Barr and Joondoph, 1983)

- Multiple white retinal lesions resembling chorioretinitis.
- Perivascular infiltrates, retinal haemorrhages, cotton wool spots and Roth spots.
- Vitreous cells.
- Optic disc oedema.
- Exudative retinal detachment.
- Features of opportunistic infections.

Cutaneous T-cell lymphoma

Cutaneous T-cell lymphoma includes conditions such as mycosis fungoides, Sézary syndrome and adult T-cell leukaemia/lymphoma.

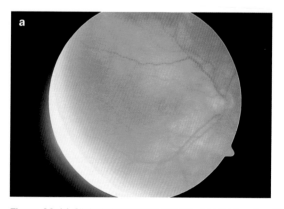
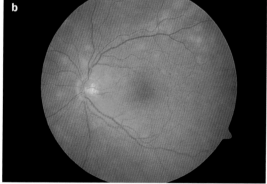

Figure 20.11 Clinical photographs of a 72-year-old female with systemic non-Hodgkin's lymphoma: (**a**) right fundus, showing a white mass superior to the fovea and (**b**) left fundus, showing regressed lesions similar to birdshot retinopathy. The tumours regressed spontaneously in both eyes, without any ocular or systemic treatment

OPHTHALMIC SIGNS (Cook *et al.*, 1999)

- Ectropion, eyelid thickening or tumour.
- Retinal infiltrate and haemorrhages.
- Keratitis.

Multiple myeloma

Although myeloma is not a lymphoma it is mentioned here for convenience.

Myeloma cells grow in bone and other sites, also secreting immunoglobulin, to cause lytic lesions, bone pain, fractures, hypercalcaemia, anaemia, renal failure and immunodeficiency with a tendency to develop bacterial infections.

OCULAR SIGNS (Knapp *et al.*, 1987)

- Retinal changes of anaemia and thrombocytopenia.
- Micro-aneurysms due to hyperviscosity.
- Corneal gammopathy.
- Exudative retinal detachment.
- Pars plana cysts.

REFERENCES

Akpek, E.K., Ahmed, I., Hochberg, F.H., Soheilian, M., Dryja, T.P., Jakobiec, F.A. and Foster, C.S. (1999a) Intraocular-central nervous system lymphoma. Clinical features, diagnosis and outcomes. *Ophthalmology*, **106**, 1805–10.

Akpek, E.K., Polcharoen, W., Ferry, J.A. and Foster, S. (1999) Conjunctival lymphoma masquerading as chronic conjunctivitis. *Ophthalmology*, **106**, 757–60.

Barr, C.C. and Joondeph, H.C. (1983) Retinal periphlebitis as the initial finding in a patient with Hodgkin's disease. *Retina*, **3**, 253–7.

Boubenider, S., Hiesse, C., Goupy, C., Kriaa, F., Marchand, S. and Charpentier, B. (1997) Incidence and consequences of post-transplantation lymphoproliferative disorders. *J. Nephrol.*, **10**, 136–45.

Brown, S.M., Jampol, L.M. and Cantrill, H.L. (1994) Intraocular lymphoma presenting as retinal vasculitis. *Surv. Ophthalmol.*, **39**, 133–40.

Buggage, R.R., Whitcup, S.M. and Nussenblatt, C.-C. (1999) Using interleukin 10 to interleukin 6 ratio to distinguish primary intraocular lymphoma and uveitis. *Invest. Ophthalmol. Vis. Sci.*, **40**, 2462–3.

Char, D.H. (1997) *Clinical Ocular Oncology.* Philadelphia: Lippincott–Raven, Ch. 7, pp. 192–202.

Chatzistefanou, K., Markomichelakis, N.N., Christen, W., Soheilian, M. and Foster, C.S. (1998) Characteristics of uveitis presenting for the first time in the elderly. *Ophthalmology*, **105**, 347–52.

Cockerham, G.C., Hidayat, A.A., Bijwaard, K.E. and Sheng, Z.M. (2000) Re-evaluation of "reactive lymphoid hyperplasia of the uvea": an immunohistochemical and molecular analysis of 10 cases. *Ophthalmology*, **107**, 151–8.

Cook, B.E. Jr., Bartley, G.B. and Pittelkow, M.R. (1999) Ophthalmic abnormalities in patients with cutaneous T-cell lymphoma. *Ophthalmology*, **106**, 1339–40.

Coupland, S.E., Krause, L., Delecluse, H.-J., Anagnostopoulos, I., Foss, H.-D., Hummel, M., Bornfeld, N., Lee, W.R. and Stein, H. (1998) Lymphoproliferative lesions of the ocular adnexa. Analysis of 112 cases. *Ophthalmology*, **105**, 1430–41.

Croley, J., Lloyd, W., Gulley, M., Chacko, B. and O'Hara, M. (1999) Personal communication; International Congress on Ocular Endoscopy, Philadelphia.

Dean, J.M., Novak, M.A., Chan, C.C. and Green, W.R. (1996) Tumor detachments of the retinal pigment epithelium in ocular/central nervous system lymphoma. *Retina*, **16**, 47–56.

Desroches, G., Abrams, G.W. and Gass, J.D.M. (1983) Reactive lymphoid hyperplasia of the uvea: a case with ultrasonographic and computed tomographic studies. *Arch. Ophthalmol.*, **101**, 725–8.

Dunbar, S.F., Linggood, R.M., Doppke, K.P., Duby, A. and Wang, C.C. (1990) Conjunctival lymphoma: results and treatment with a single anterior electron field. A lens sparing approach. *Int. J. Radiat. Oncol. Biol. Phys.*, **19**, 249–57.

Dunker, S., Reuter, U., Rosler, A. and Wiegand, W. (1996) Sehnervenbeteiligung bei chronisch-lymphatischer Leukamie der B-Zell-Reihe. *Ophthalmologe*, **93**, 351–3.

Escoffery, R.F., Bobrow, J.C. and Smith, M.E. (1985) Exudative retinal detachment secondary to orbital and intraocular benign lymphoid hyperplasia. *Retina*, **5**, 91–3.

Fishburne, B.C., Wilson, D.J., Rosenbaum, J.T. and Neuwelt, E.A. (1997) Intravitreal methotrexate as an adjunctive treatment of intraocular lymphoma. *Arch. Ophthalmol.*, **115**, 1152–6.

Freeman, L.N., Schachat, A.P., Knox, D.L., Michels, R.G. and Green, W.R. (1987) Clinical features, laboratory investigations, and survival in ocular reticulum cell sarcoma. *Ophthalmology*, **94**, 1631–9.

Freilich, R.J., Delattre, J.Y., Monjour, A. and DeAngelis, L.M. (1996) Chemotherapy without radiation therapy as initial treatment for primary CNS lymphoma in older patients. *Neurology*, **46**, 435–9.

Gass, J.D.M. (1967) Retinal detachment and narrow angle glaucoma secondary to inflammatory pseudotumor of the uveal tract. *Am. J. Ophthalmol.*, **64**, 612–21.

Gass, J.D.M., Sever, R.J., Grizzard, W.S., Clarkson, J.G., Blumenkranz, M., Wind, C.A. and Shugarman, R. (1984) Multifocal pigment epithelial detachments by reticulum cell sarcoma. A characteristic fundus picture. *Retina*, **4**, 135–43.

Gass, J.D.M., Weleber, R.G. and Johnson, D.R. (1987) Non-Hodgkin's lymphoma causing fundus picture simulating fundus flavimaculatus. Report of four cases and clinicopathologic review. *Retina*, **7**, 209–14.

Grossniklaus, H.E., Martin, D.F., Avery, R., Shields, J.A., Shields, C.L., Kuo, I.C., Green, R.L. and Rao, N.A. (1998) Uveal lymphoid infiltration. Report of four cases and clinicopathologic review. *Ophthalmology*, **105**, 1265–73.

Harris, N.L., Jaffe, E.S., Stein, H., Banks, P.M., Chan, J.K., Cleary, M.L., Delsol, G., De-Wolf-Peeters, C., Fallini, B. and Gatter, K.C. (1994) A revised European-American classification of lymphoid neoplasms: a proposal from the International Lymphoma Study Group. *Blood*, **84**, 1361–92.

Hoang-Xuan, T., Bodaghi, B., Toublanc, M., Delmer, A., Schwartz, L., D'Hermies, F. (1996) Scleritis and mucosal-associated lymphoid tissue lymphoma: a new masquerade syndrome. *Ophthalmology*, **103**, 631–5.

Jakobiec, F.A., Sacks, E., Kronish, J.W., Weiss, J. and Smith, M. (1987) Multifocal static creamy choroidal infiltrates: an early sign of lymphoid neoplasia. *Ophthalmology*, **94**, 397–406.

Jenkins, C. (1999) Ocular lymphoma. Personal communication; Course on Ocular Oncology, Royal College of Ophthalmologists, London.

Jensen, O.A., Johansen, S. and Kiss, K. (1994) Intraocular T-cell lymphoma mimicking a ring melanoma. First manifestation of systemic disease. Report of a case and survey of the literature. *Graefes Arch. Clin. Exp. Ophthalmol.*, **232**, 148–52.

Johnson, R., McDonald, H.W. and Ai, E. (1999) Personal communication; International Congress of Ocular Oncology, Philadelphia.

Knapp, A.J., Gartner, S. and Henkind, P. (1987) Multiple myeloma and its ocular manifestations. *Surv. Ophthalmol.*, **31**, 343–51.

Lutz, J.M. and Coleman, M.P. (1994) Trends in primary cerebral lymphoma. *Br. J. Cancer*, **70**, 716–18.

Medeiros, L.J. and Harris, N.L. (1990) Immunohistologic analysis of small lymphocytic infiltrates of the orbit and conjunctiva. *Hum. Pathol.*, **21**, 1126–31.

Oh, K.T., Polk, T.D., Boldt, H.C. and Turner, J.F. Jr. (1998) Systemic small noncleaved cell lymphoma presenting as a posterior choroidal mass. *Am. J. Ophthalmol.*, **125**, 560–2.

Pavan, P.R., Oteiza, E.E. and Margo, C.E. (1995) Ocular lymphoma diagnosed by internal subretinal pigment epithelium biopsy. *Arch. Ophthalmol.*, **113**, 1233–4.

Peterson, K., Gordon, K.B., Heinemann, M. and DeAngelis, L.M. (1993) The clinical spectrum of ocular lymphoma. *Cancer*, **72**, 843–9.

Rivero, M.E., Kuppermann, B.D., Wiley, C.A., Garcia, C.R., Smith, M.D., Dreilinger, A. and Freeman, W.R. (1999) Acquired immunodeficiency syndrome-related intraocular B-cell lymphoma. *Arch. Ophthalmol.*, **117**, 616–22.

Ryan, S.J., Zimmerman, L.E. and King, F.M. (1972) Reactive lymphoid hyperplasia: an unusual form of intraocular pseudotumor. *Trans. Am. Ophthalmol. Soc.*, **76**, 652–71.

Sandor, V., Stark-Vancs, V., Pearson, D., Nussenblatt, R.B., Whitcup, S.M., Brouwers, P., Patronas, N., Heiss, J., Jaffe, E., de Smet, M.D., Kohler, D., Simon, R. and Wittes, R. (1998) Phase II trial of chemotherapy alone for primary CNS and intraocular lymphoma. *J. Clin. Oncol.*, **16**, 3000–6.

Shipp, M.A., Mauch, P.M. and Harris, N.L. (1997) Non-Hodgkin's lymphomas. In: V.T. DeVita, S. Hellman Jr. and S.A. Rosenberg (eds), *Cancer. Principles and Practice of Oncology*. Philadelphia: Lippincott–Raven, Ch. 44.2, pp. 2165–220.

de Smet, M.D., Stark Vancs, V., Kohler, D.R., Smith, J., Wittes, R. and Nussenblatt, R.B. (1996) Intraocular levels of methotrexate after intravenous administration. *Am. J. Ophthalmol.*, **121**, 442–4.

Ursea, R., Heinemann, M.H., Silverman, R.H., DeAngelis, L.M., Daly, S.W. and Coleman, D.J. (1997) Ophthalmic, ultrasonographic findings in primary central nervous system lymphoma with ocular involvement. *Retina*, **17**, 118–23.

Valluri, S., Moorthy, R.S., Khan, A. and Rao, N.A. (1995) Combination treatment of intraocular lymphoma. *Retina*, **15**, 125–9.

Verbraeken, H.E., Hanssens, M., Priem, H., Lafaut, B.A. and De Laey, J.-J. (1997) Ocular non-Hodgkin's lymphoma: a clinical study of nine cases. *Br. J. Ophthalmol.*, **81**, 31–6.

Whitcup, S.M., de Smet, M.D., Rubin, B.I., Palestine, A.G., Martin, D.F., Burnier, M. Jr, Chan, C.-C. and Nussenblatt, R.B. (1993) Intraocular lymhoma. Clinical and histopathologic diagnosis. *Ophthalmology*, **100**, 1399–406.

White, W.L., Ferry, J.A., Harris, N.L. and Grove, A.S. Jr. (1995) Ocular adnexal lymphoma. A clinicopathologic study with identification of lymphomas of mucosa-associated lymphoid tissue type. *Ophthalmology*, **102**, 1994–2006.

White, V.A., Gascoyne, R.D. and Paton, K.E. (1999) Use of the polymerase chain reaction to detect B- and T-cell gene rearrangements in vitreous specimens from patients with intraocular lymphoma. *Arch. Ophthalmol.*, **117**, 761–5.

Wotherspoon, A.C., Diss, T.C., Pan, L.X., Schmid, C., Kerr-Muir, M.G., Lea, S.H. and Isaacson, P.G. (1993) Primary low-grade B-cell lymphoma of the conjunctiva: a mucosa-associated lymphoid tissue type lymphoma. *Histopathology*, **23**, 417–24.

Chapter 21

Leukaemia

A wide range of ocular abnormalities occur in most patients with leukaemia but are usually sub-clinical and often overlooked in the presence of serious systemic disease (Kincaid and Green, 1983).

Ocular manifestations can be the presenting sign of leukaemia or an indication of relapse after treatment. They generally indicate a poor prognosis for survival, with cotton wool spots being particularly significant (Abu El-Asrar *et al.*, 1996).

PATHOLOGY

1. **Chronic lymphocytic leukaemia (CLL)** is the most common type of leukaemia. It usually consists of small lymphocytic B cells, which accumulate in blood, bone marrow, lymph nodes and spleen. Patients may have a normal prognosis for survival without treatment, or may develop anaemia, thrombocytopenia and hypogammaglobulinaemia, which are fatal without appropriate chemotherapy.
2. **Chronic myelogenous leukaemia (CML)** is caused by a translocation between chromosomes 22 and 9 (Philadelphia chromosome translocation). Mature myelocytes gradually replace bone marrow until a 'blast crisis' occurs, when there is invasion of all major organs of the body, causing haemorrhage and infection.
3. **Acute lymphocytic leukaemia (ALL) and acute myelogenous leukaemia (AML)** both tend to present with clinical manifestations of anaemia and thrombocytopenia and, less commonly, hepatomegaly, splenomegaly and lymphadenopathy. ALL is the commonest childhood malignancy, whereas AML is more common in adults.

SYMPTOMS

Visual loss can occur as a result of (a) optic nerve infiltration and other ocular complications, (b) meningitis due to an opportunistic infection, and (c) chemotherapeutic agents such as vincristine and cytosine arabinoside (Ara-C), which can cause optic neuropathy.

SIGNS

The clinical signs of intraocular leukaemia are caused by (a) leukaemic deposits, (b) haematological abnormalities, and (c) opportunistic infections (Rosenthal, 1983; Schachat and Dhaliwal, 1994).

LEUKAEMIC DEPOSITS

a. Optic nerve infiltration can cause disc swelling with visual loss (Ellis and Little, 1973) (Figure 21.1).

b. Choroidal deposits are usually sub-clinical, but can cause a leopard skin RPE appearance, serous retinal detachment, RPE detachment and ciliochoroidal effusion (Kincaid and Green, 1983). After treatment, there can be residual RPE stippling (Clayman *et al.,* 1972).

c. Intraretinal deposits can cause (1) vascular sheathing, (2) discrete, white nodules obscuring the retinal blood vessels, (3) cotton wool spots, probably due to vascular occlusion by leukaemic cells, and (4) Roth spots, each consisting of a central white aggregate of leukaemic cells or platelet-fibrin emboli surrounded by a ring of red blood cells (Rosenthal, 1983). Intraretinal infiltration can also cause total retinal detachment (Primack *et al.,* 1995).

d. Vitreous infiltrates can resemble lymphoma (Swartz and Schumann, 1980).

e. Anterior disease can present as a pseudohypopyon (Abramson *et al.,* 1981; Ayliffe *et al.,* 1995) (Figure 21. 2) or ciliary body mass.

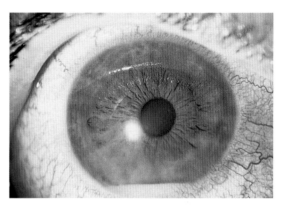

Figure 21.2 Leukaemic pseudohypopyon as the first indication of relapse in a patient with lymphocytic leukaemia. (Courtesy of A.M. Abu El-Asrar, Riyadh, Saudi Arabia)

HAEMATOLOGICAL ABNORMALITIES

a. Anaemia and thrombocytopenia may cause dot, blot and flame retinal haemorrhages (Guyer *et al.,* 1989) (Figure 21.3), and disc swelling without visual loss. The blood vessels can be yellow due to anaemia and a high white cell count.

b. Hyperviscosity can cause micro-aneurysms (Duke *et al.,* 1968), venous tortuosity, venous occlusion, retinal ischaemia and neovascularization of the optic disc (Delaney and Kinsella, 1985) or retina, forming 'sea-fans' resembling those of sickle cell retinopathy (Morse and McCready, 1971).

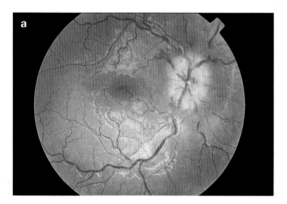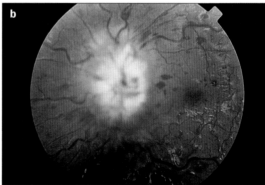

Figure 21.1 Bilateral leukaemic optic nerve infiltration in a patient with acute lymphocytic leukaemia: (**a**) right eye and (**b**) left eye. (Courtesy of A.M. Abu El-Asrar, Riyadh, Saudi Arabia)

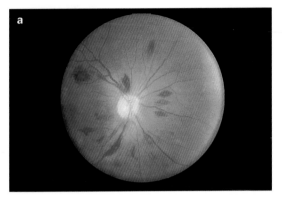 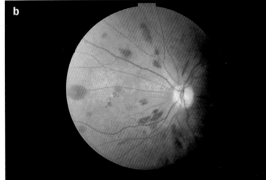

Figure 21.3 Leukaemic retinopathy in a patient with acute lymphocytic leukaemia showing flame haemorrhages, Roth spots and cotton wool spots in (**a**) right eye and (**b**) left eye. (Courtesy of A.M. Abu El-Asrar, Riyadh, Saudi Arabia)

OPPORTUNISTIC INFECTIONS

a. Cytomegalovirus retinitis forms a characteristic line of haemorrhages and yellow inflammatory infiltrates spreading in a 'bush-fire' pattern.

b. Toxoplasmosis can cause uveitis, retinochoroiditis, papillitis and CNS disease.

c. Aspergillus and cryptococcus infections cause uveitis, fluffy chorioretinal infiltrates, and occasionally Roth spots.

OTHER MANIFESTATIONS

a. Papilloedema, due to raised intracranial pressure caused by meningeal infiltration or intracranial haemorrhage.

b. Neurological deficits, such as facial nerve palsy and Horner's syndrome.

c. Proptosis, due to orbital haemorrhage or infiltration, which can precede detectable haematological or bone marrow abnormality by several months (Zimmerman and Font, 1975). The ophthalmologist can therefore play an important role in diagnosing the disease at an early stage, when chemotherapy may be more effective.

d. Herpes zoster ophthalmicus.

e. Cataract, due to chemotherapy and radiotherapy.

f. Perilimbal infiltrates (Font *et al.*, 1985) and other conjunctival leukaemic tumours (Cook and Bartley, 1997).

g. Graft-versus-host disease (GVHD), which follows allogeneic bone marrow transplantation. This causes severe kerato-conjunctivitis sicca, keratinization of conjunctiva, perforating corneal ulcers, cicatricial lagophthalmos, and opportunistic eye infections (Lopez *et al.*, 1991), as well as retinopathy (Cunningham *et al.*, 1996) and acute retinal necrosis (Lewis *et al.*, 1996).

h. Paraneoplastic cicatrizing conjunctivitis (Anhalt *et al.*, 1990), which is rare.

INVESTIGATIONS

Fluorescein angiography can show multiple, pinpoint, hyperfluorescent spots over choroidal infiltrates, which leak in the later frames. There may also be serous retinal detachment and pigment epithelial detachment.

Choroidal infiltration can cause choroidal thickening on ultrasonography and a subnormal EOG.

DIFFERENTIAL DIAGNOSIS

1. **Lymphoma**, which may have preceded the leukaemia (Chapter 20).
2. **Uveitis**, particularly in children.
3. **Metastasis** (Chapter 19).
4. **Sarcoidosis**, which can cause infiltration and swelling of the optic disc.

Leukaemic optic neuropathy may improve with steroids to mimic optic neuritis.

MANAGEMENT

Ocular infiltrates tend to respond to systemic chemotherapy, but may require external beam radiotherapy (Kincaid and Green, 1983).

Retinopathy due to anaemia and thrombocytopenia improves after transfusion whereas hyperviscosity states respond to leukapheresis (Mehta *et al.,* 1984).

Optic nerve infiltration requires urgent radiotherapy (Ridgway *et al.,* 1976) because visual loss may be irreversible.

REFERENCES

Abramson, D.H., Wachtel, A., Watson, C.W., Jereb, B. and Wollner, N. (1981) Leukemic hypopyon. *J. Pediatr. Ophthalmol. Strabismus,* **18**, 42–4.

Abu El-Asrar, A.M., Al-Momen, A.-K., Kangave, D. and Harakati, M.S. (1996) Prognostic importance of retinopathy in acute leukemia. *Doc. Ophthalmol.,* **91**, 273–81.

Anhalt, G.J., Kim, S.C., Stanley, J.R., Korman, N.J., Jabs, D.A., Kory, M., Izumi, H., Ratrie, H. 3rd, Mutasim, D. and Ariss-Abdo, L. (1990) Paraneoplastic pemphigus. An autoimmune mucocutaneous disease associated with neoplasia. *N. Engl. J. Med.,* **323**, 1729–35.

Ayliffe, W., Foster, C.S., Marcoux, P., Upton, M., Finkelstein, M., Kuperwaser, M. and Legmann, A. (1995) Relapsing acute myeloid leukemia manifesting as hypopyon uveitis. *Am. J. Ophthalmol.,* **119**, 361–4.

Clayman, H.M., Flynn, J.T., Koch, K. and Israel, C. (1972) Retinal pigment epithelial abnormalities in leukemic disease. *Am. J. Ophthalmol.,* **74**, 416–19.

Cook, B.E. Jr. and Bartley, G.B. (1997) Acute lymphoblastic leukemia manifesting in an adult as a conjunctival mass. *Am. J. Ophthalmol.,* **124**, 104–5.

Cunningham, E.T. Jr., Irvine, A.R. and Rugo, H.S. (1996) Bone marrow transplantation retinopathy in the absence of radiation therapy. *Am. J. Ophthalmol.,* **122**, 268–70.

Delaney, W.V. Jr and Kinsella, G. (1985) Optic disc neovascularizatoin in leukemia. *Am. J. Ophthalmol.,* **99**, 212–13.

Duke, J.R., Wilkinson, C.P. and Sigelman, S. (1968) Retinal microaneurysms in leukaemia. *Br. J. Ophthalmol.,* **52**, 368–74.

Ellis, W. and Little, H.L. (1973) Leukemic infiltration of the optic nerve head. *Am. J. Ophthalmol.,* **75**, 867–71.

Font, R.L., McKay, B. and Tang, R. (1985) Acute monocytic leukemia recurring as bilateral perilimbal infiltrates. Immunohistochemical and ultrastructural confirmation. *Ophthalmology,* **92**, 1681–5.

Guyer, D.R., Schachat, A.P., Vitale, S., Markowitz, J.A., Braine, H., Burke, P.J., Karp, J.E. and Graham, M. (1989) Leukemic retinopathy: relationship between fundus lesions and hematologic parameters at diagnosis. *Ophthalmology,* **96**, 860–4.

Kincaid, M.C. and Green, W.R. (1983) Ocular and orbital involvement in leukemia. *Surv. Ophthalmol.,* **27**, 211–32.

Lewis, J.M., Nagae, Y. and Tano, Y. (1996) Progressive outer retinal necrosis after bone marrow transplantation. *Am. J. Ophthalmol.,* **122**, 892–5.

Lopez, P.F., Sternberg, P. Jr., Dabbs, C.K., Vogler, W.R., Crocker, I. and Kalin, N.S. (1991) Bone marrow transplant retinopathy. *Am. J. Ophthalmol.,* **112**, 635–46.

Mehta, A.B., Goldman, J.M. and Kohner, E. (1984) Hyperleucocytic retinopathy in chronic granulocytic leukaemia: the role of intensive leucapheresis. *Br. J. Haematol.,* **56**, 661–7.

Morse, P.H. and McCready, J.L. (1971) Peripheral retinal neovascularization in chronic myelocytic leukemia. *Am. J. Ophthalmol.,* **72**, 975–8.

Primack, J.D., Smith, M.E. and Tychsen, L. (1995) Retinal detachment in a child as the first sign of leukemic relapse: histopathology, MRI findings, treatment, and tumor-free follow up. *J. Pediatr. Ophthalmol. Strabismus,* **32**, 253–6.

Ridgway, E.W., Jaffe, N. and Walton, D.S. (1976) Leukemic ophthalmopathy in children. *Cancer,* **38**, 1744–9.

Rosenthal, A.R. (1983) Ocular manifestations of leukemia. A review. *Ophthalmology,* **90**, 899–905.

Schachat, A.P. and Dhaliwal, R.S. (1994) Leukemias and lymphomas. In: S.J. Ryan (ed.), *Retina.* St Louis: Mosby, Vol. 1, Ch. 56, pp. 873–90.

Swartz, M. and Schumann, B. (1980) Acute leukemic infiltration of the vitreous diagnosed by pars plana aspiration. *Am. J. Ophthalmol.,* **90**, 326–30.

Zimmerman, L.E. and Font, R.L. (1975) Ophthalmologic manifestations of granulocytic sarcoma (myeloid sarcoma or chloroma). The third Pan American Association of Ophthalmology and American Journal of Ophthalmology Lecture. *Am. J. Ophthalmol.,* **80**, 975–90.

Chapter 22

Paraneoplastic syndromes

Paraneoplastic syndromes describe abnormalities remote from the primary tumour and any associated metastases (John *et al.*, 1997).

There are several mechanisms, which include the following:

a. Hormones and growth factors secreted by the tumour (e.g., ectopic Cushing's syndrome caused by adrenocorticotropin produced by lung cancer).
b. Antibodies and proteins secreted by the body in response to the tumour (e.g., tumour necrosis factor, which is believed to cause cachexia).

Recognition of a paraneoplastic syndrome may allow early detection and treatment of the underlying neoplasm.

Cancer-associated retinopathy (CAR)

This syndrome is believed to be an autoimmune disease caused by antibodies reacting with a variety of retinal antigens to cause loss of photoreceptors and cells in the outer nuclear layer.

CAR has been associated with the following malignancies:

- Bronchial carcinoma.
- Gynaecological cancers (Ohkawa *et al.*, 1996).
- Breast carcinoma.
- Cutaneous melanoma. This condition is called 'melanoma-associated retinopathy (MAR)' (Kim *et al.*, 1994) and primarily affects the bipolar cells (Gittinger and Smith, 1999).

SYMPTOMS

a. Visual loss, including ring-like scotomas, perhaps progressing to light perception.
b. Night blindness.
c. Photopsia.

The ocular symptoms of CAR usually precede the development of systemic malignancy by several months. In contrast, MAR tends to occur years after treatment of the primary cutaneous melanoma and is usually associated with clinical metastatic disease (Keltner and Thirkill, 1998).

SIGNS

- A normal fundus in the early stages of the disease.
- RPE stippling.
- Slight attenuation of the retinal vessels, perhaps with sheathing.
- Optic atrophy in some patients.
- Vitiligo and uveal depigmentation (i.e., 'acute Vogt–Koyanagi–Harada-like syndrome') in patients with MAR (Gass, 1987).
- Rarely, cells in the vitreous and anterior chamber (Klingele *et al.,* 1984).

INVESTIGATIONS

a. ERG demonstrates abnormalities usually affecting both rods and cones, or occasionally only cones (Jacobson and Thirkill, 1995).

b. Serum studies may reveal antibodies reacting with recoverin, a 23-kDa calcium-binding protein in retinal cells (Thirkill *et al.,* 1993) or other antigens (Murphy *et al.,* 1997) (Figure 22.1).

TREATMENT OPTIONS

- Treatment of the primary tumour.
- Systemic steroids (Keltner *et al.,* 1983).
- Plasmapheresis.

- Intravenous immunoglobulin (Guy and Aptsiauri, 1997).

The results of treatment are unpredictable.

Bilateral diffuse uveal melanocytic proliferation (BDUMP)

The main feature is a diffuse proliferation of pigmented and amelanotic melanocytes developing simultaneously in the uvea of both eyes, with areas of RPE hyper- and hypopigmentation (Borruat *et al.,* 1992; Mooy *et al.,* 1994). The proliferating cells can be benign (Barr *et al.,* 1982) or malignant (Prause *et al.,* 1984; Margo *et al.,* 1987) or both (Mooy *et al.,* 1994) (Figure 22.2).

A variety of systemic malignancies have developed in patients with BDUMP, usually several months after presentation with ocular signs.

SIGNS (Lafaut *et al.,* 1994; Gass *et al.,* 1990; Leys *et al.,* 1991)

- Diffuse uveal thickening.
- Several pigmented and non-pigmented, slightly elevated tumours (Figure 22.2).
- Multiple red/grey patches in the RPE, perhaps with a reticular appearance.
- Cysts of the ciliary body and iris.
- Cells in the vitreous and anterior chamber.

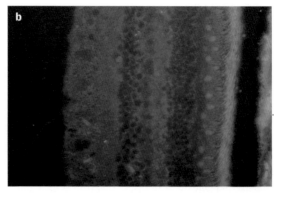

Figure 22.1 Indirect immunofluorescence demonstrating anti-recoverin antibodies in a patient with small cell carcinoma and CAR: (**a**) positive reaction in outer retina in sections of rhesus monkey retina, which were first incubated with patient serum (at 1:500) and then stained with goat anti-human polyvalent gamma globulins conjugated to fluorescein isothiocyanate; (**b**) negative reaction with normal serum control (1:100). (Courtesy of C.E. Thirkill, UC Davis Ophthalmology Research, Davis, California, USA)

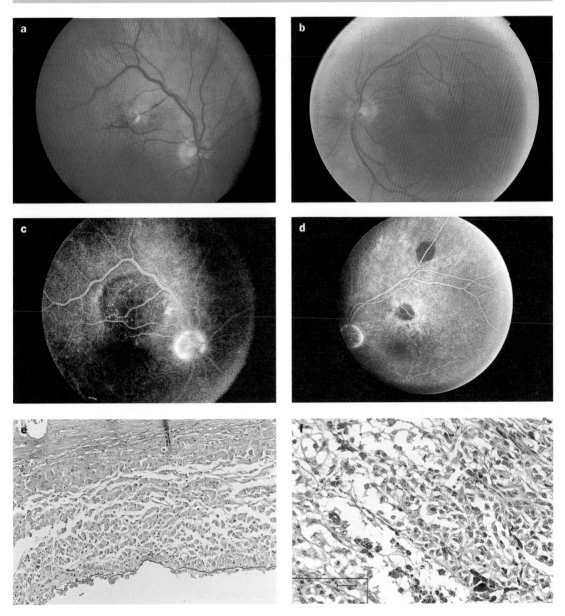

Figure 22.2 BDUMP in an 82-year-old man: (**a**) pigmented tumour with 'orange pigment' at the right macula, (**b**) pigmented and depigmented lesions in the left eye (present bilaterally), (**c**) fluorescein angiogram of the right macula, showing hypofluorescent lesion, (**d**) fluorescein angiogram of the left eye showing hypofluorescent lesions, with some showing marginal diffuse hyperfluorescence. The patient developed a bronchial carcinoma and died. Postmortem ocular examination showed (**e**) melanocytoma cells (identifiable after bleaching) in the pigmented lesions and (**f**) malignant melanoma cells forming a circumferential ciliary body tumour in each eye, with episcleral extension in the right eye. (Courtesy of C.M. Mooy, Erasmus University, Rotterdam)(Case report published in the *Br. J. Ophthalmol.*, 1994, **78**, 483–4)

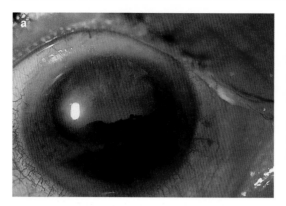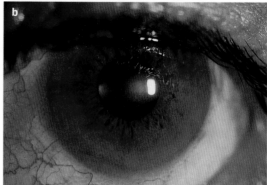

Figure 22.3 Bilateral, pigmented ciliary body and iris tumours in a 47-year-old man with carcinoma of the lung: (**a**) right eye and (**b**) left eye. (Courtesy of W.S. Foulds, Glasgow, UK)

- Ciliary body and iris tumours (Figure 22.3).
- Episcleral tumour nodules.

COMPLICATIONS

- Exudative retinal detachment.
- Cataract.
- Angle closure glaucoma.

FLUORESCEIN ANGIOGRAPHY

Fluorescein angiography shows masking of choroidal fluorescence by the pigmented tumours and extensive hyperfluorescent pinpoint lesions in the RPE (Figure 22.4)

TREATMENT

The ocular manifestations of BDUMP are generally regarded as untreatable, although visual improvement with systemic steroids has been reported (Lafaut *et al.,* 1994).

Miscellaneous syndromes

a. Optic neuritis (Boghen *et al.,* 1988).
b. Opsoclonus (Luque *et al.,* 1991).
c. Loss of saccades (Baloh *et al.,* 1993).
d. Eaton–Lambert syndrome, usually in patients with lung cancer, which is charac-

terized by muscle weakness, particularly affecting the thigh, but which can include ptosis and diplopia.
e. Dermatomyositis, with a purple discoloration of the eyelids, which is associated with a variety of cancers.
f. Cicatricial conjunctivitis and other oculomucocutaneous diseases, which can occur in conditions such as lymphoma (Lam *et al.,* 1992; Kreutzer *et al.,* 1996).
g. Erythrocytosis in von Hippel–Lindau disease, due to cerebellar haemangioblastoma or a renal tumour.
h. Exophthalmos similar to thyroid disease due to testicular seminoma (Mann, 1967).
i. Purtscher retinopathy due to pancreatic cancer (Tabandeh *et al.,* 1999).
j. Steroid-induced glaucoma due to carcinoid tumour (Blumenthal *et al.,* 1999).

REFERENCES

Baloh, R.W., DeRossett, S.E., Cloughesy, T.F., Kuncl, R.W., Miller, N.R., Merrill, J. and Posner, J.B. (1993) Novel brainstem syndrome associated with prostate carcinoma. *Neurology,* **43**, 2591–6.

Barr, C.C., Zimmerman, L.E., Curtin, V.T. and Font, R.L. (1982) Bilateral diffuse melanocytic uveal tumors associated with systemic malignant neoplasms: a recently recognized syndrome. *Arch. Ophthalmol.,* **100**, 249–55.

Blumenthal, E.Z., Muszkat, M., Pe'er, J. and Ticho, U. (1999) Corticosteroid-induced glaucoma attributa-

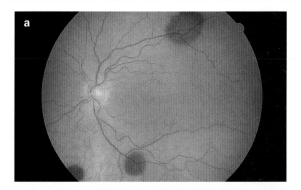

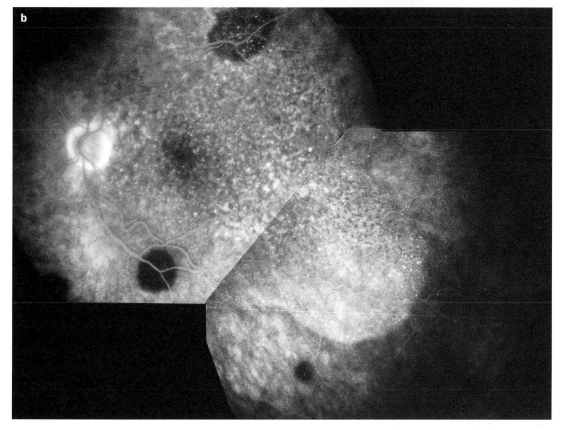

Figure 22.4 Left eye of a 63-year-old woman with BDUMP and ovarian carcinoma: (**a**) colour photograph showing multiple pigmented choroidal tumours and faint RPE lesions; (**b**) fluorescein angiogram showing masking of choroidal fluorescence by pigmented tumours and extensive pinpoint hyperfluorescence corresponding to RPE lesions. (Courtesy of A.M. Leys, Leuven, Belgium)(Case report published in *Arch. Ophthalmol.,* 1991, **109**, 1590–4)

ble to an adrenocorticotrophin-secreting malignant carcinoid tumor of the thymus. *Am. J. Ophthalmol.*, **128**, 100–1.

Boghen, D., Sebag, M. and Michaud, J. (1988) Paraneoplastic optic neuritis and encephalomyelitis. Report of a case. *Arch. Neurol.*, **45**, 353–6.

Borruat, F.X., Othenin-Girard, P., Uffer, S., Othenin-Girard, B., Regli, F. and Hurlimann, J. (1992) Natural history of diffuse uveal melanocytic proliferation. Case report. *Ophthalmology*, **99**, 1698–704.

Gass, J.D.M. (1987) *Stereoscopic Atlas of Macular Diseases: Diagnosis and Treatment.* St Louis: Mosby–Year Book.

Gass, J.D.M., Gieser, R.G., Wilkinson, C.P., Beahm, D.E. and Pautler, S.E. (1990) Bilateral diffuse uveal melanocytic proliferation in patients with occult carcinoma. *Arch. Ophthalmol.*, **108**, 527–33.

Gittinger, J.W. and Smith, T.W. (1999) Cutaneous melanoma-associated paraneoplastic retinopathy: histopathologic correlations. *Am. J. Ophthalmol.*, **127**, 612–14.

Guy, J. and Aptsiauri, N. (1999) Treatment of paraneoplastic visual loss with intravenous immunoglobulin: report of 3 cases. *Arch. Ophthalmol.*, **117**, 471–7.

Jacobson, D.M. and Thirkill, C.E. (1995) Paraneoplastic cone dysfunction: an unusual visual remote effect of cancer. *Arch. Ophthalmol.*, **113**, 1580–2.

John, W.J., Foon, K.A. and Patchell, R.A. (1997) Paraneoplastic syndromes. In: V.T. De Vita Jr., S. Hellman and A. Rosenberg (eds), *Cancer. Principles and Practice of Oncology.* Fifth edn. Philadelphia: J.B. Lippincott, pp. 2397–2422.

Keltner, J.L., Roth, A.M. and Chang, R.S. (1983) Photoreceptor degeneration: possible autoimmune disorder. *Arch. Ophthalmol.*, **101**, 564–9.

Keltner, J.L. and Thirkill, C.E. (1998) Cancer-associated retinopathy vs recoverin associated retinopathy. *Am. J. Ophthalmol.*, **126**, 296–302.

Kim, R.Y., Retsas, S., Fitzke, F.W., Arden, G.B. and Bird, A.C. (1994) Cutaneous melanoma-associated retinopathy. *Ophthalmology*, **101**, 1837–43.

Klingele, T.G., Burde, R.M., Rappazzo, J.A., Isserman, M.J., Burgess, D. and Kantor, O. (1984) Paraneoplastic retinopathy. *J. Clin. Neuroophthalmol.*, **4**, 239–45.

Kreutzer, B., Stubiger, N., Thiel, H.J. and Zierhut, M. (1996) Oculomucocutaneous changes as paraneoplastic syndromes. *Ger. J. Ophthalmol.*, **5**, 176–81.

Lafaut, B.A., Bourgoignie, K.B., Sallet, G. and De Laey J.-J. (1994) Prolifération bilatérale diffuse des méla-nocytes uvéaux. A propos d'un cas particulier. *J. Fr. Ophtalmol.*, **17**, 208–13.

Lam, S., Stone, M.S., Goeken, J.A., Massicotte, S.J., Smith, A.C., Folberg, R. and Krachmer, J.H. (1992) Paraneoplastic pemphigus, cicatricial conjunctivitis, and acanthosis nigricans with pachydermatoglyphy in a patient with bronchogenic squamous cell carcinoma. *Ophthalmology*, **99**, 108–13.

Leys, A.M., Dierick, H.G. and Sciot, R.M. (1991) Early lesions of bilateral diffuse melanocytic proliferation. *Arch. Ophthalmol.*, **109**, 1590–4.

Luque, F.A., Furneaux, H.M., Ferziger, R., Rosenblum, M.K., Wray, S.H., Schold, S.C. Jr., Glantz, M.J., Jaeckle, K.A., Biran, H. and Lesser, M. *et al.* (1991) Anti-Ri: an antibody associated with paraneoplastic opsoclonus and breast cancer. *Ann. Neurol.*, **29**, 241–51.

Mann, A.S. (1967) Bilateral exophthalmos in seminoma. *Am. J. Ophthalmol.*, **27**, 1500–2.

Margo, C.E., Pavan, P.R., Gendelman, D. and Gragoudas, E. (1987) Bilateral melanocytic uveal tumors associated with systemic non-ocular malignancy. Malignant melanomas or benign paraneoplastic syndrome? *Retina*, **7**, 137–41.

Mooy, C.M., de Jong, P.T. and Strous, C. (1994) Proliferative activity in bilateral paraneoplastic melanocytic proliferation and bilateral uveal melanoma. *Br. J. Ophthalmol.*, **78**, 483–4.

Murphy, M.A., Thirkill, C.E. and Hart, W.M. Jr. (1997) Paraneoplastic retinopathy: a novel autoantibody reaction associated with small-cell lung carcinoma. *J. Neuro-ophthalmol.*, **17**, 77–83.

Ohkawa, T., Kawashima, H., Makino, S., Shimizu, Y., Shimizu, H., Sekiguchi, I. and Tsuchida, S. (1996) Cancer-associated retinopathy in a patient with endometrial cancer. *Am. J. Ophthalmol.*, **122**, 740–2.

Prause, J.U., Jensen, O.A., Eisgart, F., Hansen, U. and Kieffer, M. (1984) Bilateral diffuse malignant melanoma of the uvea associated with large cell carcinoma, giant cell type, of the lung. Case report of a newly described syndrome. *Ophthalmologica*, **189**, 221–8.

Tabandeh, H., Rosenfeld, P.J., Alexandrakis, G., Kronish, J.P. and Chaudhry, N.A. (1999) Purtscher-like retinopathy associated with pancreatic adenocarcinoma. *Am. J. Ophthalmol.*, **128**, 650–2.

Thirkill, C.E., Keltner, J.L., Tyler, N.K. and Roth, A.M. (1993) Antibody reactions with retina and cancer-associated antigens in 10 patients with cancer-associated retinopathy. *Arch. Ophthalmol.*, **111**, 931–7.

TREATMENT

Chapter 23

Radiotherapy

Radiosensitivity

Radiation can cause (a) immediate cell death, (b) delayed cell death, which occurs when the cell attempts to divide, and (c) cellular sterilization, with prolonged survival but without the ability to divide.

The proportion of cells surviving radiation varies with dose (Figure 23.1). At moderate and high doses, the survival fraction diminishes linearly as dose is increased, with the slope being proportional to the radiosensitivity of the cells. At low doses, the cells repair the mildly damaged DNA (i.e., 'sub-lethal damage repair') and survive, so that the survival curve is flatter (i.e., has 'a shoulder').

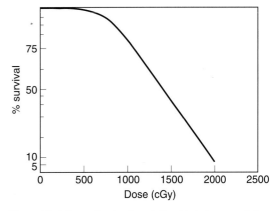

Figure 23.1 Curve showing the relationship between radiation dose and cell survival

FACTORS INCREASING RADIOSENSITIVITY

a. Oxygenation (which encourages free radicals).
b. Hyperthermia.
c. High dose-rate.
d. Pharmacological agents, such as bromodeoxyuridine (BUDR).

Radioresponsiveness

The radioresponsiveness of a tumour depends on the lifespan of the neoplastic cells, with rapidly proliferating tumours shrinking rapidly after radiotherapy. For this reason, fast growing tumours, such as metastases and retinoblastomas, tend to regress more quickly than melanomas.

Brachytherapy

Brachytherapy is radiotherapy delivered by radio-active sources placed close to the target tissues.

INDICATIONS

a. Small to medium sized uveal melanomas.
b. Medium sized retinoblastomas.
c. Small uveal metastases ((Shields *et al.*, 1997).
d. Selected iris melanomas (Shields *et al.*, 1995).
e. Selected vascular uveal and retinal tumours.
f. Selected malignant conjunctival tumours.
g. Treatment of choroidal melanoma as an adjunct to local resection (Damato *et al.*, 1997) or transpupillary thermotherapy (Oosterhuis *et al.*, 1995).

APPLICATORS

^{106}RUTHENIUM PLAQUE

The main features of ruthenium plaques (BEBIG, GmbH, Berlin, Germany) are the following:

a. An outer silver shell, 0.9 mm thick (Figure 23.2).
b. A layer of ^{106}Ru painted on the inner surface of the shell and sealed with a 0.1 mm coating of silver.
c. Half-life of 368 days, making it possible for the same plaque to be used many times over a one-year period.
d. Emission of electrons with an average energy of 3.3 MeV.
e. The availability of notched plaques for juxta-papillary tumours and ciliary body tumours.

^{125}IODINE PLAQUE

a. Gold or steel shell (e.g., ROPES, Australia), shielding orbital structures (Figure 23.3).
b. An appropriate number of iodine seeds, usually about 13. The number and location can be altered so as to tailor the dose to a particular tumour.
c. Emission of low-energy gamma irradiation, with a mean energy of 28.3 keV (range

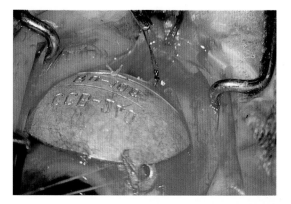

Figure 23.2 The ruthenium plaque

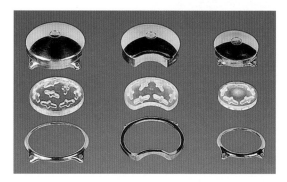

Figure 23.3 The iodine plaque. (Courtesy of C. Karolis, Radiation Oncology Physics and Engineering Services Pty Ltd, St Paul's, N.S.W., Australia)

27.4–35.5 keV). This means that if 100 Gy is delivered to a 5 mm thick tumour then the retina diagonally opposite receives about 15% of the dose and a structure such as disc or fovea located 5 mm laterally from the edge of the plaque receives about 40% of the dose.

d. Silastic insert or resin, for holding the seeds in a particular distribution.
e. Lip at the shell margin, to reduce side-scatter.
f. A 1 mm thick absorber between seeds and sclera to reduce the dose to sclera for a specified tumour apex dose (because of the inverse-square law).
g. Half-life of about 60 days.
h. Notched applicators for juxtapapillary and ciliary body tumours.

OTHER ISOTOPES

Other isotopes used for brachytherapy include [90]strontium, [103]palladium (Finger *et al.,* 1999) and [192]iridium (Valcárcel *et al.,* 1994). [60]Cobalt plaques have largely been superseded by less energetic plaques.

SURGICAL TECHNIQUE

1. Any overlying rectus or oblique muscles are temporarily disinserted or pulled to one side with a suture sling (Figure 23.4**a**).
2. The uveal tumour is localized by transillumination or by binocular indirect ophthalmo-

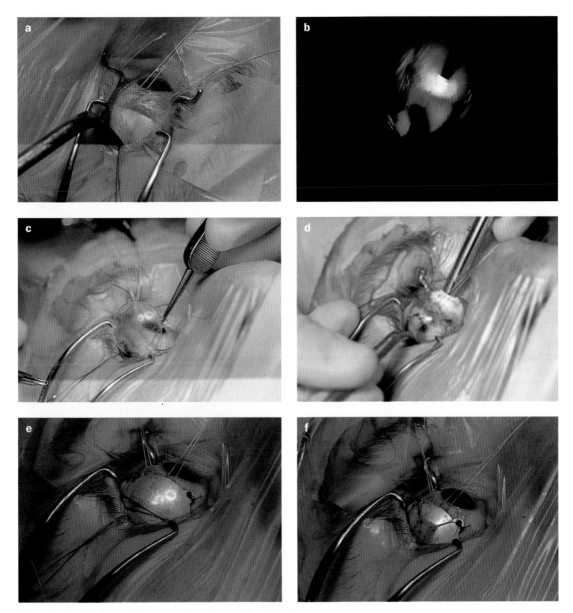

Figure 23.4 Technique of plaque insertion (see text for details)

scopy with indentation and its margins are marked on the sclera with a pen or diathermy (Figure 23.4**b**).

3. A plaque having a diameter 4 mm greater than the tumour diameter is generally recommended so as to achieve a safety margin of 2 mm all around the tumour.

4. A template consisting of a transparent plastic dummy or metal ring with eyelets is sutured to the sclera, tying each suture with a releasable bow (Figure 23.4**c**).

5. The position of this template can be checked by transillumination (Figure 23.4**d**) or by performing indirect ophthalmoscopy while indenting the eye with the template. An alternative approach is to perform intraoperative ultrasonography.

6. Once the template is in the correct position, the sutures are loosened and used to secure the radioactive plaque. Special care is taken to ensure that the entire plaque margin is firmly in contact with the sclera, either by

suturing additional eyelets or, in the case of a ruthenium implant, by placing a mattress suture over the plaque (Figure 23.4**e**). A technique for achieving good apposition with juxtapapillary plaques involves a sling passed under the rectus muscles and sutured to the sclera near the cornea (Abdel-Dayem and Trese, 1999).

7. The extraocular muscles are attached to their original insertions or to sclera by a sling so that they lie in the normal anatomical position (Figure 23.4**f**).

8. Dosimetry is performed using computerized software, which creates a three-dimensional model of the eye and tumour using measurements derived from ultrasonography or CT scans (Astrahan *et al.*, 1990) (Figure 23.5). The time required to deliver a specified dose to the sclera or tumour apex is calculated, together with the total doses received by lens, macula and optic nerve.

9. Once the appropriate dose has been delivered, usually within 3–7 days, the conjunctiva is opened and the plaque is removed, temporarily disinserting any overlying extraocular muscles if necessary. If the obli-

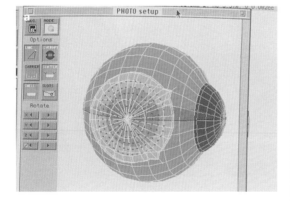

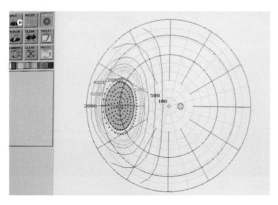

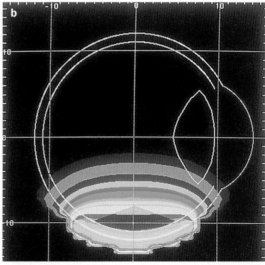

Figure 23.5 Dosimetry for plaque radiotherapy: (**a**) three-dimensional model of the eye, (**b**) section showing plaque, tumour and normal ocular structures and (**c**) retinal diagram showing isodose curves

que muscle has been lying in its correct anatomical position, it should have become adherent to episclera so that re-suturing is not required.

Charged particle radiotherapy

Proton beam radiotherapy is to some extent based on the principle that protons induce most tissue damage at the depth at which they slow down, with relative sparing of superficial tissues (i.e., Bragg peak) (Figure 23.6).

There are presently about a dozen cyclotron units worldwide that are capable of proton beam radiotherapy of ocular tumours. The indications and contraindications vary from centre to centre.

INDICATIONS

a. Choroidal melanomas that cannot easily be treated with a plaque because of large size or posterior location.
b. Iris melanomas, as a means of avoiding a surgical defect and photophobia.
c. Choroidal haemangiomas.
d. Conjunctival tumours not amenable to other treatment.

METHOD

1. Before surgery, ultrasonographic measurements are obtained of ocular and tumour dimensions.
2. Under local or general anaesthesia, four or five radio-opaque, tantalum markers are sutured to the sclera at known distances from the tumour margins (Figure 23.7).
3. Once the postoperative inflammation has settled, a face-mask and a bite-block are moulded, which will help immobilize the patient during treatment. In addition, a computerized three-dimensional model of the eye is generated using fundus photographs, ultrasonographic data, intraoperative measurements, and radiographs showing the marker positions (Figure 23.8). This information is used to calculate (a) beam range and profile, (b) ideal eye position and (c) radiation doses to important ocular structures.
4. Four fractions of radiotherapy are delivered over five days. The patient is seated in a mechanized chair with the head immobilized in a frame by means of the face-mask and bite-block (Figure 23.9). The eye is positioned by looking at an adjustable fixation target. Proper positioning of the eye is confirmed by localizing the tantalum markers

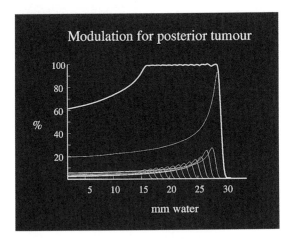

Figure 23.6 Ionization curve of a proton beam, showing the Bragg peak, with a surface tissue dose of approximately 20%. Such surface sparing is diminished when the tumour is thick or anterior. (Courtesy of A. Kaçperek, Clatterbridge, UK)

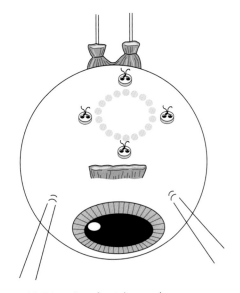

Figure 23.7 Insertion of tantalum markers

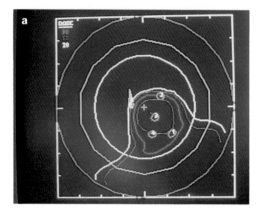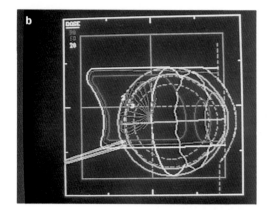

Figure 23.8 Dosimetry for proton beam radiotherapy: (**a**) beam's eye view, (**b**) horizontal section. (Courtesy of A. Kaçperek, Clatterbridge, UK)

radiographically (Figure 23.10). During each treatment, which lasts 30–40 seconds, the eye position is monitored visually, using a high-magnification video camera.

External beam radiotherapy

INDICATIONS

a. Uveal metastases.
b. Choroidal haemangioma.
c. Residual orbital tumour after enucleation.
d. Selected retinoblastomas, not treatable by other methods.

METHOD

Treatment planning is performed using a radiation simulator. The radiation fields are checked using portal films and light localizers. Temporary marks are placed on the skin to facilitate positioning. In infants, immobilization is achieved using a transparent face-mask and by administering the treatment under general anaesthesia.

RADIATIONAL FIELDS

a. The 'classic', D-shaped ipsilateral temporal field has its anterior margin level with the lateral bony canthus and equator of the eye.

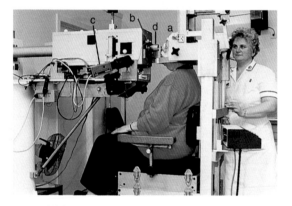

Figure 23.9 Positioning of the patient during proton beam radiotherapy. Note (**a**) head fixation with a mask and dental bite, (**b**) visual target for maintaining direction of gaze of treated eye, (**c**) TV camera for monitoring eye position and (**d**) collimator. (Courtesy of A. Kaçperek, Clatterbridge, UK)

This can be angled vertically and horizontally to spare the fellow eye (Figure 23.11).

b. The Schipper technique is an ipsilateral temporal field delivered with a 6–8 MeV beam, which is highly collimated with a penumbra of 1.5 mm (Schipper, Imhoff and Tan, 1997) (Figure 23.12). The beam is aimed with an accuracy of 0.3 mm by attaching the collimator to a rod, which rests gently on a corneal contact lens. The anterior margin of the beam is level either with the posterior lens surface or a point 3 mm anteriorly.

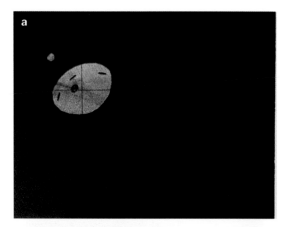

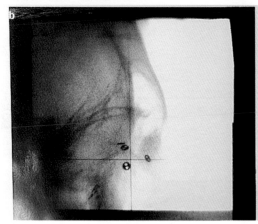

Figure 23.10 Radiographs showing position of markers: (**a**) beam's eye view and (**b**) lateral view

c. The anterior field completely spares the fellow eye and is delivered with or without lens shielding (Figure 23.13).
d. Various split-field techniques combine an ipsilateral temporal field with an anterior field, usually using a lens shield (Weiss *et al.*, 1975; McCormick *et al.*, 1988).

Stereotactic irradiation

With this method, the radiation is focused on the tumour by directing multiple, highly collimated beams converging on the tumour from different locations around the eye, either concurrently or sequentially.

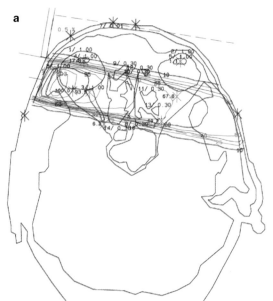

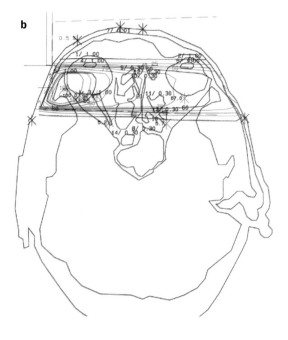

Figure 23.11 Lateral field (**a**) with and (**b**) without sparing of the fellow eye. (Courtesy of R.D. Errington, Clatterbridge, UK)

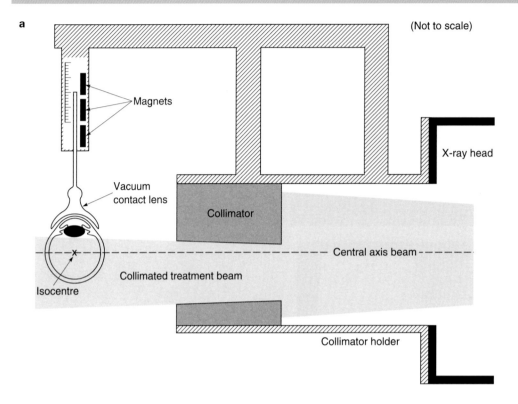

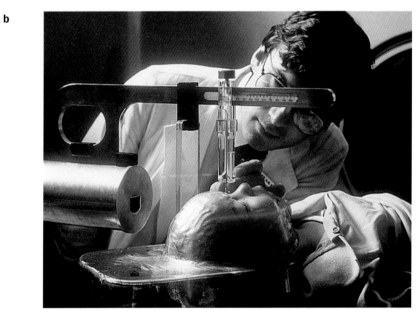

Figure 23.12 The Schipper technique: (**a**) diagram showing attachment of the collimator to a rod, which rests gently on a corneal contact lens so that a highly collimated beam is accurately directed at the eye (courtesy of J. Schipper, Arnhem, The Netherlands); (**b**) actual model in operation (courtesy of A. Harnett, Glasgow, UK)

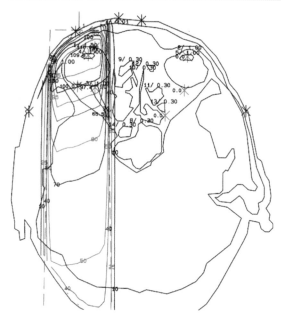

Figure 23.13 Anterior field, showing significant radiation of the brain. (Courtesy of R.D. Errington, Clatterbridge, UK)

INDICATIONS

This is a new technique so that the indications and contraindications have not yet been fully defined. It may be an alternative to proton beam radiotherapy when brachytherapy is not possible.

METHOD

1. CT and MRI scans are obtained while the patient's head is immobilized in a stereotactic head frame.
2. A three-dimensional plan of the target volume is prepared, which includes a 2 mm safety margin.
3. The radiotherapy is delivered using the same head frame and immobilizing the eye either with a visual target or a suction device. The eye is monitored with a TV camera.
4. The treatment is given either in several fractions (i.e., 'stereotactic radiotherapy') or in a single fraction (i.e., 'radiosurgery').

STEREOTACTIC DELIVERY SYSTEMS

a. The Leksell Gamma Knife has 201 cobalt-60 sources arranged in a hemispherical array, with the radiational beams collimated towards a single focus by means of a collimator helmet (Zehetmayer *et al.*, 1997).
b. The modified linear accelerator (LINAC) delivers photons using a micro-multileaf collimator to shape the final dose volume (Debus *et al.*, 1997) (Figure 23.14). A total dose of 60–70 Gy is delivered in five fractions over 8–10 days.

Complications

NON-RADIATIONAL

a. Rhegmatogenous retinal detachment, if a retinal tear is created while suturing a plaque or marker to the sclera.
b. Choroidal detachment, caused by compression of a vortex vein by a plaque.
c. Diplopia, if an extraocular muscle is not repositioned accurately after temporary disinsertion. The diplopia usually resolves spontaneously, but may occasionally be persistent, particularly if due to a disturbance of a vertical rectus or oblique muscle.

EARLY RADIATIONAL

a. Eyelid erythema, ulceration and crusting after external radiotherapy. These develop in the first weeks (Figure 23.15) and heal over 1 or 2 months.
b. Conjunctivitis with hyperaemia and a mucopurulent discharge.
c. Acute exudative retinal detachment, which can follow the use of a new, 'hot' plaque. It tends to resolve spontaneously within 6 months.
d. Choroidal detachment if a high dose of radiotherapy is delivered within a short time, as with a hot plaque. This complication can cause secondary angle closure glaucoma (Figure 23.16).
e. Superficial punctate keratitis.

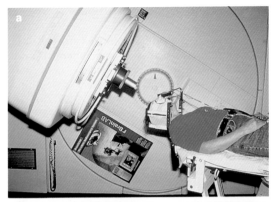

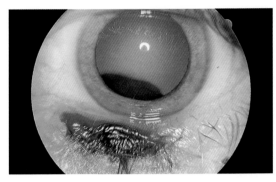

Figure 23.15 Acute eyelid damage after proton beam radiotherapy. This heals after a few weeks leaving an area of atrophy with loss of lashes

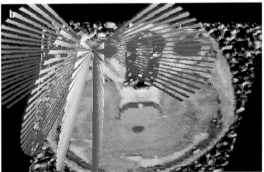

LATE RADIATIONAL

a. Eyelid damage, such as depigmentation, loss of lashes or eyebrows, and atrophic scars.
b. Lacrimal gland atrophy, after high doses of irradiation, causing a dry eye if the accessory glands are also irradiated.
c. Canalicular irradiation causes obstruction and intractable epiphora (Figure 23.17).
d. Conjunctival telangiectasia causes a cosmetic deficit whereas epithelial abnormalities result in an unstable tear film, with irritation, and cold intolerance (Figure 23.18). Ocular discomfort is increased by keratinization, especially if this occurs in the superior palpebral conjunctiva.

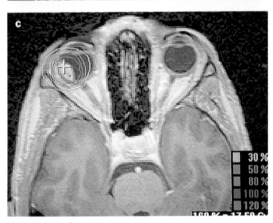

Figure 23.14 The modified linear accelerator (LINAC): (**a**) photograph of a patient receiving treatment, (**b**) diagram showing convergence of the radiational beams onto the tumour and (**c**) isodose curves superimposed on merged CT and MRI scans. (Courtesy of M. Zehetmayer, Vienna, Austria)

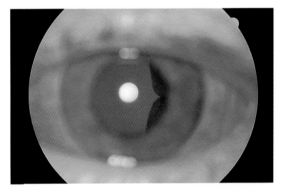

Figure 23.16 Choroidal detachment during ruthenium plaque radiotherapy, with secondary angle closure glaucoma, which resolved after a short period of medical therapy

f. Iritis is not usually a problem unless high-dose radiotherapy has been delivered.

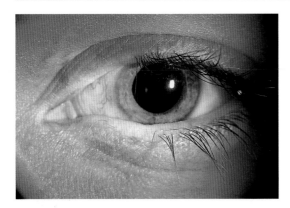

Figure 23.17 Canalicular obstruction after proton beam radiotherapy. Note also the loss of lashes and depigmentation of eyelid skin

23.19). There may also be hard exudates and oedema arising from the regressing tumour (Figure 23.20). Retinal neovascularization may respond to pan-retinal photocoagulation, thereby preventing vitreous haemorrhage (Archer *et al.*, 1991).

i. Optic neuropathy is likely if the tumour extends to within a disc diameter of the optic disc margin (Figure 23.21). Between 1 and 3 years after the radiotherapy, the disc initially becomes swollen and hyperaemic, often with surrounding exudates and haemorrhages and occasionally with new vessels. The end result is optic atrophy and poor vision, usually ranging from 6/60 to No Light Perception.

j. Chronic retinal detachment often follows treatment of large choroidal melanomas and

e. Keratitis is usually due to dry eye or radiational damage to the upper eyelid margin. A neurotrophic ulcer can develop, possibly leading to corneal perforation.

f. Scleral perforation can rarely follow plaque radiotherapy over ciliary body or behind a rectus muscle insertion.

g. Cataract tends to develop from the second year onwards after radiotherapy, either because of direct radiation of the lens or because of other ocular complications.

h. Retinopathy usually develops 2 or 3 years after radiotherapy. It consists of retinal vasculopathy, with telangiectasia, capillary closure, cotton wool spots, hard exudates, oedema, and neovascularization (Figure

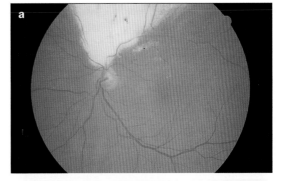

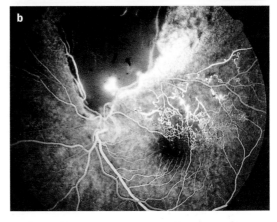

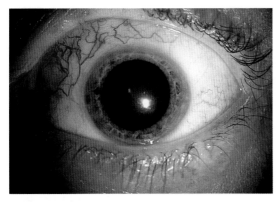

Figure 23.18 Conjunctival telangiectasia after proton beam radiotherapy

Figure 23.19 Radiation retinopathy with cotton wool spots, retinal telangiectasia and capillary closure after ruthenium plaque radiotherapy and photocoagulation of a melanoma

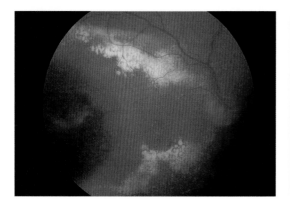

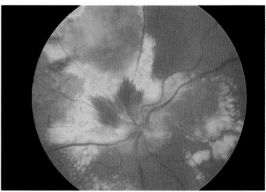

Figure 23.20 Macular exudation after plaque radiotherapy

Figure 23.21 Optic neuropathy after proton beam radiotherapy

is possibly due to radiational vasculopathy within the tumour.

k. Neovascular glaucoma usually complicates severe and prolonged exudative retinal detachment, possibly because the outer retina becomes ischaemic when it is separated from the choriocapillaris. Rubeosis can also occur as a consequence of optic neuropathy or extensive ciliary body irradiation (Kim *et al.*, 1986).

l. Choroidal atrophy contributes to visual loss but is useful in demonstrating where the radiotherapy has been delivered (Figure 23.22). After ruthenium plaque radiotherapy with a minimum dose of 350 Gy to the choroid, a pepper and salt appearance develops in the irradiated area within 2 or 3 months, and this eventually progresses to total choroidal atrophy, often with peripheral cobblestone degeneration (Figure 23.22**b**). With iodine plaque radiotherapy, stereotactic radiotherapy and proton beam radiotherapy, these changes occur more slowly.

m. Orbital bone growth arrest can occur after external beam radiotherapy, especially if treatment is given in the first year of life.

n. Epilepsy and hypopituitarism may follow external beam radiotherapy with an anterior field.

o. Malignant neoplasms can develop in a dose-related fashion in healthy individuals, the risk increasing greatly in patients with germ-

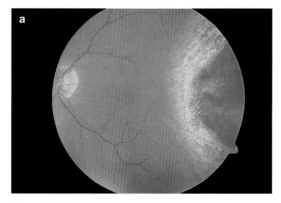

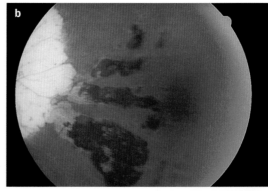

Figure 23.22 Choroidal atrophy after ruthenium plaque radiotherapy: (**a**) posterior margin and (**b**) anterior margin showing hyperpigmented cobblestone-type atrophy due to vascular closure

line RB1 mutations, especially if the radiotherapy is delivered in the first year of life (Figure 13.15) (Abramson and Frank, 1998).

'Threshold' doses for radiational ocular complications have been estimated (Sagerman *et al.,* 1993; Alberti, 1997) but are not included here because they vary greatly according to numerous factors. These include the following:

a. Fractionation of the total radiation dose into several small doses (e.g., 1.8–2.0 Gy) so that a higher total dose of radiation can be given without causing excessive acute complications.

b. Hyperthermia, which increases radiosensitivity so that a lower total dose is required (Finger, 1997).

c. Diabetes mellitus and other causes of vasculitis, which are aggravated by radiation (Viebahn *et al.,* 1991; Gragoudas *et al.,* 1999).

d. Concurrent chemotherapy (Parsons *et al.,* 1994), which increases radiational complications.

e. Tumour volume, which is related to the incidence of complications.

f. Old age, which contributes to the development of cataract.

g. Infancy, which increases the risk of orbital bone growth arrest.

REFERENCES

Abdel-Dayem, H.K. and Trese, M.T. (1999) A technique for suturing peripapillary radioactive plaques. *Am. J. Ophthalmol.*, **127**, 224–6.

Abramson, D.H. and Frank, C.M. (1998) Second nonocular tumors in survivors of bilateral retinoblastoma: a possible age effect on radiation-related risk. *Ophthalmology*, **105**, 573–9.

Alberti, W. (1997) Acute and late side effects of radiotherapy for ocular disease: an overview. In: T. Wiegel, N. Bornfeld, M.H. Foerster and W. Hinkelbein (eds), *Radiotherapy of Ocular Disease.* Basel: Karger, pp. 281–6.

Archer, D.B., Amoaku, W.M.K. and Gardiner, T.A. (1991) Radiation retinopathy: clinical, histopathological, ultrastructural and experimental correlations. *Eye*, **5**, 239–51.

Astrahan, M.A., Luxton, G., Jozsef, G., Kampp, T.D., Liggett, P.E., Sapozink, M.D. and Petrovich, Z. (1990) An interactive treatment planning system for ophthalmic plaque radiotherapy. *Int. J. Radiat. Oncol. Biol. Phys.*, **18**, 679–87.

Damato, B.E. (1997) Adjunctive plaque radiotherapy after local resection of uveal melanoma. *Front. Radiat. Ther. Oncol.*, **30**, 123–32.

Debus, J., Engenhart-Cabillic, R., Holz, F.G., Pastyr, O., Rhein, B., Bortfeld, T. and Wannenmacher, M. (1997) Stereotactic precision radiotherapy in the treatment of intraocular malignancies with a micromultileaf collimator. In: T. Wiegel, N. Bornfeld, M.H. Foerster and W. Hinkelbein (eds), *Radiotherapy of Ocular Disease.* Basel: Karger, pp. 39–46.

Finger, P.T. (1997) Microwave thermotherapy for uveal melanoma: results of a 10-year study. *Ophthalmology*, **104**, 1794–1803.

Finger, P.T., Berson, A. and Szechter, A. (1999) Palladium-103 plaque radiotherapy for choroidal melanoma. Results of a 7-year study. *Ophthalmology*, **106**, 606–13.

Gragoudas, E.S., Li, W., Lane, A.-M., Munzenrider, J. and Egan, K.M. (1999) Risk factors for radiation maculopathy and papillopathy after intraocular irradiation. *Ophthalmology*, **106**, 1571–8.

Kim, M.K., Char, D.H., Castro, J.L., Saunders, W.M., Chen, G.T. and Stone, R.D. (1986) Neovascular glaucoma after helium ion irradiation for uveal melanoma. *Ophthalmology*, **93**, 189–93.

McCormick, B., Ellsworth, R., Abramson, D., Haik, B., Tome, M., Grabowski, E. and LoSasso, T. (1988) Radiation therapy for retinoblastoma: comparison of results with lens-sparing versus lateral beam techniques. *Int. J. Radiat. Oncol. Biol. Phys.*, **15**, 567–74.

Oosterhuis, J.A., Journée de Korver, H.G., Kakebeeke Kemme, H.M. and Bleeker, J.C. (1995) Transpupillary thermotherapy in choroidal melanomas. *Arch. Ophthalmol.*, **113**, 315–21.

Parsons, J.T., Bova, F.J., Fitzgerald, C.R., Mendenhall, W.M. and Million, R.R. (1994) Radiation retinopathy after external-beam irradiation: analysis of time–dose factors. *Int. J. Radiat. Oncol. Biol. Phys.*, **30**, 765–73.

Sagerman, R.H., Chung, C.T. and Alberti, W.E. (1993) Radiosensitivity of ocular and orbital structures. In: W.E. Alberti and R.H. Sagerman (eds), *Radiotherapy of Intraocular and Orbital Tumors.* Berlin: Springer-Verlag, Ch. 38, pp. 375–85.

Schipper, J., Imhoff, S.M. and Tan, K.E.W.P. (1997) Precision megavoltage external beam radiation therapy for retinoblastoma. *Front. Radiat. Ther. Oncol.*, **30**, 65–80.

Shields, C.L., Shields, J.A., De Potter, P., Quaranta, M., Freire, J., Brady, L.W. and Barrett, J. (1997) Plaque radiotherapy for the management of uveal metastasis. *Arch. Ophthalmol.*, **115**, 203–9.

Shields, C.L., Shields, J.A., De Potter, P., Singh, A.D., Hernandez, C. and Brady, L.W. (1995) Treatment of non-resectable malignant iris tumours with custom designed plaque radiotherapy. *Br. J. Ophthalmol.*, **79**, 306–12.

Valcárcel, F., Valverde, S., Caŕdenes, H., Cajigal, C., de la Torre, A., Magallón, R., Regueiro, C., Encinas, J.L. and Aragón, G. (1994) Episcleral iridium-192 wire therapy for choroidal melanomas. *Int. J. Radiat. Oncol. Biol. Phys.*, **30**, 1091–7.

Viebahn, M., Barricks, M.E. and Osterloh, M.D. (1991) Synergism between diabetic and radiation retinopa-thy: case report and review. *Br. J. Ophthalmol.*, **75**, 629–32.

Weiss, D.R., Cassady, J.R. and Petersen, R. (1975) Retinoblastoma: a modification in radiation therapy technique. *Radiology*, **114**, 705–8.

Zehetmayer, M., Menapace, R., Kitz, K., Ertl, A., Strenn, K. and Ruhswurm, I. (1997) Stereotactic irradiation of uveal melanoma with the Leksell Gamma Unit. In: T. Wiegel, B. Bornfeld, M.H. Foerster and W. Hinkelbein (eds), *Radiotherapy of Ocular Disease*. Basle: Karger, pp. 47–55.

Chapter 24

Surgery

Local resection of conjunctival tumours

INDICATIONS

a. Diagnosis and treatment of nodular melanoma, squamous cell carcinoma and other
discrete conjunctival tumours.
b. Localized primary acquired melanosis.
c. Recurrent conjunctival tumours.

1. The conjunctival and episcleral vessels
around the tumour are cauterized, to prevent
bleeding (Shields *et al.,* 1998) (Figure 24.1).
2. The conjunctiva and episclera are divided
with scissors, clearing the tumour margin
by at least 3 mm.
3. These tissues are then dissected from the
sclera, maintaining haemostasis with cautery. If the tumour is adherent to sclera then
the superficial sclera is included in the block

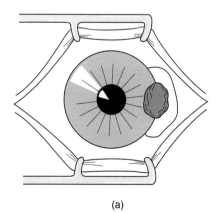
(a)

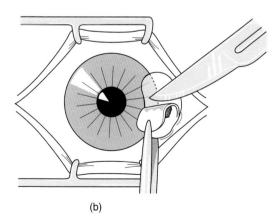
(b)

Figure 24.1 Local resection of conjunctival tumour

resection. To prevent seeding of tumour cells, the 'no touch technique' is used. This involves handling only normal tissue around the tumour, without letting the instruments touch the tumour itself. Other precautions against tumour seeding are not irrigating the eye, not re-using swabs and using fresh instruments for closure.

4. If the tumour extends to the limbus, the adjacent corneal epithelium is included in the specimen. If possible, Bowman's layer is left intact as it is a barrier to tumour invasion. Separation of the corneal epithelium from Bowman's layer is facilitated by swabbing the cornea with absolute alcohol.

5. The specimen is gently laid flat onto a piece of paper, taking care to avoid crush artifact, and placed in fixative.

6. Local tumour recurrence is prevented by applying cryotherapy to the surrounding conjunctiva. Some surgeons prefer to use a retinal cryoprobe placed underneath the conjunctiva (Shields *et al.*, 1998) and others use liquid nitrogen spray. The double or triple freeze–thaw technique is used, lowering the temperature to approximately −20° C. An alternative to cryotherapy is radiotherapy, usually delivered with a beta emitter such as the strontium applicator or a ruthenium plaque.

7. The conjunctival defect can either be closed surgically or left to heal by second intention.

COMPLICATIONS

a. Local tumour recurrence from invisible microscopic deposits months or years after treatment.

b. Scleral necrosis and perforation following radiotherapy or, rarely, cryotherapy (Tucker *et al.*, 1993).

Iridectomy

INDICATIONS

Iridectomy is indicated for melanomas involving less than about four clock hours of iris but not extending to the angle.

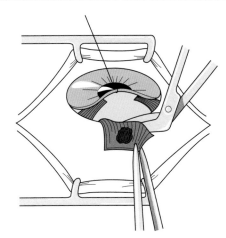

Figure 24.2 Iridectomy, performed through limbal incision

TECHNIQUE

Iridectomy is performed through a limbal incision with wide margins (Figure 24.2).

COMPLICATIONS

An inevitable complication is the iris defect, which can cause photophobia, refractive errors and cosmetic problems (Figure 24.3). These may be remediable with a painted contact lens or an artificial iris implant if the eye is pseudophakic.

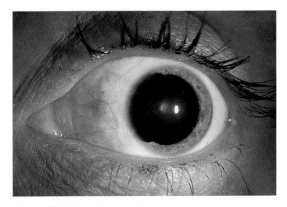

Figure 24.3 Iris coloboma after local resection

Iridocyclectomy

INDICATIONS

Iridocyclectomy is indicated when a tumour such as melanoma or adenocarcinoma involves the angle or ciliary body but not more than a third of these structures.

TECHNIQUE

1. A lamellar scleral flap is prepared, hinged at the limbus and with the posterior incision over the region of the ora serrata (Figure 24.4**a**).

2. Deep scleral incisions are then made 1–2 mm within the superficial scleral incision (Figure 24.4**b**).

3. The tumour is removed together with the deep scleral lamella, if possible avoiding damage to lens and vitreous base (Figure 24.4**c**).

4. The scleral flap is closed with interrupted sutures (Figure 24.4**d**). An alternative approach is to perform full thickness corneoscleral excision with grafting (Naumann and Rummelt, 1996).

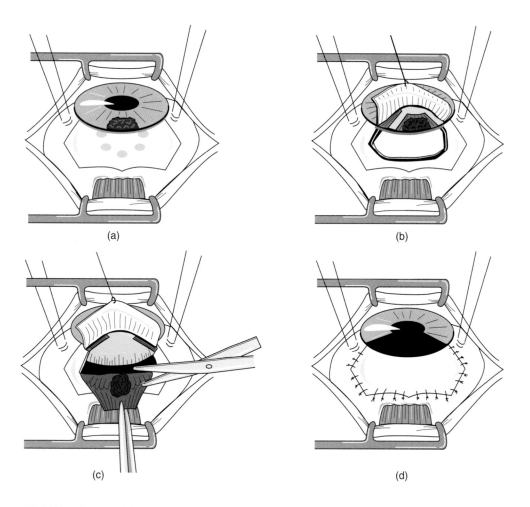

(a)

(b)

(c)

(d)

Figure 24.4 Iridocyclectomy: (**a**) superficial scleral flap, hinged at limbus, (**b**) deep scleral incision, (**c**) iridocyclectomy and (**d**) closure of flap

COMPLICATIONS

a. Local tumour recurrence if the clearance margins are inadequate.
b. Ocular hypotony or phthisis if more than a third of ciliary body is removed.
c. Subluxation of the lens and cataract if more than a third of the ciliary body is excised.
d. Aqueous misdirection and malignant glaucoma is a rare problem and is most likely to occur if an intact vitreous face is preserved.
e. Cyclodialysis with secondary hypotony and macular oedema may require surgical treatment to close the cleft.

Choroidectomy and cyclo-choroidectomy

Trans-scleral local resection of choroidal melanomas is difficult and therefore not widely performed (Peyman and Gremillion, 1989; Shields *et al.*, 1991; Damato and Foulds, 1994).

INDICATIONS

a. Choroidal melanomas considered too thick for radiotherapy.
b. Benign uveal tumours, such as leiomyoma and neurilemmoma.

CONTRAINDICATIONS

a. Basal tumour diameter exceeding 16 mm.
b. Tumour extension to within 1–2 DD of optic nerve head, unless the increased risks of residual tumour are acceptable.
c. Involvement of more than 2–3 clock hours of the ciliary body or angle.
d. Retinal invasion, unless vitreoretinal surgery is acceptable.
e. Scleral perforation, unless full-thickness scleral grafting or other measures are possible.

TECHNIQUE

1. The tumour is localized by transillumination.

2. A lamellar scleral flap is dissected, hinged posteriorly, applying diathermy to any intervening vortex veins or posterior ciliary vessels (Figure 24.5**a**).
3. The intraocular pressure is lowered by pars plana vitrectomy, to prevent prolapse of the retina through the scleral window.
4. The deep sclera is incised with scissors around the tumour, creating a stepped wound edge (Figure 24.5**a**).
5. The tumour is resected together with deep scleral lamella, avoiding retinal damage if possible (Figure 24.5**b**).
6. Using fresh instruments, the scleral window is closed with interrupted 8-0 nylon sutures (Figure 24.5**c**).
7. The eye is reformed with an intra-vitreal injection of Balanced Salt Solution.
8. If possible, the margins of the choroidal coloboma are treated with a double row of binocular indirect laser photocoagulation. Adjunctive plaque radiotherapy is routinely administered by some surgeons to prevent local tumour recurrence (Damato *et al.*, 1996) (Figure 24.5**d**).
9. Intraoperative haemorrhage is minimized by lowering the systolic blood pressure to approximately 40 mm Hg (Todd and Colvin, 1991). This is administered by a highly skilled anaesthetist, using an intra-arterial line to measure the blood pressure, and with continuous cardiac and cerebral monitoring. It is also helpful to cauterize long and short posterior ciliary vessels as well as choroidal vessels around the tumour.

COMPLICATIONS

a. Incomplete tumour excision results in either clinically visible residual tumour at the end of the operation, or microscopic, sub-clinical tumour deposits, which develop into clinically detectable recurrent tumour after months or years (Damato *et al.*, 1996) (Chapter 7).
b. Retinal tears are unusual unless the tumour is adherent to retina.
c. Retinal detachment develops only if there is a retinal tear or a large retinal dialysis.

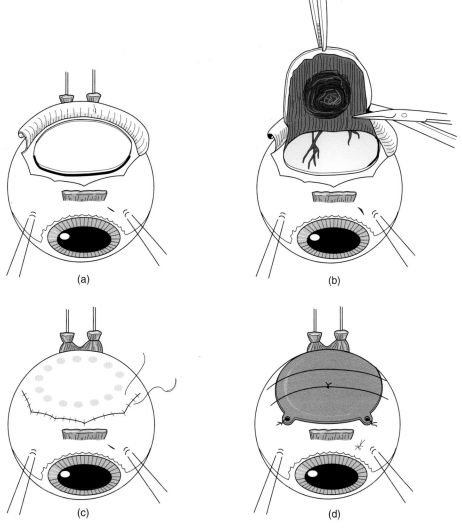

Figure 24.5 Choroidectomy: (**a**) superficial scleral flap, deep scleral incision and sclerotomy for core vitrectomy, (**b**) choroidectomy, (**c**) closure of scleral flap and (**d**) adjunctive plaque radiotherapy

d. Uncontrolled haemorrhage can sometimes occur despite hypotensive anaesthesia.

e. Vitreous haemorrhage is possible only if there is a retinal break.

f. Ocular hypotension and phthisis can occur if more than 2–3 clock hours of the ciliary body is excised.

g. Choroidal tears can be caused by excessive traction while excising the tumour (Figure 24.6)

h. Disciform macular scarring can develop from choroidal neovascularization arising at the margins of the coloboma (Figure 24.7).

i. Anaesthetic complications, such as myocardial infarction and cerebrovascular accident, should not occur if the hypotensive anaesthesia is administered by a skilled anaesthetist with appropriate cardiac and cerebral monitoring.

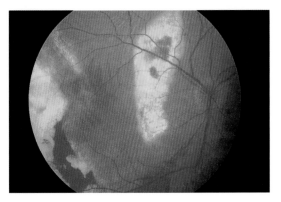

Figure 24.6 Choroidal tear after trans-scleral local resection

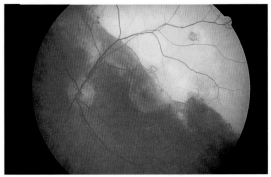

Figure 24.7 Disciform macular scar after trans-scleral local resection

Endoresection

This procedure is controversial and is performed only by a small number of surgeons (Lee *et al.*, 1993; Damato *et al.*, 1998). The indications and contraindications are therefore only tentative.

INDICATIONS

a. Extension of a choroidal melanoma to within 1 DD of the optic disc.
b. Recurrent choroidal melanoma after radiotherapy or phototherapy.

CONTRAINDICATIONS

a. Involvement of more than a third of optic disc margin, because the potential for conserving vision is limited.
b. Basal tumour diameter greater than 10–11 mm, because of the risk of hypotony.
c. Diffuse melanoma, because of the increased risk of recurrence.
d. Tumour treatable by more conventional methods.

TECHNIQUE

1. If possible, the endoresection is immediately preceded by transpupillary thermotherapy (Chapter 25).
2. Total vitrectomy is performed, inducing posterior vitreous detachment and removing vitreous near entry sites.
3. The tumour is removed piecemeal with the vitrector, either through a retinotomy (Figure 24.8a) or after folding back a retinal flap.
4. Endo-diathermy is applied to the scleral bed and the margins of the coloboma to prevent bleeding and tumour recurrence.
5. Fluid–air exchange is performed to flatten the retina (Figure 24.8b).
6. Endo-laser photocoagulation is applied to destroy residual tumours and to create retinal adhesion around the coloboma (Figure 24.8c).
7. The eye is filled with silicone oil (Figure 24.8d).
8. The sclerotomies are closed and treated with cryotherapy.
9. Incomplete or uncertain tumour excision is treated with adjunctive plaque radiotherapy. Trans-scleral diode laser phototherapy is also possible, using a right-angled probe placed behind the eye.
10. The oil is removed after 10–12 weeks.

COMPLICATIONS

a. Local tumour recurrence can develop at the margin of the coloboma and within the sclera. Subconjunctival seedlings have been reported (Bechrakis, 1999). Longer follow-up studies are required to determine

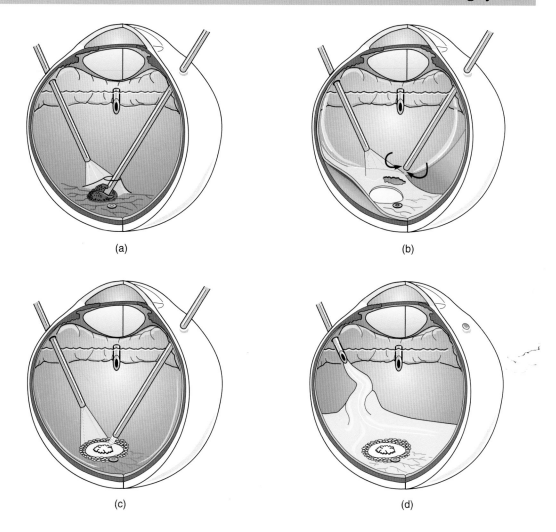

Figure 24.8 Endoresection: (**a**) tumour resection through retinotomy, (**b**) fluid–air exchange, (**c**) endo-laser photocoagulation and (**d**) air–silicone exchange

whether there are late recurrences from seeding to other parts of the eye.

b. Retinal detachment can be due to entry site tears, inadequate retinopexy around the margins of any retinotomies, and retinal traction by vitreous bands.

c. Cataract eventually develops in almost all eyes due to the use of silicone oil.

d. Ocular hypertension occasionally occurs in the immediate postoperative period. It is usually transient and responsive to medical therapy.

Enucleation

INDICATIONS

a. Inability to conserve safely what the patient (or the parent) considers to be a useful eye.

b. High probability of incomplete control of a primary malignant tumour.

c. Poorly motivated patient.

d. Blind painful eye after local therapy.

e. Untreatable local tumour recurrence after conservative therapy.

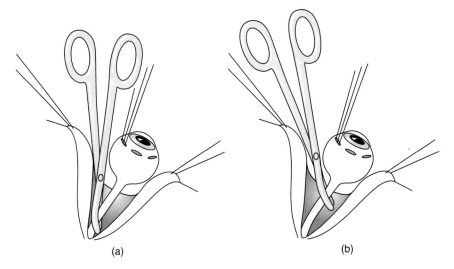

Figure 24.9 Enucleation, with (**a**) correct and (**b**) incorrect angulation of scissors, if long optic nerve stump is required

f. Opaque media preventing proper monitoring after conservative therapy.

The main contraindication to enucleation is lack of informed consent, if the patient has not been made aware of possible conservative therapies.

TECHNIQUE

1. To eliminate any possibility of enucleating the wrong eye, it is essential to visualize the tumour before starting the operation but *after* taping the other eye shut and draping the patient.
2. A retrobulbar injection of about 10 ml of 0.75% bupivacaine with 1:100 000 adrenaline can be given to prevent (a) intraoperative haemorrhage, (b) the oculo-cardiac reflex, and (c) postoperative pain. This injection also pushes the globe forward, facilitating transection of the nerve.
3. The enucleation is performed as gently as possible. When it is necessary to obtain a long optic nerve stump, the eye is pulled gently from the socket before the stretched nerve is divided at the orbital apex using scissors introduced along the medial orbital wall (Figure 24.9**a**), without being tilted laterally (Figure 24.9**b**). Instead of scissors, it is possible to use a snare, which reduces haemorrhage but which may also reduce the quality of histological examination by squeezing myelin into the eye (i.e., 'toothpaste artifact').

4. The surgeon's preferred orbital implant is used, taking appropriate measures to avoid extrusion.
5. A pressure bandage is applied to prevent a periorbital haematoma.

COMPLICATIONS

a. A short optic nerve stump, which increases the risk of residual retinoblastoma.
b. Postoperative pain, which can be severe.
c. Orbital haematoma, due to an inadequate pressure bandage.
d. Orbital cellulitis.
e. Extrusion of the implant, due to inadequate suturing of Tenon's capsule.
f. Ptosis, which is multifactorial.
g. Upper eyelid sulcus, due to loss of orbital volume and migration of the orbital implant.
h. Sagging of lower eyelid, caused by the weight of the ocular prosthesis.
i. Orbital growth retardation after enucleation in early childhood does not occur if an orbital implant is used (Fountain *et al.*, 1999).

Exenteration

Exenteration is performed less frequently than in previous years, and is reserved for tumours that cannot be locally resected.

REFERENCES

Bechrakis, N. (1999) Personal communication. International Congress of Ocular Oncology, Philadelphia.

Damato, B.E. and Foulds, W.S. (1994) Surgical resection of choroidal melanomas. In: S.J. Ryan (ed.), *Retina.* St Louis: Mosby, Vol. 1, Ch. 47, pp. 795–807.

Damato, B.E., Groenewald, C., McGalliard, J. and Wong, D. (1998) Endoresection of choroidal melanoma. *Br. J. Ophthalmol.*, **82**, 213–18.

Damato, B.E., Paul, J. and Foulds, W.S. (1996) Risk factors for residual and recurrent uveal melanoma after trans-scleral local resection. *Br. J. Ophthalmol.*, **80**, 102–8.

Fountain, T.R., Goldberger, S. and Murphree, A.L. (1999) Orbital development after enucleation in early childhood. *Ophthal. Plast. Reconstr. Surg.*, **15**, 32–6.

Lee, K.J., Peyman, G.A. and Raichand, S. (1993) Internal eye wall resection for posterior uveal melanoma. *Jpn J. Ophthalmol.*, **37**, 287–92.

Naumann, G.O.H. and Rummelt, V. (1996) Block excision of tumors of the anterior uvea. *Ophthalmology*, **103**, 2017–28.

Peyman, G.A. and Gremillion, C.M. (1989) Eye wall resection in the management of uveal neoplasms. *Jpn J. Ophthalmol.*, **33**, 458–71.

Shields, J.A., Shields, C.L. and De Potter, P. (1998) Surgical management of circumscribed conjunctival melanomas. *Ophthal. Plast. Reconstr. Surg.*, **14**, 208–15.

Shields, J.A., Shields, C.L., Shah, P. and Sivalingam, V. (1991) Partial lamellar sclerouvectomy for ciliary body and choroidal tumors. *Ophthalmology*, **98**, 971–83.

Todd, J.G. and Colvin, J.R. (1991) Ophthalmic surgery. In: W.R. MacRae and J.A.W. Wildsmith (eds), *Induced Hypotension.* London: Elsevier Science, Ch. 8, pp. 257–69.

Tucker, S.M., Hurwitz, J.J., Pavlin, C.J., Howarth, D.J. and Nianiaris, N. (1993) Scleral melt after cryotherapy for conjunctival melanoma. *Ophthalmology*, **100**, 574–7.

Chapter 25

Phototherapy

An increasing variety of wavelengths are available for phototherapy (Figure 25.1).

Photocoagulation

Photocoagulation raises the tissue temperature above 60°C, to cause coagulation of proteins and immediate cell death.

INDICATIONS

The use of photocoagulation as a primary form of treatment for choroidal melanoma, choroidal hae-mangioma, and retinoblastoma has largely been superseded by other methods.

TECHNIQUE

CHOROIDAL MELANOMA

A variety of techniques have been described over the years (Bornfeld and Wessing, 1994).

Low-energy, long-exposure photocoagulation (Foulds and Damato, 1986) is performed in three stages.

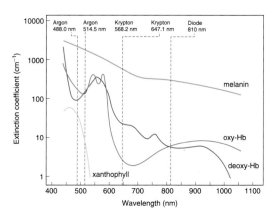

Figure 25.1 Graph showing pigments and lasers. (Adapted from Mainster, M.A. (1986) Wavelength selection in macular photocoagulation. *Ophthalmology*, **93**, 952)

1. At the first session, two or three confluent rows of moderate 500 μm, 0.5 s argon burns are placed all around the tumour margins (Figure 25.2**b**). This creates a wide zone of choroidal atrophy, preventing lateral tumour spread and avoiding retinal traction when the tumour is later treated. At the next session, heavy, white 500 μm burns are

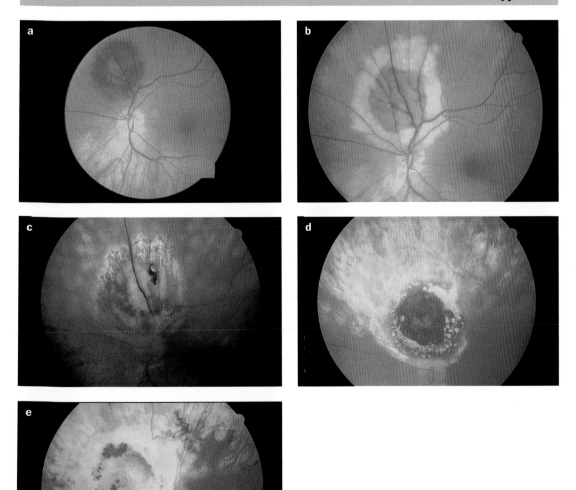

Figure 25.2 Photocoagulation technique: (**a**) pre-treatment photograph, (**b**) retinal and choroidal burns around the tumour margin, (**c**) retinal burns over tumour applied when choroidal scarring has developed around the tumour, (**d**) scleral exposure after deliberate 'explosions' in residual tumour and (**e**) final appearance

placed over the entire tumour surface to cause retinal atrophy, thereby preventing retinal blanching from interfering with direct treatment of the tumour in subsequent sessions (Figure 25.2c).

2. Once retinal atrophy over the tumour and choroidal atrophy and retinal adhesion around the tumour margins have developed, the tumour is treated directly with low-dose, long-duration krypton burns.

Confluent, 500 μm burns, each 10–30 seconds long, are placed over the entire tumour, keeping the power just low enough to prevent explosions. This treatment is repeated at monthly intervals until a flat or slightly elevated, pigmented, fibrotic scar remains.

3. In case there is any active tumour under the fibrotic scar, explosions can be created over the residual pigmented area, keeping well within the surrounding retinopexy (Figure

25.2**d**). The explosions are achieved by increasing the power to approximately 0.5 W. The final result should be an extensive area of bare sclera (Figure 25.2**e**).

RETINOBLASTOMA

High intensity laser burns created on the surface of the retinoblastoma can cause explosions with seeding of tumour cells into the vitreous and other parts of the eye. The aim of treatment is therefore to deprive the tumour of its retinal blood supply by placing heavy, confluent, white, 500 μm argon burns all around the tumour (Murphree and Munier, 1994) (see Figure 13.26).

CHOROIDAL HAEMANGIOMA

The objective of photocoagulation is to create adhesions between the RPE and retina. Tumour destruction is not attempted. Heavy white argon burns are placed over the entire tumour surface. An alternative procedure is to create a confluent line of burns between the edge of the tumour and the fovea, so as to prevent macular oedema (Shields and Shields, 1992). The laser treatment may need to be repeated several times.

RETINAL HAEMANGIOBLASTOMA

The lesion is covered with 0.2 second, 200 μm argon blue–green burns at an energy sufficient to blanch the tumour surface (i.e., approximately 0.5 W). Intravenous fluorescein injection has been used to enhance light absorption. The treatment is repeated every one or two weeks until the tumour appears white and shrunken, with resolution of retinal exudates and a return of the feeder vessels to the normal size (Lane *et al.*, 1989).

Transpupillary thermotherapy (TTT)

The objective is to cause tumour cell death by raising the temperature to between 45°C and 60°C for about one minute. Histological studies

suggest that a single treatment causes tumour necrosis to a depth of 3–4 mm, and this is believed to occur because the tumour blood vessels remain patent, transferring heat to the deeper parts of the tumour (Journée de Korver *et al.*, 1997).

INDICATIONS

TTT is reserved for small choroidal melanomas and retinoblastomas as a means of avoiding optic nerve and macular damage by radiotherapy.

TECHNIQUE

CHOROIDAL MELANOMA

Infra-red diode laser (810 nm) applications, 3.0 mm in diameter, are placed over the entire tumour surface (Figure 25.3**a**). Each exposure is about 60 seconds long, with the power adjusted so that the treated area begins to blanch after 40 seconds, developing a light grey appearance at the end of each application (Figure 25.3**b**). The power should not be high enough to close the retinal vessels. About 1.5–2.0 mm of clinically normal choroid around the tumour is treated to prevent marginal recurrence. Between two and four sessions of treatment are required to destroy the entire tumour (Oosterhuis *et al.*, 1998; Shields *et al.*, 1998) (Figure 25.3**c**). Some workers recommend adjunctive plaque radiotherapy (i.e., 'sandwich' technique) (Oosterhuis *et al.*, 1998). Indocyanine green, injected intravenously a few minutes before the phototherapy, can be used to enhance the light absorption in amelanotic tumours.

RETINOBLASTOMA

Similar methods of TTT are used with retinoblastoma. In some cases, the thermotherapy is applied after prior chemotherapy has reduced the tumour size (i.e., chemoreduction) (Shields *et al.*, 1996). In addition to transpupillary phototherapy, it is possible to deliver diode laser trans-sclerally (Abramson *et al.*, 1998).

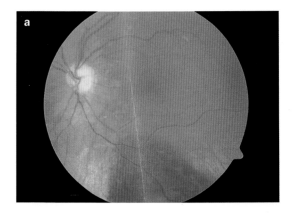

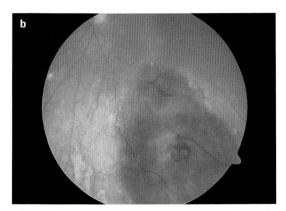

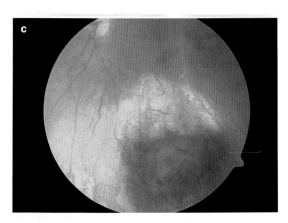

Figure 25.3 Transpupillary thermotherapy technique: (**a**) suspected residual tumour 15 months after ruthenium plaque radiotherapy of a choroidal melanoma in the left eye, (**b**) light grey phototherapy reaction over posterior part of tumour and (**c**) atrophic area 6 months later

VASCULAR TUMOURS

Choroidal haemangiomas can be treated with long exposures using methods similar to those described for amelanotic choroidal melanoma (Othmane *et al.*, 1999).

Photodynamic therapy

Light of an appropriate wavelength is used to activate a photosensitizer, thereby releasing toxic free radicals, which destroy adjacent tumour cells and cause vaso-occlusion (Foster *et al.*, 1997). Various agents have been used, which include:

a. Haematoporphyrin derivative (HPD) (Bruce, 1984). This has largely been superseded by sensitizers that have less tendency to cause sunburn.
b. Benzoporphyrin derivative (BPD), which gives encouraging results in animal studies (Kim *et al.*, 1996). Its main absorption peaks occur at 450 nm and 692 nm so that it can be activated by a variety of light sources according to the depth of the required effect, with red light inducing the deepest activation.

Thermochemotherapy

Thermochemotherapy of retinoblastoma is based on the finding that the cytotoxicity of carboplatin is enhanced by hyperthermia of 6–9°C (Herman and Teicher, 1994).

According to one method, carboplatin is administered intravenously over a 1-hour period (Murphree *et al.*, 1996). Several hours later, hyperthermia is generated by diode laser (810 nm) delivered through an operating microscope with a three-mirror Goldmann type lens taped to the child's face. A spot with a diameter of 0.8–2.0 mm is delivered at a power of 300–700 mW for 10–30 minutes so that the tumour develops some whitening, with micro-haemorrhages. Blanching of the retina adjacent to the tumour is avoided by reducing the power or the duration. This treatment can be preceded by chemoreduction and followed by various forms of local therapy.

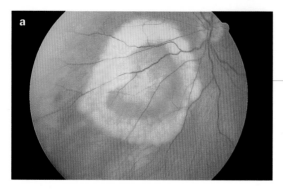 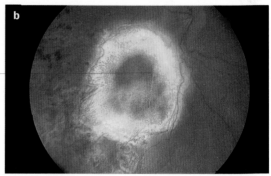

Figure 25.4 Retinal traction after photocoagulation. Left fundus (**a**) immediately after photocoagulation of an inferonasal choroidal melanoma and (**b**) 6 months later. Note the displacement of the inferior retinal vessels

Complications of phototherapy

a. Uveal melanoma can recur at its margins, from unrecognized lateral tumour extensions, and extraocularly, because of inadequate treatment centrally. Recurrences can develop many years after treatment, making life-long follow-up essential. Retinoblastoma can recur centrally, due to inadequate tumour destruction, and improper technique can result in tumour seeding to other parts of the eye.

b. Retinal traction, due to overzealous treatment, can cause macular oedema, retinal folds and tears as well as rhegmatogenous retinal detachment (Figure 25.4).

c. Retinal vein occlusion can result in disc neovascularization and vitreous haemorrhage.

d. Rupture of Bruch's membrane can lead to choroidal neovascularization and vitreous haemorrhage (Figure 25.5).

e. Iris burns can occur if the pupil is not well dilated, leading to uveitis, posterior synechiae and cataract.

f. Systemic agents for photodynamic therapy and thermochemotherapy can cause a variety of complications.

REFERENCES

Abramson, D.H., Servodidio, C.A. and Nissen, M. (1998) Treatment of retinoblastoma with the transscleral diode laser. *Am. J. Ophthalmol.*, **126**, 733–5.

Bornfeld, N. and Wessing, A. (1994) Photocoagulation of choroidal melanoma. In: S.J. Ryan (ed.), *Retina*. St Louis: Mosby, Vol. 1, Ch. 49, pp. 815–23.

Bruce, R.A., Jr. (1984) Evaluation of hematoporphyrin photoradiation therapy to treat choroidal melanomas. *Lasers Surg. Med.*, **4**, 59–64.

Foster, B.S., Gragoudas, E.S. and Young, L.H. (1997) Photodynamic therapy of choroidal melanoma. *Int. Ophthalmol. Clin.*, **37**, 117–26.

Foulds, W.S. and Damato, B.E. (1986) Low-energy long-exposure laser therapy in the management of choroidal melanoma. *Graefes Arch. Clin. Exp. Ophthalmol.*, **224**, 26–31.

Herman, T.S. and Teicher, B.A. (1994) Summary of studies adding systemic chemotherapy to local hyperthermia and radiation. *Int. J. Hyperthermia*, **10**, 443–9.

Figure 25.5 Choroidal neovascularization with retrohyaloid haemorrhage after photocoagulation of an inferior choroidal melanoma in the left eye

Journée de Korver, J.G., Oosterhuis, J.A., de Wolff-Rouendaal, D. and Kemme, H. (1997) Histopathological findings in human choroidal melanomas after transpupillary thermotherapy. *Br. J. Ophthalmol.*, **81**, 234–9.

Kim, R.Y., Hu, L.-K., Foster, B.S., Gragoudas, E.S. and Young, L.H.Y. (1996) Photodynamic therapy of pigmented choroidal melanomas of greater than 3 mm thickness. *Ophthalmology*, **103**, 2029–36.

Lane, C.M., Turner, G., Gregor, Z.J. and Bird, A.C. (1989) Laser treatment of retinal angiomatosis. *Eye*, **3**, 33–8.

Murphree, A.L. and Munier, F.L. (1994) Retinoblastoma. In: S.J. Ryan (ed.), *Retina*. St Louis: Mosby, Vol. 1, Ch. 27, pp. 571–626.

Murphree, A.L., Villablanca, J.G., Deegan, W.F. IIIrd, Sato, J.K., Malogolowkin, M., Fisher, A., Parker, R., Reed, E. and Gomer, C.J. (1996) Chemotherapy plus local treatment in the management of intraocular retinoblastoma. *Arch. Ophthalmol.*, **114**, 1348–56.

Oosterhuis, J.A., Journée de Korver, H.G. and Keunen, J.E. (1998) Transpupillary thermotherapy: results in 50 patients with choroidal melanoma. *Arch. Ophthalmol.*, **116**, 157–62.

Othmane, I.S., Shields, C.L., Shields, J.A., Gündüz, K. and Mercado, G. (1999) Circumscribed choroidal hemangioma managed by transpupillary thermotherapy. *Arch. Ophthalmol.*, **117**, 136–7.

Shields, C.L., De Potter, P., Himelstein, B.P., Shields, J.A., Meadows, A.T. and Maris, J.M. (1996) Chemoreduction in the initial management of intraocular retinoblastoma. *Arch. Ophthalmol.*, **114**, 1330–8.

Shields, C.L., Shields, J.A., Cater, J., Lois, N., Edelstein, C., Gündüz, K. and Mercado, G. (1998) Transpupillary thermotherapy for choroidal melanoma: tumor control and visual results in 100 consecutive cases. *Ophthalmology*, **105**, 581–90.

Shields, J.A. and Shields, C.L. (1992) *Intraocular Tumors. A Text and Atlas*. Philadelphia: W.B. Saunders.

Chapter 26

Counselling

The management of ocular tumours, and indeed any condition, requires good communication between the practitioner and the patient. In addition, it is essential to address psychological problems in patients and their families.

COMMUNICATING WITH PATIENTS

TOPICS FOR DISCUSSION

a. Basic ocular anatomy.
b. The nature of the disease (i.e., what might happen without treatment).
c. The objectives of treatment (i.e., prevention of metastatic disease, conservation of the eye and vision, avoidance of pain etc.).
d. All the management options, together with the risks and benefits of each form of treatment.
e. The logistics of the preferred form of management (i.e., time in hospital etc.).
f. Likely outcomes and possible complications.
g. Plans for after-care and long-term follow-up.
h. Possible impact on occupation, driving and other activities, for example, if vision is lost.
i. Family implications, if the disease is hereditary.

Some patients express resentment at not being told about their condition by their own general ophthalmologist when their tumour was first diagnosed. It is therefore important for them to have some idea of the possible diagnosis and its significance. This knowledge may also help patients to prevent unnecessary delays in treatment if any administrative errors occur, for example, if a letter of referral does not reach its destination.

AIDS TO COUNSELLING

a. A quiet space, with comfortable seating.
b. The presence of a close relative or friend.
c. The help of a trained, sympathetic nurse.
d. A model of the eye.
e. Illustrated information leaflets.
f. A 'bank' of patients, who have been through a similar experience and who are prepared to speak to new patients by telephone or in person.
g. An understanding about whether or not the patient wishes to know about a poor prognosis.
h. Sufficient time for proper discussion to take place.

Patients and their relatives tend to remember little of what is said at their consultation. For several years, the author has given each new patient an audio-cassette tape recording of their consultation, with marked improvement in communication (Ah-Fat *et al.*, 1998). Information leaflets can be helpful, if prepared following certain guidelines (Coulter *et al.*, 1999). Some patients may be using denial as a subconscious defence mechanism and this is acceptable as long as it does not seem to get in the way of what is deemed to be the proper treatment.

In an increasing number of countries it is no longer considered correct to leave patients uninformed about their condition. Attempts by well-intentioned relatives to have secret conversations with the doctor should be resisted.

TREATMENT SELECTION

The patient's priorities (i.e., 'utilities') that need to be considered when planning management include the following:

a. Peace of mind about local tumour control and the prevention of metastatic disease. Some patients are able to accept a certain risk of local tumour recurrence whereas others prefer to have the eye removed.
b. Conservation of a cosmetically satisfactory eye, with vision being only of secondary importance. Patients may worry about how young children might react to an artificial eye, particularly if they are teachers, parents or grandparents.
c. Conservation of visual acuity or field, with the eye being useless to them in their occupation unless such vision is retained.
d. A quick, definitive treatment without the possibility of prolonged absences from home or work. Some patients, particularly if elderly, 'can't be bothered' to travel extensively for treatment and follow-up.

FACTORS ASSISTING PROPER TREATMENT SELECTION

a. Guidance from the doctor about what is the best form of treatment for each patient's particular situation. This is because even after prolonged explanation, many patients have only a limited understanding of their disease and its treatment.
b. Giving patients the opportunity of contributing to the decision making, as this is known to make it easier for them to cope with their condition in the long term (Fallowfield *et al.*, 1990).
c. The doctor's approval of the treatment that has been selected (provided that the doctor agrees with the decision taken). This helps to prevent patients from blaming themselves for any complications.

PSYCHOLOGICAL PROBLEMS DUE TO CANCER

a. Fear of death.
b. Hypochondriacism, attributing every minor ailment to recurrent disease.
c. Guilt about surviving.
d. Difficulty resuming normal life.
e. Denial of the condition.
f. Depression, anxiety and other psychiatric disease, which may not necessarily be precipitated by the diagnosis of cancer.
g. Problems with concentration, memory, sexual dysfunction and alcohol abuse.

The diagnosis of cancer is particularly difficult for patients to cope with psychologically if a close relative or friend has suffered from a similar illness or if there are other concurrent problems, for example, related to work or marital relationships. Relatives may develop difficulties, also requiring assistance.

PSYCHOLOGICAL PROBLEMS DUE TO OCULAR DISEASE

Psychological problems caused by the loss of the eye or vision (Maguire and Parkes, 1998) include:

a. Loss of self-image.
b. Visual handicap.
c. Grief at the loss of physical attractiveness or the inability to function as before.
d. Depression, anxiety and loss of libido.

These problems can develop immediately or after a delay, if the patient has initially repressed any emotions.

MANAGEMENT OF PSYCHOLOGICAL PROBLEMS

a. Recognize problems by asking direct questions.
b. Discuss any problems that are anticipated.
c. Reassure patients about the normality of their psychological responses, if appropriate.
d. Establish how well the family is coping.
e. Help patients to get in touch with others who have previously had similar treatment.
f. Organize pharmacological treatment of anxiety or depression.

HELPFUL RESOURCES

a. Encouragement from the surgeon, which may be more effective than support provided by other staff.
b. Support from relatives and friends.
c. Religious support.
d. Patients support groups.
e. Psychological counselling from trained carers.

f. Psychiatric evaluation, with pharmacological treatment if necessary.

Patients seem to adjust especially well to their condition when they feel that some good has come out of their crisis, for example, discovering what is or is not important in their life.

REFERENCES

Ah-Fat, F.G., Sharma, M.C. and Damato, B.E. (1998) Taping outpatient consultations: a survey of attitudes and responses of adult patients with ocular malignancy. *Eye*, **12**, 789–91.

Coulter, A., Entwistle, V. and Gilbert, D. (1999) Sharing decisions with patients: is the information good enough? *Br. Med. J.*, **318**, 318–22.

Fallowfield, L.J., Hall, A., Maguire, G.P. and Baum, M. (1990) Psychological outcomes of different treatment policies in women with early breast cancer outside a clinical trial. *Br. Med. J.*, **301**, 575–80.

Maguire, P. and Parkes, C.M. (1998) Coping with loss. Surgery and loss of body parts. *Br. Med. J.*, **316**, 1086–8.

Glossary

Adenoma and adenocarcinoma. Benign and malignant neoplasms respectively, which arise from glandular epithelium or which show glandular differentiation (e.g., RPE, ciliary epithelium or iris epithelium).

Acanthosis. Thickening of the prickle cell layer (i.e., *stratum Malpighii*) of the epithelium.

Anaplasia. Total loss of cellular specialization so that there is no structural or functional resemblance to the parent tissue.

Aneuploidy. Any chromosome number that is not an exact multiple of the haploid number.

Angiogenesis. The development of a vasculature under the influence of growth factors such as vascular endothelial growth factor (VEGF) and inhibitory factors such as thrombospondin and angiostatin. Angiogenesis is believed to determine whether a micrometastasis remains dormant or whether it grows to cause clinical disease.

Apoptosis. Programmed cell death, which unlike necrosis occurs without an inflammatory response.

Atypia. Features suggestive of malignant transformation, which include the presence of a large, irregular, 'vesicular' nucleus with one or more prominent nucleoli, and cellular pleomorphism.

BCL-2. A 'B cell lymphoma' gene, which blocks apoptosis.

Becquerel. A unit of radioactivity. One becquerel (1 Bq) is one disintegration per second.

Cancer. A disease in which a clone of mutant cells grows in an uncontrolled fashion, with the cells losing their differentiated structure and function, invading surrounding tissues and possibly spreading to other parts of the body.

Carcinoma. A malignant neoplasm arising from epithelium.

Cell-doubling time. The time between one mitosis and the next.

Choristoma. A malformation present at birth and forming a tumour containing structures of different origins (e.g., lacrimal gland and muscle), which are not normally present at the site of the tumour.

Differentiation. The degree of specialization of a cell, described in terms of histological appearance, and immunohistochemical profile, which reflects the ability of the cell to function and collaborate with adjacent normal cells.

Diploid. The normal number of chromosomes in somatic cells.

Dysplasia. Partial loss of cellular specialization or an altered appearance suggesting a precancerous change.

Dyskeratosis. Abnormally deep keratinization of epidermal cells.

Familial. Any condition that is commoner in the patient's relatives than in the general population.

Gray. A unit describing the amount of radioactive energy absorbed by tissue. One gray (1 Gy) is equal to 1 joule of energy absorbed by one kilogramme of tissue. This unit has replaced the rad (i.e., 1 Gy = 100 rad = 100 cGy).

Hamartoma. A malformation present at birth composed of cells normally present in the tissue of origin.

Haploid. The number of chromosomes in gametes.

Hereditary. The transmission of characteristics and diseases to descendants.

Heterogeneity. Although derived from a single clone, cells within the same tumour evolve in different directions as they compete with each other for survival so that a heterogenous population develops. If an external influence such as chemotherapy occurs, the more resistant cells will outgrow the sensitive cells to become predominant.

Hypertrophy. Enlargement of cells within a tissue.

Hyperplasia. Increase in number of cells within a tissue.

In situ carcinoma or melanoma. Intra-epithelial proliferation of malignant cells without stromal invasion.

Invasion. Direct spread of neoplastic cells into adjacent tissues, a process involving cellular proliferation, adhesion (mediated by integrins etc.), proteolysis (mediated by metalloproteinases etc.) and migration (mediated by a variety of cytokines).

Isomerization. The loss of electrons from target atoms under the influence of radioactive emissions.

Keratosis. Excessive epithelial keratinization, usually referred to as hyperkeratosis.

Knudson's two-hit hypothesis. This states that in conditions such as retinoblastoma and von Hippel–Lindau syndrome, both the maternal and paternal alleles of a tumour suppressor gene must be abnormal for tumour formation to occur.

Leukoplakia. A clinical term referring to the development of a white plaque on a mucous membrane.

Malformation. A primary error of normal development of a tissue or organ.

Melanosis. Increased melanin concentration in a tissue, caused by over-production of melanin by individual cells or the presence of excessive numbers of melanocytes.

Mesectodermal. Arising from embryonic mesenchyme (i.e., 'packing cells' lying between epithelium and mesothelium) of neural crest origin (e.g., ciliary muscle is mesectodermal, but the sphincter pupillae differentiate from the ectoderm of the optic cup).

Metaplasia. The transformation of one type of differentiated tissue into another.

Metastasis. A complicated process whereby neoplastic cells colonize organs distant from the primary tumour. For a metastasis to develop, the neoplastic cell must be capable of invading a blood vessel or lymphatic channel, circulating around the body without being destroyed by immunological surveillance mechanisms, adhering to vascular endothelial cells in the target organ, extravasating, and activating angiogenesis.

Micrometastasis. A tiny, sub-clinical mass of metastatic tumour cells in the target organ.

Microvascular density. The number of tumour vessels within a specified area of neoplasm, a feature indicating the prognosis for survival.

Monosomy. Loss of one of a pair of chromosomes.

Mosaic. An individual with cells of more than one genotype.

Neoplasm. A new growth formed as a result of an abnormal proliferation of cells.

Oncogenes. These are mutated versions of genes normally involved in a variety of cellular functions. Oncogenes include (a) growth factors, (b) receptors, (c) intracellular signal transduction systems, (d) DNA binding nuclear proteins and (e) cell cycle regulators, such as cyclins, cyclin dependent kinases and kinase inhibitors.

p53. A tumour suppressor gene, located on chromosome 17p. In the presence of DNA damage, this gene is activated to arrest the cell cycle until the damage is repaired. If DNA repair is not possible, then p53 induces apoptosis to prevent malignancy.

Pagetoid spread. Spread of neoplastic cells within an epithelium.

Phakomatosis. A confusing term referring to a group of syndromes (i.e., tuberous sclerosis, neurofibromatosis, and von Hippel–Lindau syndrome), which are characterized by multiple hamartomas and neoplasms (benign and malignant) in various organs (particularly the skin, eye and nervous system). Some authors also include other conditions, such as the Sturge–Weber syndrome, Wyburn–Mason syndrome, retinal cavernous haemangioma and ataxia–telangiectasia.

Pleomorphism. Variation in structure.

Polyploidy. An abnormal increase in the number of chromosomes that is an exact multiple of the haploid number.

Sarcoma. A malignant non-epithelial tumour derived from connective tissue cells.

Sporadic. Not having any known genetic basis.

'Suicide' gene therapy. Destruction of cancerous cells by introducing a foreign gene encoding an enzyme that converts a prodrug into a cytotoxic agent (e.g. treatment of murine retinoblastoma with herpes simplex virus thymidine kinase followed by ganciclovir).

TNM classification. TNM (an acronym from 'Tumour', 'Nodes' and 'Metastasis') is a method of classifying neoplastic tumours according to their size, differentiation and spread. It was developed by the American Joint Committee on Cancer and the International Union Against Cancer.

Topoisomerases. These enzymes uncoil and disentagle DNA, allowing transcription and other vital processes to occur. Inactivation of topoisomerases by drugs such as etoposide results in cellular necrosis or apoptosis.

Tumour. A swelling or mass, which can be solid or cystic, neoplastic or non-neoplastic, benign or malignant.

Tumour doubling time. The time taken for a tumour to double in volume, which depends on (a) the cell doubling time, (b) the fraction of cells proliferating and (c) the fraction of cells being lost from the tumour. Theoretically, if a tumour is composed of 10 μm cells, and if all cells proliferate and survive, it should reach a size of 1 cubic millimetre (10^6 cells) after 20 cell doublings and a size of 1 cubic centimetre (10^9 cells) after another 10 cell doublings. A tumour of this size should develop in about 8 years if the cell cycle time is 100 days.

Vascular pattern. Morphological characteristics of the tumour vasculature, some of which are of prognostic value. For example, the presence of at least one closed vascular loop in a uveal melanoma is associated with an increased incidence of metastatic death.

Index